BROCHERT'S
CRUSH STEP 3

THE ULTIMATE USMLE
STEP 3 REVIEW

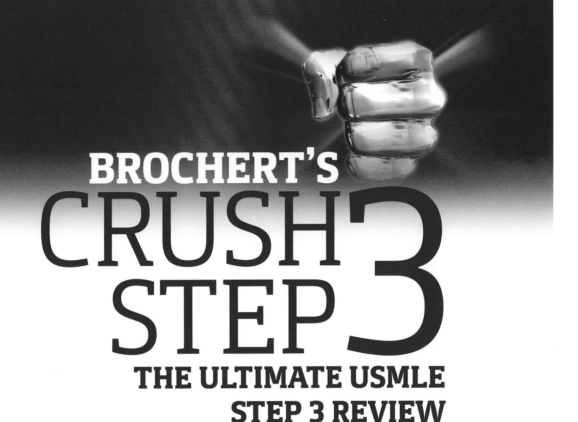

BROCHERT'S
CRUSH STEP 3
THE ULTIMATE USMLE
STEP 3 REVIEW

Fourth Edition

Mayur K. Movalia, MD

Head of Clinical Pathology, Eastern Maine Medical Center, Bangor, Maine;
Medical Director, Affiliated Laboratories, Bangor, Maine;
Medical Director, Flow Cytometry Laboratory, Dahl-Chase Diagnostic Services, Bangor, Maine;
Medical Director, Cancer Care of Maine Laboratory, Brewer, Maine;
Medical Director, Mount Desert Island Hospital Laboratory, Bar Harbor, Maine;
Partner Physician, Hematopathologist, Dahl-Chase Pathology Associates, Bangor Maine;
Faculty, University of Maine, Orono, Maine

Theodore X. O'Connell, MD

Program Director, Family Medicine Residency Program,
Kaiser Permanente Woodland Hills, Woodland Hills, California;
Assistant Clinical Professor, Department of Family Medicine,
David Geffen School of Medicine at UCLA, Los Angeles, California;
Partner Physician, Southern California Permanente Medical Group,
Woodland Hills, California

ELSEVIER
SAUNDERS

ELSEVIER
SAUNDERS

1600 John F. Kennedy Blvd.
Ste 1800
Philadelphia, PA 19103-2899

CRUSH STEP 3: THE ULTIMATE USMLE STEP 3 CS REVIEW   ISBN: 978-1-4557-0310-4
Copyright © 2013, 2008, 2004, 2001 by Saunders, an imprint of Elsevier Inc.

Notices

Knowledge and best practice in this field are constantly changing. As new research and experience broaden our understanding, changes in research methods, professional practices, or medical treatment may become necessary.

Practitioners and researchers must always rely on their own experience and knowledge in evaluating and using any information, methods, compounds, or experiments described herein. In using such information or methods they should be mindful of their own safety and the safety of others, including parties for whom they have a professional responsibility.

With respect to any drug or pharmaceutical products identified, readers are advised to check the most current information provided (i) on procedures featured or (ii) by the manufacturer of each product to be administered, to verify the recommended dose or formula, the method and duration of administration, and contraindications. It is the responsibility of practitioners, relying on their own experience and knowledge of their patients, to make diagnoses, to determine dosages and the best treatment for each individual patient, and to take all appropriate safety precautions.

To the fullest extent of the law, neither the Publisher nor the authors, contributors, or editors assume any liability for any injury and/or damage to persons or property as a matter of products liability, negligence or otherwise, or from any use or operation of any methods, products, instructions, or ideas contained in the material herein.

Library of Congress Cataloging-in-Publication Data
Movalia, Mayur.
  Brochert's crush step 3 : the ultimate USMLE step 3 CS review / Mayur
K. Movalia, Theodore X. O'Connell.—4th ed.
     p. ; cm.
  Crush step 3
  Rev. ed. of: Crush step 3 / Adam Brochert. 3rd ed. c2008.
  Includes index.
  ISBN 978-1-4557-0310-4 (pbk.)
  I. O'Connell, Theodore X. II. Brochert, Adam, 1971- Crush step 3. III.
Title. IV. Title: Crush step 3.
  [DNLM: 1. Medicine—Examination Questions. W 18.2]
  610.76—dc23   2012029640

Senior Content Strategist: James Merritt
Content Development Manager: Lucia Gunzel
Content Development Specialist: Andrea Vosburgh
Publishing Services Manager: Anne Altepeter
Project Manager: Kiruthiga Kasthuriswamy
Designer: Steve Stave

Working together to grow
libraries in developing countries

www.elsevier.com | www.bookaid.org | www.sabre.org

ELSEVIER   BOOK AID International   Sabre Foundation

Printed in China

Last digit is the print number: 9 8 7 6 5 4 3 2 1

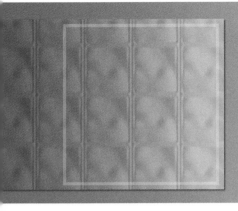

RESIDENT REVIEW BOARD

Each of the following reviewers scored above the 90th percentile on USMLE Step 3, with most scoring at the 99th percentile.

The authors and publisher express sincerest gratitude to these physicians for their many helpful comments, suggestions, and recommendations for improving the text that appears in this book.

Jessica Kraeft, MD
Radiology Resident
Mount Auburn Hospital
Harvard Medical School
Cambridge, Massachusetts

Captain Jason Michael Johnson, MD, USAFR
Clinical Fellow in Neuroradiology
Massachusetts General Hospital
Harvard Medical School
MA Clinical Instructor in Radiology
Boston, Massachusetts

Linda Hall, MD
Family Medicine Resident PGY3
Kaiser Permanente Woodland Hills Medical Center
Woodland Hills, California

Joseph Nezgoda, MD, MBA
Case Affiliated Hospitals Residency Program in Ophthalmology
University Hospitals Case Medical Center
Cleveland, Ohio

Yewlin E. Chee, MD
Ophthalmology Resident
Massachusetts Eye and Ear Infirmary
Harvard Medical School
Boston, Massachusetts

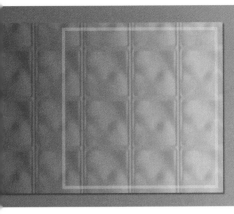

PREFACE

This book was written because we believed there was no good, quick, high-yield review book for the USMLE Step 3. If you're interested in this book, you're probably a busy resident with little free time. This book is designed for you. You already know how to take USMLE exams and (hopefully) feel somewhat comfortable with the types of things you'll be asked. Step 3 covers a lot of information, and this book was written to touch on important concepts in a format that can be read quickly. If you know all the concepts in this book, you should do much better than just pass: You should *Crush Step 3!*

Step 3 has the same level of difficulty as Steps 1 and 2, but the questions are more relevant to the day-to-day management of patients in inpatient and outpatient settings. Step 3 stresses the things that a general practitioner should know. Knowing how to diagnose, manage, and treat common diseases is stressed. In addition, common emergencies must be recognized.

Knowing how to manage exotic or rare conditions is low yield. Usually, when the examiners ask about a rare disease, they simply want you to recognize it from a classic presentation.

The topics in Step 3 are broad based and cover all subspecialties. Most of the exam contains standard multiple-choice questions (MCQs) related to variable-length passages. The exam is 2 days, with 8 hours to complete the testing on each day. The first day includes 336 MCQs divided into 7 blocks of 48 questions over 60 minutes each. You have about 1 minute and 15 seconds per question. The second day includes 144 MCQs in 4 blocks of 36 questions over 45 minutes each and 9 to 12 computer-based case simulations (CCS) over 4 hours. This can seem like a long and grueling 2 days. If you think fatigue and stamina may affect your concentration, consider practicing online question banks such as usmleconsult.com to build up tolerance to sitting through hours of MCQs and CCS cases.

It is extremely important that the examinee practices the CCS case scenario format using the Primum software available for download from the official usmle.org website. Six CCS cases are currently available for practice with basic explanations. Without prior familiarity, the examinee could easily flunk this section of the exam simply because of a lack of ability to use the program effectively. Only after spending several hours practicing the software will this part of the exam test your clinical knowledge—as opposed to your software and computer skills!.

Studying for Step 3 can seem like an overwhelming task—in a sense, anything is fair game. Given the time constraints of residents, most need a concise review of the commonly tested topics. It is our hope that *Crush Step 3* will meet your needs in this regard.

We have compiled a list of "10 Commandments" for taking the Step 3 exam that should prevent you from missing easy points:

1. It is just as important to know when something is normal or only needs observation as it is to know when to jump in and be a hero. If the patient is not crashing in front of your eyes, always consider delaying intervention and taking the conservative "wait and see approach" or ordering the most noninvasive tests if you're not certain of the diagnosis. (Surgery residents, are you paying attention?) However, when a patient is truly crashing in front of you, take action! In other words, get the crash cart, intubate, put in a chest tube, etc. (Pathology residents, are you paying attention?)

2. A presentation may be normal (especially in pediatrics and psychiatry) and need no treatment or simple reassurance.

3. If you're going to take the time to study for Step 3, study outside your field. In other words, if you're a medicine resident, don't spend too much time studying medicine for Step 3; study everything else. After 6 months to a year as a resident within a specific specialty, you probably know what you need to know for Step 3 purposes in that field.

4. You need to know common cutoff values for the treatment of common conditions. In other words: What laboratory values define diabetes? What blood pressure defines hypertension? When do you treat hypercholesterolemia? and so on. This book provides updates you need in this regard.

5. Subspecialties are fair game. We've all heard about or experienced the exam with "a million" dermatology or orthopedic questions. You never know what field may seem to be stressed in a particular exam administration.

6. Be a patient advocate. Don't yell at your patients, don't harshly judge them, don't refuse to be their doctor if they don't want treatment or tell you they're going to take some tree root for their cancer. Protect them when you can, and respect their autonomy. Work with them and ask them "why" whenever their actions puzzle you.

7. Don't be afraid to consult a specialist if you've made a diagnosis that you know is not commonly treated by a general practitioner. For example, if you think a patient may have a ruptured aortic aneurysm, look for an option that discusses consulting a vascular surgeon.

8. This may sound simple—but answer every question! If the passage is very long, consider reading the question at the end first. The question can sometimes be answered without reading the passage, or you may save time when you read the passage because you know what important points to look for. Don't waste 5 minutes on one difficult question that may leave you no time to read and answer the last 5 questions, which may be easy.

9. Never forget health maintenance. If a 35-year-old woman presents with a migraine headache and hasn't seen a doctor in 10 years, the correct answer of what to do next may be a Pap smear because of routine health maintenance!

10. Don't even think about taking the exam before you've practiced the CCS case format using Primum software, available for download from usmle.org. (Have we made our point on this issue yet?) In fact, preparing for the CCS cases is so important that a separate *Crush Step 3* book focusing on the CCS cases has been developed.

We wish you the best on the exam and in all your future endeavors.

Mayur Movalia, MD
Theodore O'Connell, MD
Adam Brochert, MD

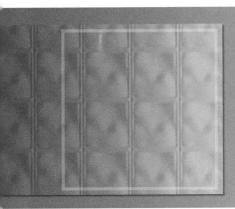

CONTENTS

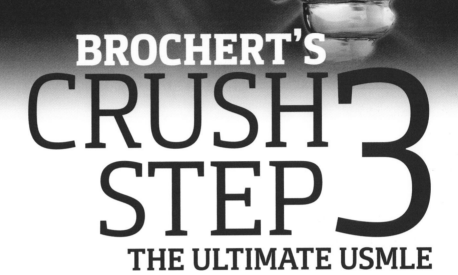

BROCHERT'S
CRUSH STEP 3
THE ULTIMATE USMLE STEP 3 REVIEW

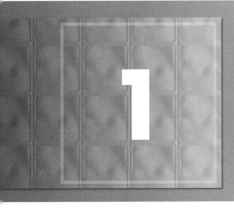

PREVENTIVE MEDICINE AND BIOSTATISTICS

ADULT SCREENING GUIDELINES

The U.S. Preventive Services Task Force (USPSTF) Clinical Guidelines for prevention and care management and American Cancer Society guidelines for cancer screening in asymptomatic patients are shown in Tables 1-1 and 1-2.

TABLE 1-1 USPSTF Clinical Guidelines for Prevention and Care Management

AAA	Men age 65-75 who have ever smoked: one-time ultrasound examination
Blood pressure	Men and women age >18: every 1-2 yr
Diabetes mellitus	Adults with hypertension or hyperlipidemia: fasting plasma glucose every 3 yr
Lipids	Men ≥35, Women ≥45: every 5 yr including total cholesterol and HDL
Osteoporosis	Women ≥65: DEXA scan of the hip and lumbar spine
Vision	Age ≥65: visual acuity test

Data from U.S. Preventive Services Task Force: Recommendations for Adults, 2011. Available at http://www.uspreventiveservicestask force.org/adultrec.htm.
AAA, Abdominal aortic aneurysm; *BMI,* body mass index; *DEXA,* dual-energy x-ray absorptiometry; *HDL,* high-density lipoprotein; *HIV,* human immunodeficiency virus; *STI,* sexually transmitted infection; *USPSTF,* U.S. Preventive Services Task Force.
Also screen for the following at routine visits: height/weight (BMI), depression, HIV risk factors, tobacco use, alcohol use, diet, injury prevention, STI risk.

TABLE 1-2 American Cancer Society Guidelines for Cancer Screening in Asymptomatic Patients*

CANCER	AGE (yr)	PROCEDURE/FREQUENCY
Colorectal	>50 for all studies[†]	Colonoscopy every 10 yr or Flexible sigmoidoscopy every 5 yr or Double-contrast barium enema every 5 yr or CT colonography every 5 yr or Fecal occult blood test yearly[§] or Fecal immunochemical test yearly or Stool DNA test (interval undetermined)
Prostate	>50[‡]	Prostate-specific antigen and digital rectal examination annually (do not screen if life expectancy is <10 yr)
Cervical	Age 21, regardless of sexual activity	Regular Pap smear yearly or liquid-based Pap test every 2 yr At age 30, screen every 2-3 yr if the patient has had three normal Pap tests. If Pap smear and HPV test combined, test every 3 yr At age 70, if 3 or more Pap tests in a row are normal in the last 10 yr, patient can choose to stop
Gynecologic	21–64 ≥65	Pelvic examination annually. Every 2-3 yr after 3 normal examinations Annually; when to stop is not clearly established
Breast	20-40 >40	Clinical (physician) breast examination every 3 yr (self breast examination no longer recommended) Mammography and clinical breast examination annually

Data from American Cancer Society Guidelines for the Early Detection of Cancer (2011). Available at http://www.cancer.org/Healthy/ FindCancerEarly/CancerScreeningGuidelines/american-cancer-society-guidelines-for-the-early-detection-of-cancer.
CT, Computed tomography; *DNA,* deoxyribonucleic acid.
*This table is for screening of asymptomatic, healthy patients. Other guidelines exist, but you will be fine if you follow this table for boards (controversial areas are generally not tested).
[†]Individuals with a family history of colon cancer, a personal history of inflammatory bowel disease, and certain inheritable syndromes such as familial adenomatous polyposis should be screened earlier.
[‡]American Cancer Society recommends men make an informed decision with their doctors, as the potential benefits of screening and treatments have not been entirely proved. Start at age 45 in African-Americans or in men with a first-degree relative who was diagnosed with prostate cancer before age 65.
[§]The multiple stool take-home test should be used. One test done by the doctor in the office is not adequate for testing. A colonoscopy should be done if the test is positive.

🗀 **CASE SCENARIO:** What should you do to screen for lung cancer in a high-risk, asymptomatic patient? Nothing. No definite benefit has been shown so far.

No cancer screening: In general, urinalysis (screening for urinary tract cancer, which is associated with hematuria); alpha fetoprotein (liver/gonadal cancer); CA-125 (ovarian cancer); and other serum markers are not appropriate for screening asymptomatic people with no physical findings, but look for these abnormal laboratory values as a clue to diagnosis. In high-risk individuals, screening with serum markers may be appropriate, but this is an evolving area. For example, patients with cirrhosis and chronic viral hepatitis may be screened for hepatocellular carcinoma with alpha fetoprotein and liver ultrasound every 6 months.

ADULT IMMUNIZATIONS (Table 1-3)

TABLE 1-3 Summary of Adult Immunizations

VACCINE	AGE	RECOMMENDATION
Hepatitis B	All adolescents and adults at risk	People at increased risk for the development of hepatitis B virus infection (including health care workers)
Herpes zoster	Adults 60 yr of age and older	Approved to help reduce the risk of developing zoster (shingles)
Human papillomavirus (HPV)	Females aged 9-26 yr Males aged 9-18 yr	Quadrivalent human papillomavirus recombinant vaccine is FDA-approved in females aged 9-26 to prevent cervical cancer, vaginal and vulvar cancer, precancerous genital lesions, and genital warts. It is also approved for use in males aged 9-18 yr to prevent genital warts
Influenza	Age >6 mo	People who should get vaccinated each year include: Children aged 6 mo to 18 yr Women who will be pregnant during the flu season People who are immunosuppressed Adults aged 50 and older and their household contacts People with chronic medical conditions (pulmonary, cardiovascular, renal, hepatic, hematologic, or metabolic disorders including diabetes) People who live in nursing homes and long-term care facilities Health care personnel Household contacts and caregivers of children aged <5 yr
Pneumococcus	All adults ≥65 yr of age	Also, people 2-64 yr old with chronic cardiovascular disease, chronic pulmonary disease, diabetes mellitus, functional or anatomic asplenia, alcoholism, chronic liver disease, or cerebrospinal fluid leak
Rubella	All women of child-bearing age who lack immunity	Do not give to pregnant women or immunocompromised patients (except HIV-positive patients). Women should avoid pregnancy for 4 wk after the vaccine. Also give to health care workers (to protect pregnant women's unborn children)
Td and Tdap	All adults should be given a tetanus booster (Td) every 10 yr (DTap and DT are given to children <7 yr of age, Tdap and Td are given to older children and adults.)	Give tetanus prophylaxis for any wound if vaccination history is unknown or patient has received <3 total doses Give tetanus booster in people with full vaccination history if more than 5 yr has passed since last dose for all wounds other than clean, minor wounds (including burns) Give tetanus immunoglobulin with vaccine for patients with unknown/incomplete vaccination and nonclean/major wounds Adults ≥65 yr of age should get Td (not Tdap) every 10 yr Tdap should be given to adults who have or anticipate having close contact with an infant age <12 mo, women before conception or in the immediate postpartum period, health care workers
Varicella	12 mo of age and older	Contraindications include pregnancy, immunosuppressant therapy, leukemia, lymphoma, active untreated tuberculosis, and immunodeficiency states such as AIDS

AIDS, Acquired immunodeficiency syndrome; *FDA,* U.S. Food and Drug Administration; *HIV,* human immunodeficiency virus; *TD and Tdap,* tetanus.

VITAMINS AND MINERALS

Deficiency of fat-soluble vitamins (A, D, E, K) is often due to *malabsorption* (e.g., cystic fibrosis, cirrhosis, celiac disease [sprue], pancreatic insufficiency). Parenteral supplementation may be necessary if high-dose oral supplements fail to correct the problem (Tables 1-4 and 1-5).

Table 1-4 Vitamins

VITAMIN	SIGNS AND SYMPTOMS	
	DEFICIENCY	**TOXICITY**
A	Night blindness, scaly rash, xerophthalmia (dry eyes), Bitot spots (debris on conjunctiva); increased infections	Brittle nails, alopecia, hypercalcemia, pseudotumor cerebri, bone thickening, teratogenicity
D	Rickets, osteomalacia, hypocalcemia	Hypercalcemia, nausea/vomiting, renal stone
E	Anemia, peripheral neuropathy, ataxia	Necrotizing enterocolitis in infants, easy bruising, diplopia, increased risk of hemorrhagic stroke
K	Hemorrhage, prolonged prothrombin time	Hemolysis (kernicterus)
B_1 (thiamine)	Wet beriberi (high-output cardiac failure), dry beriberi (peripheral neuropathy), Wernicke-Korsakoff syndrome (eye movement disorders, ataxia and impaired memory)	
B_2 (riboflavin)	Cheilosis, angular stomatitis, dermatitis	
B_3 (niacin)	Pellagra (dementia, dermatitis, diarrhea, death), stomatitis	Flushing, vasodilation, pruritus, hepatotoxicity
B_6 (pyridoxine)	Peripheral neuropathy, cheilosis, stomatitis, convulsions in infants, microcytic anemia, seborrheic dermatitis	"Stocking-glove" peripheral neuropathy, depressed deep tendon reflexes
B_{12} (cobalamin)	Megaloblastic anemia *plus* neurologic symptoms	
Folic acid	Megaloblastic anemia *without* neurologic symptoms	
C	Scurvy (hemorrhages—skin petechiae, bone, gums; loose teeth; gingivitis); poor wound healing; hyperkeratotic hair follicles; bone pain (from periosteal hemorrhages)	Hemolytic syndromes, renal stones

Table 1-5 Minerals

MINERAL	SIGNS AND SYMPTOMS	
	DEFICIENCY SIGNS AND SYMPTOMS	**TOXICITY**
Iodine	Goiter, cretinism, hypothyroidism	Myxedema
Fluoride	Dental caries (cavities)	Fluorosis with mottling of teeth/bone exostoses
Zinc	Hypogeusia (decreased taste), rash, slow wound healing	
Copper	Menke's disease (X-linked; kinky hair and mental retardation)	Wilson disease
Selenium	Cardiomyopathy and muscle pain	Loss of hair and nails
Manganese		"Manganese madness" in miners of ore
Chromium	Impaired glucose tolerance	

Rickets is associated with interesting physical and x-ray findings: craniotabes (skull is poorly mineralized and bones feel like the surface of a ping-pong ball), rachitic rosary (costochondral beading; small round masses on anterior rib cage), delayed fontanelle closure, bossing of the skull, kyphoscoliosis, bowleg, and knock-knee. Bone changes first appear at the lower ends of the radius and ulna.

🗀 **CASE SCENARIO:** A 29-year-old woman with vitiligo develops numbness in her feet with decreased vibratory sense and megaloblastic anemia. She most likely has what condition? *Pernicious anemia,* the most common cause of vitamin B_{12} deficiency. Pernicious anemia can be associated with autoimmune disorders such as vitiligo, hypothyroidism, and hypoadrenalism. Removal of the ileum and parasitic infection with the tapeworm *Diphyllobothrium latum* are rare causes of B_{12} deficiency.

🗀 **CASE SCENARIO:** A person on a strict vegan diet who does not eat meat or animal products (milk, eggs, cheese) and does not take regular multivitamin tablets is most at risk for which vitamin deficiency? Vitamin B_{12}. In some patients it may take 10 to 15 years before vitamin B_{12} deficiency due to diet becomes clinically apparent.

🗀 **CASE SCENARIO:** A 34-year-old man is put on a 6-month course of isoniazid for purified protein derivative skin test conversion. He develops tingling in his hands and feet. What vitamin deficiency might he have? Vitamin B_6 (pyridoxine)—remember to always give vitamin B_6 if prescribing isoniazid.

📁 **CASE SCENARIO:** What test does a 22-year-old woman need before starting oral isotretinoin for acne? *Pregnancy test.* Vitamin A and its derivatives are teratogenic. She must be placed on some form of birth control and given periodic pregnancy tests. Counsel about the risks of teratogenicity.

📁 **CASE SCENARIO:** An infant born at home with no perinatal care develops bleeding problems shortly after birth. What is the likely cause? *Hemorrhagic disease of the newborn.* Vitamin K is given to all newborns for prophylaxis against this condition. Vitamin K is necessary for the synthesis of factors II, VII, IX, and X, as well as proteins C and S.

📁 **CASE SCENARIO:** A patient with end-stage cirrhosis has a markedly prolonged prothrombin time. How should you treat it? With fresh frozen plasma. *Vitamin K does not work in the setting of liver failure* because the liver cannot synthesize clotting proteins.

📁 **CASE SCENARIO:** A 45-year-old man with mild macrocytic anemia has a borderline-normal serum vitamin B_{12} level. What is the most appropriate next test to evaluate for vitamin B_{12} deficiency? Methylmalonic acid (MMA). MMA levels are elevated in more than 90% of patients with vitamin B_{12} deficiency.

EPIDEMIOLOGY

Per-year rates that are commonly used to compare groups should be known:
- Birth rate: live births/1000 population
- Fertility rate: live births/1000 population of females aged 15–45
- Death rate: deaths/1000 population
- Neonatal mortality rate: neonatal deaths (in first 28 days)/1000 live births
- Perinatal mortality rate: neonatal deaths + stillbirths/1000 total births. The major cause of perinatal death is prematurity. Rates are higher in nonwhites than in whites.

Note / A stillbirth (fetal death) is a prenatal or natal (during birth) death after 20 weeks' gestation.

- Infant mortality rate: deaths (0–1 year old)/1000 live births. The top three causes, in descending order, are congenital abnormalities, low birth weight/prematurity, and sudden infant death syndrome.
- Maternal mortality rate: maternal pregnancy-related deaths (deaths during pregnancy or in the first 42 days after delivery)/100,000 live births. The top three causes are pulmonary embolism; hypertension (e.g., pregnancy-induced hypertension, eclampsia); and hemorrhage. The rate increases with age and is higher in Blacks.

Medicare is health insurance for people who are eligible for Social Security (primarily people 65 years old and older, as well as permanently/totally disabled people, and people with end-stage renal disease). Nursing home care is paid by Medicare only for a short term after a hospital admission; then it is paid by the patient (if the person has no money, the state usually pays via Medicaid).

Medicaid covers indigent persons who are deemed eligible by the individual states.

BIOSTATISTICS

Get in the habit of drawing a 2 × 2 table to make calculations easier. Be sure to know how to calculate the common biostatistic parameters listed in Figure 1-1. On the boards, watch out for columns or rows being switched around.

Sensitivity: Ability to detect disease; mathematically, the number of true positives divided by the number of people with the disease. Tests with high sensitivity are used for *screening;* they may have false-positive results but do not miss many people with the disease (low false-negative rate).

Specificity: Ability to detect health (nondisease); mathematically, the number of true negatives divided by the number of people without the disease. Tests with high specificity are used for *disease confirmation;* they may yield false-negative results but do not label as sick anyone who is actually healthy (low false-positive rate). The ideal confirmatory test must have high sensitivity and high specificity. Otherwise, people with the disease may be called healthy.

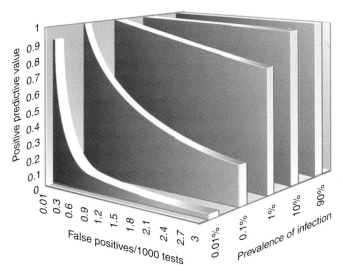

	Disease present	Disease absent
Exposure present	a	b
Exposure absent	c	d

Sensitivity = a/(a + c)
Specificity = d/(b + d)
PPV = a/(a + b)
NPV = d/(c + d)
Odds ratio = (a × d)/(b × c)
Relative risk = [a/(a +b)]/[c/(c + d)]

FIGURE 1-1 Biostatistic parameters. *NPV,* Negative predictive value; *PPV,* positive predictive value. *(From Mandell G, Bennett J, Dolin R: Mandell, Douglas, and Bennett's Principles and Practice of Infectious Disease, 7th ed. Philadelphia, Churchill Livingstone, 2009.)*

FIGURE 1-2 Positive predictive value (PPV) of a human immunodeficiency virus (HIV) confirmatory assay. The PPV is a function of disease prevalence. At very low disease prevalence (0.01%), the PPV of testing declines sharply with any false-positive test results. As the prevalence of infection increases, the PPV improves. HIV screening eliminates a majority of HIV-negative individuals for further confirmation, and the prevalence of the population of samples referred for confirmatory assay increases dramatically and will be in the range of 90%. The PPV for the sequential strategy remains high despite any false-positive results. *(From Mandell G, Bennett J, Dolin R: Mandell, Douglas, and Bennett's Principles and Practice of Infectious Disease, 7th ed. Philadelphia, Churchill Livingstone, 2009.)*

▢ **CASE SCENARIO:** A researcher says that the cutoff fasting glucose value for the diagnosis of diabetes should be lowered from 126 mg/dL to 110 mg/dL. How would this change affect the test's number of false-negative and false-positive results? Fewer false negatives, more false positives. If the cutoff value is raised, fewer people will be called diabetic (more false negatives, fewer false positives).

Positive predictive value (PPV): when a test is positive for disease, the PPV measures how likely it is that the patient has the disease (probability of having a condition, given a positive test). Mathematically, the number of true positives is divided by the number of people with a positive test. *PPV depends on the prevalence of the disease and the sensitivity/specificity of the test* (e.g., an overly sensitive test that gives more false positives has a lower PPV).

▢ **CASE SCENARIO:** How does prevalence affect the PPV? The higher the prevalence, the greater the PPV. See Figure 1-2.

Negative predictive value (NPV): When a test is negative for disease, the NPV measures how likely it is that the patient is healthy (probability of not having a condition, given a negative test). Mathematically, the number of true negatives is divided by the number of people with a negative test. Like PPV, *NPV depends on the prevalence of the disease and the sensitivity/specificity of the test* (the higher the prevalence, the lower the NPV).

▢ **CASE SCENARIO:** How does sensitivity affect NPV? The more sensitive the test, the fewer the number of false negatives and the higher the NPV.

Attributable risk: Number of cases attributable to one risk factor (put another way, the amount you would expect the incidence to decrease if a risk factor were removed). For example, if the incidence rate of lung cancer in the general population is 1/100 and in smokers it is 10/100, the attributable risk of smoking in causing lung cancer is 9/100, assuming a properly matched control (i.e., 10/100 − 1/100 = 9/100).

Relative risk: Compares the disease risk in the exposed population to the disease risk in the unexposed population. *Relative risk can be calculated only after a prospective or experimental study.* Any value for relative risk other than 1 is clinically significant. For example, if the relative risk is 2.0, a person is twice as likely to develop the condition if exposed to the factor in question. If the relative risk is 0.5, the person is only half as likely to develop the condition when exposed to the factor; in other words, the factor protects the person from developing the disease.

📁 **CASE SCENARIO:** After completing a chart and autopsy record review, a researcher finds that pancreatic cancer occurred in 5/1000 smokers and 1/1000 nonsmokers. What is the relative risk of pancreatic cancer in smokers? The relative risk cannot be calculated because this is a retrospective study. Choose "none of the above/can't be calculated."

Odds ratio: Used only for *retrospective studies* (e.g., case-control). The odds ratio compares the odds of having disease versus not having disease in exposed populations versus the odds of having disease versus not having disease in unexposed populations. There should be more disease in exposed than unexposed populations and more nondisease in unexposed than exposed populations. The odds ratio is a less-than-perfect way to estimate relative risk from retrospective data.

📁 **CASE SCENARIO:** A retrospective study finds that pancreatic cancer occurred in 5/1000 smokers and 1/1000 nonsmokers. What is the odds ratio for pancreatic cancer in smokers? 5/995 divided by 1/999, or 5.02.

Standard deviation (SD): With a normal or bell-shaped distribution, 1 SD holds 68% of values, 2 SDs hold 95% of values, and 3 SDs hold 99.7% of values. In a normal distribution, the mean = median = mode (mean is the average value, median is the middle value, and mode is the most common value).

📁 **CASE SCENARIO:** A child scores 140 on an IQ test. A review of the literature reveals that the mean IQ in the child's community is 100, with an SD of 20. How does the child's score compare with that of other children? The child did better on the examination than 97.5% of children in the community. The child scored 2 standard deviations above the mean, which holds 95% of the values. Because 2.5% fall on each end of the bell-shaped curve, the child did better on the examination than 97.5% of children in the community.

Skewed distribution: A *positive skew* is asymmetry with an excess of high values (tail on right, mean > median > mode); a *negative skew* is asymmetry with an excess of low values (tail on left, mean < median < mode). Because positive and negative skews (Fig. 1-3) are not normal distributions, standard deviation and mean are less meaningful values.

Test reliability (synonymous with *precision*) measures the reproducibility and consistency of a test (e.g., the concept of interrater reliability: if two different people administer the same test, the examinee will get the same score if the test is reliable). *Random error reduces reliability/precision* (e.g., limitation in significant figures).

Test validity (synonymous with *accuracy*) measures the trueness of measurement—whether the test measures what it claims to measure (e.g., if you give a valid IQ test to a genius, the test should not indicate that person has a mental disability). *Systematic error reduces validity/accuracy* (e.g., miscalibrated equipment).

Correlation coefficient measures how related two values are. The range of the coefficient is −1 to +1. The important point in determining the strength of the relationship between two variables is how far the number is from zero (i.e., *absolute value*). Zero equals no association whatsoever, +1 equals a perfect positive correlation (when one goes up, so does the other), and −1 equals a perfect negative correlation (Fig. 1-4).

📁 **CASE SCENARIO:** Which is a stronger correlation, +0.3 or −0.3? They are equal.

Confidence interval: When you take a set of data and calculate a mean, you want to say that the result is equivalent to the mean of the whole population, but usually the two values are not exactly equal. The confidence interval (usually set at 95%) says that you are 95% confident that the mean of the population is within a certain range (generally within 2 SD of your

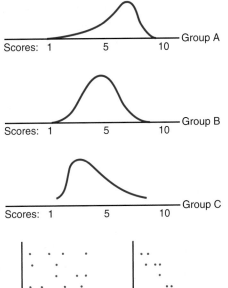

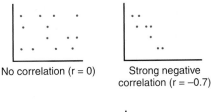

FIGURE 1-3 Group A demonstrates a negative skew *(tail on the left)*, group B has a normal distribution, and group C has a positive skew *(tail on the right)*.

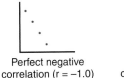

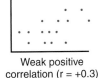

FIGURE 1-4 Correlation graphs.

experimental or derived mean using an adjustment for the sample size). A confidence interval (confidence limits) expressed as $76 < X < 84 = 0.95$ means that you are 95% certain that the mean for the whole population (X) is between 76 and 84.

Different types of studies (listed in decreasing order of quality and desirability):

1. **Experimental study/randomized controlled trial:** the gold standard type of study. Compares two equal groups in which one variable is manipulated and its effect is measured. Remember to check for double-blinding (or at least single-blinding) and well-matched control subjects.
2. **Prospective/longitudinal/cohort/incidence/follow-up study:** choose a sample population, divide it into two groups on the basis of the presence or absence of a risk factor, and follow the groups over time to see what diseases they develop. This approach is sometimes called an *observational study* because all you do is observe. For example, you may follow people with and without asymptomatic hypercholesterolemia to determine whether people with hypercholesterolemia have a higher incidence of myocardial infarction later in life. You can calculate relative risk and incidence. This type of study is time-consuming, expensive, and good for common diseases, whereas retrospective studies are less expensive, less time-consuming, and good for rare diseases.
3. **Retrospective/case-control study:** samples are chosen after the fact on the basis of the presence (cases) or absence (controls) of disease. Then information can be collected about risk factors. For example, you may look at people with lung cancer versus people without lung cancer to determine if the people with lung cancer smoke more.
4. **Case series:** good for extremely rare diseases. You simply describe the clinical presentation of people with a certain disease. Case series may suggest the need for a retrospective study.
5. **Prevalence survey/cross-sectional survey:** looks at the prevalence of a disease and prevalence of risk factors. When two different cultures are compared, you may get an idea for the cause of a disease, which can be tested with a prospective study (e.g., more colon cancer and higher-fat diet in the United States versus less colon cancer and low-fat diet in Japan).

Incidence: the number of new cases of disease in a unit of time (generally in 1 year, but any time frame can be used). The *incidence rate is equal to the absolute risk* (as opposed to relative or attributable risk). In an *epidemic,* the observed incidence greatly exceeds the expected incidence.

Prevalence: the total number of cases of disease (new or old).

■ **CASE SCENARIO:** If a widely used new form of chemotherapy allows patients with lung cancer to survive an extra 2 to 3 years without curing the disease, what will happen to the incidence and prevalence of lung cancer? Nothing happens to the incidence, but the prevalence will increase because people live longer.

■ **CASE SCENARIO:** For influenza, which is higher—incidence or prevalence? In short-term diseases (like the flu), the incidence is often higher than the prevalence (opposite of chronic diseases).

Comparison of data:
1. **Chi-squared test:** used to compare percentages or proportions (nonnumeric or nominal data)
2. **T-test:** used to compare two means
3. **Analysis of variance (ANOVA):** used to compare three or more means

P value: If someone gives you data and tells you that *P* <.05 (commonly used as the cutoff for statistical significance), there is less than a 5% chance (0.05 = 5%) that the data were obtained by random error or chance. If you read that the blood pressure (BP) in a control group is 180/100 mm Hg, but the BP after use of drug X is 120/70 mm Hg with *P* <.10, there is less than a 10% chance that the difference in BP is due to random error or chance (or up to a 9.99% chance that the result is due to chance). Keep three points in mind: (1) The study still may have serious flaws; (2) a low *P* value does *not* imply causation; and (3) a study that has statistical significance does not always have clinical significance (if drug X can lower the BP from 130/80 to 129/80 with *P* <.001, you still would not use drug X because the amount it lowers the blood pressure is negligible).

The *P* value also ties into the null hypothesis (the hypothesis of no difference). For example, in a drug study of hypertension, the null hypothesis is that the drug does not work (any difference in BP is due to random error or chance). When the drug works beautifully and lowers the BP by 60 points, the null hypothesis must be rejected, because clearly the drug works. When *P* <.05, you can confidently reject the null hypothesis because the *P* value says that there is less than a 5% chance that the null hypothesis is correct. To reject the null hypothesis is to say that the difference in BP is not due to chance; it is due to the drug.

The *P* value also represents the chance of making a type I error (concluding that there is an effect or difference when there is not or rejecting the null hypothesis when it is true).

A type II error is to accept the null hypothesis when it is false (the drug works, but you say it does not).

Power: The probability of rejecting the null hypothesis when it is false (a good thing).

■ **CASE SCENARIO:** What is the best way to increase the power of a study? Increase the sample size.

Bias and errors
1. **Recall bias:** a risk for retrospective studies. When patients cannot remember things, they may inadvertently overestimate or underestimate risk factors. For example, John died of lung cancer, and his angry wife remembers him smoking "like a chimney," whereas Mike died of a non–smoking-related disease, and his loving wife denies that he smoked much. In reality, both men smoked one pack per day.
2. **Interviewer bias:** occurs when there is no blinding. When a scientist receives big money to do a study and wants to find a difference between cases and controls, he or she may inadvertently interpret the same patient comment or outcome as "not significant" in the control group and "significant" in the treatment group.
3. **Unacceptability bias:** Patients do not admit to embarrassing behavior. They claim to exercise more than they do to please the interviewer, or they may claim to take experimental drugs when they spit them out.

■ **CASE SCENARIO:** An experimenter measures the number of ashtrays owned and the incidence of lung cancer and finds that people with lung cancer have more ashtrays. He concludes that ashtrays cause lung cancer. What is the flaw in the study? *Confounding variable* (smoking tobacco is the confounding variable because it causes the increase in both ashtrays and lung cancer).

📁 **CASE SCENARIO:** The mortality data for city A, a retirement community, and city B, a college town, are compared. The rate for A is much higher than that for B, and the researcher says that pollution or other toxic exposure must be the cause. What is the error? *Nonrandom or nonstratified sampling.* Of course city A will have a higher mortality rate (due to age differences) if the groups are not stratified into appropriate age-specific comparisons.

📁 **CASE SCENARIO:** A phone survey of 100 people finds 30 people who smoke and 20 who do not. The other 50 people did not answer the phone. The researcher concludes that the community has a smoking prevalence of 60%. What is the error? *Nonresponse bias.* In this case, the first step to try to salvage the results is repeated attempts to reach the nonresponders. If this approach is unsuccessful, list the nonresponders as unknown in the data analysis and see if any results can be salvaged. Never make up or assume responses.

📁 **CASE SCENARIO:** A prostate cancer screening test claims to prolong survival when compared with older survival data, using the same standard treatment as before. The researcher claims that earlier detection improves mortality from prostate cancer. What is the error? *Lead-time bias,* which is due to time differentials. The difference in survival is due only to earlier detection, not improved treatment or prolonged survival.

📁 **CASE SCENARIO:** In-hospital death rates for myocardial infarction (MI) are compared between hospitals A and B. Hospital A has a higher in-hospital mortality rate. Hospital A also has a cardiac catheterization lab and dedicated coronary care unit; hospital B has neither and transfers patients to hospital A if they need a catheterization lab or coronary care unit. The researcher concludes that hospital B provides better care. What is the error? *Admission rate bias.* If you take on the tough cases (hospital B does not), you are sure to have higher mortality rates. The same error also can apply to surgical mortality/morbidity rates if the surgeon takes only tough cases.

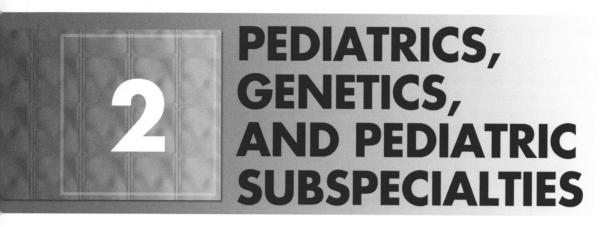

2 PEDIATRICS, GENETICS, AND PEDIATRIC SUBSPECIALTIES

GENERAL PEDIATRICS

Screening and preventive care

Height, weight, blood pressure, developmental/behavioral assessment, history/physical examination, and anticipatory guidance (counseling/discussion about age-appropriate concerns) should be done at every pediatric visit. Also, remember the following:

1. **Congenital screening:** All states screen for hypothyroidism, phenylketonuria, and galactosemia at birth (must be done within the first month). Most states screen for cystic fibrosis and sickle cell disease. As of 2010, 30 disorders are recommended for screening by the U.S. Department of Health and Human Services.

☐ **CASE SCENARIO:** A newborn screening test is positive for phenylketonuria. What should you do next? Order a confirmatory test to make sure that the screen gave you a true positive.

2. **Anticipatory guidance.** Keep the water heater at 110–120°F; use car restraints; put the baby to sleep on his or her *back* on a firm sleeping surface with light (i.e., not too heavy) clothing to help prevent sudden infant death syndrome (SIDS); do not use infant walkers, which cause fall injuries; watch out for small objects that the baby may aspirate; do not give cow's milk or honey (may contain botulism spores) before 1 year of age; introduce solid foods gradually, starting at about 6 months; supervise children in any open body of water such as a bathtub or swimming pool; and keep chemicals out of reach.

3. **Height, weight, and head circumference.** Head circumference (HC) should be measured routinely in the first 2 years; height and weight should be measured routinely until adulthood. All three are markers of general well-being. The pattern of growth along plotted growth curves tells you more than any raw number. If a patient has always been low or high compared with peers, the pattern is generally benign. If a child changes from a normal curve to an abnormal one, the pattern is much more worrisome. The classic situation involves parents who bring in a child with delayed physical growth or delayed puberty: You must know when to reassure them and when to investigate further after looking at a plotted growth curve (Fig. 2-1).

 *Increased HC may mean hydrocephalus or tumor; decreased HC may mean microcephaly due to intrauterine and/or perinatal infection with one of the **TORCH** infections—**t**oxoplasmosis, **o**ther infections (e.g., congenital syphilis, human immunodeficiency virus [HIV] infection, varicella-zoster virus infection), **r**ubella, **c**ytomegalovirus, or **h**erpes simplex virus.*

☐ **CASE SCENARIO:** What should you suspect as the cause of obesity? Obesity is usually due to overeating and lack of exercise combined with as yet undefined genetic/familial tendencies. Less than 5% of cases are due to specific organic causes (e.g., Cushing syndrome, Prader-Willi syndrome).

☐ **CASE SCENARIO:** What is the most common cause of failure to thrive? Defined as growth below the 5th percentile for age, failure to thrive is most commonly due to psychosocial or functional problems (watch for child abuse or neglect). Organic causes should have specific clues to trigger your suspicion.

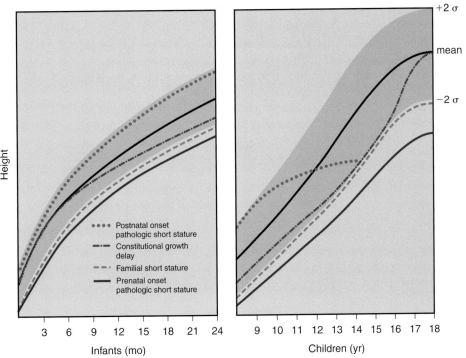

FIGURE 2-1 Height-for-age curves for the four general causes of proportional short stature: postnatal onset pathologic short stature, constitutional growth delay, familial short stature, and prenatal onset short stature. *(From Kliegman RM, Stanton BMD, St. Geme J, et al: Nelson Textbook of Pediatrics, 19th ed. Philadelphia, Saunders, 2011.)*

4. **Hearing and vision.** Hearing should be measured objectively at birth. Hearing and vision should be measured objectively at least every 2–3 years starting at the age of 4 (until late adolescence). Measure more often if history dictates.

 *Check the red reflex at birth and routinely thereafter to detect congenital cataracts (classically due to congenital rubella/TORCH or galactosemia) or **retinoblastoma** (causes leukocoria, or absence of the red reflex from the retina of the eye due to the underlying tumor).*

▭ **CASE SCENARIO:** Until what age is a "lazy eye" normal? Consistent eye deviation (strabismus) is not normal at any age. Occasional misalignment of one eye may be normal until 3 months of age. After 3 months, refer to an ophthalmologist to prevent *amblyopia* (see ophthalmology section).

▭ **CASE SCENARIO:** What two classic infectious diseases are associated with acquired hearing loss in children? *Meningitis* and *recurrent otitis media*.

5. **Anemia.** Recommendations for routine screening for anemia vary and are changing. Hemoglobin and hematocrit measurement is recommended at 12 months of age but may be required at other times as dictated by history and risk assessment (e.g., prematurity, low birth weight, use of cow's milk before 12 months, poor dietary intake). All infants except full-term infants who are exclusively breast-fed may be candidates for prophylactic iron supplements. Start iron supplements in full-term infants at 4–6 months of age and in preterm infants at 2 months of age. Most infant formulas and cereals contain iron, so separate supplements usually are not required. Menstruating adolescent females are also at risk for iron deficiency anemia—consider screening if given the option or patients have vague fatigue symptoms.

6. **Lead.** Exposure to lead can cause neurologic damage ranging from mild learning disabilities or hyperactivity to mental retardation. Routine screening is now controversial and usually only recommended for high-risk children (e.g., the child lives in an old building and is a paint-chip eater or lives near a battery recycling plant). If the level is greater than 10 mg/dL, closer follow-up and intervention are necessary. The best first course of action is to *stop the exposure*. Lead chelation therapy may be necessary with *succimer (preferred in children)* or dimercaprol (for more severe cases)

for lead levels greater than 45 µg/dL. Levels greater than 70 µg/dL require hospitalization with intravenous (IV) chelation.

7. **Fluoride.** Most children need no supplementation because fluoride is in most tap water. Supplementation is necessary in the first few years of life if water is inadequately fluoridated (primarily in rural areas relying on well water). Too much fluoride can cause mottled bones and teeth. An initial dentist appointment is recommended by 3 years of age.

8. **Vitamin D.** The American Academy of Pediatrics recommends that exclusively and partially breast-fed infants receive vitamin D supplements shortly after birth and continue until they are weaned from breast milk and consume either formula or whole milk. Formula-fed infants do not require supplements in the United States because all formulas contain vitamin D supplements.

9. **Tuberculosis (TB).** Do not screen for TB unless there are risk factors or symptoms. Screen annually at any age if risk factors are present (e.g., HIV infection, incarceration). If the only risk factor is that the child lives in a high-risk area or is the offspring of an immigrant, screen once at 4–6 years of age and once at 11–16 years of age.

10. **Urinalysis.** Universal screening is not recommended. However, screen for congenital/anatomic abnormalities after a urinary tract infection (UTI) in children 2 months to 2 years of age by getting an ultrasound and voiding cystourethrogram (VCUG). Screening in older children after a UTI is more controversial unless the UTIs are recurrent.

11. **Immunizations.** Things have become more complex as combination vaccines have been introduced, and different manufacturers may produce the same vaccine with slightly different schedules. You need to know rough ages and administration, but precise schedule memorization is low yield. A routine immunization schedule for healthy children with no specific risk factors is shown in Table 2-1; indications and contraindications are given in Table 2-2.

TABLE 2-1 Routine Vaccination Schedule

	BIRTH	2 mo	4 mo	6 mo	12-15 mo	15-18 mo	4-6 yr	11-12 yr
Hepatitis B	#1	#2		#3				
Diphtheria, tetanus, pertussis (DTP)		#1	#2	#3		#4	#5	Tdap Booster
Haemophilus influenzae type b		#1	#2	#3	#4			
Pneumococcus		#1	#2	#3	#4			
Polio, inactivated		#1	#2	#3 (6-18 mo)			#4	
Measles, mumps, rubella (MMR)					#1		#2	
Hepatitis A					#1 (12-18 mo)	#2 (6 mo after #1)		
Varicella					#1 (12-18 mo)		#2	
Meningococcal								#1
Rotavirus		#1	#2	#3				
Influenza*				#1 (yearly after)				

*Influenza vaccine should be given yearly beginning at the age of 6 months.
Human papillomavirus: 3 doses beginning around age 11 and up to age 26 years in females.
HPV4 may be given in a 3-dose series to males aged 9-26 years to reduce the likelihood of acquiring genital warts.

TABLE 2-2 Vaccine Indications and Contraindications

VACCINE	INDICATIONS AND CONTRAINDICATIONS
Rotavirus	Be aware of possible risk of intussusception after vaccination and avoid in those with history of intussusception and those who are immunocompromised
Measles, mumps, rubella (MMR)	Avoid in children with anaphylactic reaction to eggs or neomycin, avoid in those with severe immunodeficiency (HIV-infected patients without clinically significant AIDS should receive this vaccine)

TABLE 2-2 Vaccine Indications and Contraindications—cont'd

VACCINE	INDICATIONS AND CONTRAINDICATIONS
Hepatitis B	Give first dose at birth with hepatitis B immune globulin if mother has active hepatitis B
Polio	Avoid in those with anaphylaxis to neomycin or streptomycin
Varicella	Avoid in those with immunodeficiency or anaphylaxis to neomycin
Influenza	Starting at age 6, give to children with immunodeficiency, with cardiovascular or respiratory disease, or on chronic aspirin therapy (to prevent Reye syndrome), or close contacts of high-risk person; avoid in those with anaphylaxis to eggs
Meningococcus	Give to children 2-10 yr of age with terminal complement deficiencies, other immunodeficiency, or anatomic/functional asplenia
Pneumococcus	Give to children older than 2 yr of age who have not been vaccinated if they have immunodeficiency of any kind or surgical/functional asplenia (sickle cell)
Rabies	Postexposure, administer rabies immunoglobulin plus 4 doses of vaccine in immunocompetent patients; administer immunoglobulin plus 5 doses of vaccine in immunocompromised patients

CASE SCENARIO: A 1-year-old boy presents for routine evaluation. He has a history of severe wheezing, shortness of breath, and allergy (rash) to eggs. What vaccine should be avoided? Influenza vaccine. Immediate hypersensitivity reaction to eggs is a contraindication to the influenza vaccine.

Infants

Apgar score. The Apgar score is assessed 1 and 5 minutes after birth. Immediate intervention (e.g., intubation) for a neonate in distress should not be delayed for Apgar scoring. The scale consists of five categories with a maximum score of 2 points per category, for a maximum total of 10 points. Resuscitation and close monitoring are usually performed until the child gets a score greater than 7 or goes to the intensive care unit (Table 2-3).

TABLE 2-3 Apgar Score

PARAMETER	0	1	2
Heart rate (beats/min)	Absent	<100	>100
Respiratory effort	None	Slow, weak cry	Good, strong cry
Muscle tone	Limp	Some flexion of extremities	Active motion
Color	Pale, blue	Pink body, blue extremities	Completely pink
Reflex/irritability*	None	Grimace	Grimace and strong cry/cough/sneeze

*Done by checking the response to stimulation of the sole of foot or a catheter put in the nose.

Umbilical cord. Check the umbilical cord at birth for two arteries and one vein. If only one umbilical artery is present, consider the possibility of *congenital renal malformations*.

Caput succedaneum is diffuse swelling/edema of the scalp at birth that *crosses the midline* and is benign (no further testing necessary). Cephalohematomas are subperiosteal hemorrhages that are sharply limited by sutures and *do not cross the midline*. Both result from birth trauma. Cephalohematomas are usually benign and self-resolving, but in rare cases they may indicate an underlying skull fracture (consider ordering computed tomography [CT] scan without contrast to rule out a fracture).

Infantile hemangioma. First noticed a few days after birth, the tumor increases in size after birth and then gradually resolves within the first few years. Most hemangiomas (65%) in infancy are capillary hemangiomas, whereas 15% are cavernous hemangiomas. If they are on the face/lid and obscure the visual axis, they need to be treated to prevent amblyopia; otherwise, they can be watched. If the hemangioma is large and the infant has petechiae, consider Kasabach-Merritt syndrome with platelet sequestration in the hemangioma and thrombocytopenia.

The anterior fontanelle usually closes by 18 months. A large anterior fontanelle or delayed closure may indicate *hypothyroidism, hydrocephalus*, rickets, or intrauterine growth retardation (IUGR).

Moro and palmar grasp reflexes usually disappear by 6 months. An absent or inadequate Moro reflex (sudden loss of support) on one side is characteristic in infants with hemiplegia, brachial plexus palsy, or a fractured clavicle. Persistence of the Moro response beyond the age of 6 months is noted in infants with severe neurologic defects such as cerebral palsy.

Milestones and miscellaneous issues

Among many developmental milestones, the commonly tested ones are listed in Table 2-4. The exact age is not as important as the overall pattern when you are looking for dysfunctional development. When in doubt, use a formal developmental test. Table 2-4 gives rough average ages when milestones are achieved:

TABLE 2-4 Developmental Milestones			
MILESTONE	**AGE***	**MILESTONE**	**AGE***
Social smile	1-2 mo	Voluntary grasp with voluntary release	10 mo
Cooing sounds	2-4 mo	Waves "bye-bye"	10 mo
While prone, lifts head up 90 degrees	3-4 mo	Separation anxiety	12-15 mo
Rolls front to back	4-5 mo	Walks without help	13 mo
Voluntary grasp (no release)	5 mo	Can build tower of 2 cubes	13-15 mo
Stranger anxiety	6-9 mo	Understand one step commands (no gesture)	15 mo
Sits with no support	7 mo	Good use of cup and spoon	15-18 mo
Pulls to stand	9 mo	Runs well	2 yr
Plays pat-a-cake	9-10 mo	Can build tower of 6 cubes	2 yr
First words	9-12 mo	Ties shoelaces	5 yr
Imitates others' sounds	9-12 mo		

*Remember that the age of a premature patient is reduced in the first 2 years in assessments of development (e.g., a premature child born after 6 months' gestation will have 3 months subtracted from his or her chronologic age; thus, when 9 months old, the infant is expected to perform only at the 6-month-old level).

Tanner stages. Stage I is preadolescent; stage V is adult. Increasing stages are assigned for testicular and penile growth in males and for breast growth in females; both also use pubic hair development. Average age at puberty (when the patient first changes from stage I status) is 11.5 years in boys, usually with *testicular enlargement* as the first event, and 10.5 years in girls, usually with *breast development* as the first event.

Delayed puberty becomes evident when there is no testicular enlargement in boys by the age of 14 years and no breast development or pubic hair in girls by the age of 13 years. The delay usually is a *constitutional delay*, which is a normal variant. Parents often have a similar history, and the growth curve lags behind that for peers of the same age but is a consistent curve. Delayed puberty is rarely due to primary testicular failure (e.g., *Klinefelter syndrome*, cryptorchidism, history of chemotherapy, gonadal dysgenesis) or ovarian failure (e.g., *Turner syndrome*, gonadal dysgenesis). It also is rarely due to hypothalamic/pituitary defect such as a tumor.

Precocious puberty is usually idiopathic. Rare causes include *McCune-Albright syndrome* (café-au-lait spots, fibrous dysplasia, and precocious puberty in girls); ovarian tumors (granulosa cell or theca cell, which can secrete estrogen); testicular tumors (Leydig cell, which can secrete testosterone); central nervous system (CNS) disease or trauma (e.g., pineal gland or hypothalamus affected); adrenal neoplasm; and *congenital adrenal hyperplasia* (in boys, usually 21-hydroxylase deficiency; in girls, associated with ambiguous genitalia). Most patients with uncorrectable, idiopathic precocious puberty are given long-acting *gonadotropin-releasing hormone* (GnRH) agonists to suppress progression of puberty and thus prevent premature epiphyseal closure.

Child abuse. Watch for failure to thrive; multiple fractures, bruises, or injuries in different stages of healing—order a skeletal survey; "shaken baby syndrome" (subdural hematomas and retinal hemorrhages with no external trauma signs; get a dilated fundus exam); behavioral, emotional, and interaction problems; sexually transmitted diseases; and multiple personality disorder (sexual abuse). Metaphyseal "bucket handle"/metaphyseal "corner" fractures, fractures of long bones, and/or posterior rib fractures on radiograph are essentially pathognomonic for child abuse (Fig. 2-2). *Consider abuse whenever the injury does not fit the story.*

▢ **CASE SCENARIO:** You suspect child abuse but are not sure. Should you report your suspicion to the authorities? Reporting any child abuse suspicion is mandatory. You do not need proof and cannot be sued for reporting your suspicion.

GENETICS

Chromosomal disorders

1. **Down syndrome (trisomy 21):** the most common known cause of mental retardation. The major risk factor is the age of the mother (1/1500 offspring of 16-year-old mothers, 1/25 offspring of 45-year-old mothers). At birth look for hypotonia, transverse palmar crease, and characteristic facies. *Congenital cardiac defects* (especially ventricular septal defect) are common and often affect prognosis. Patients

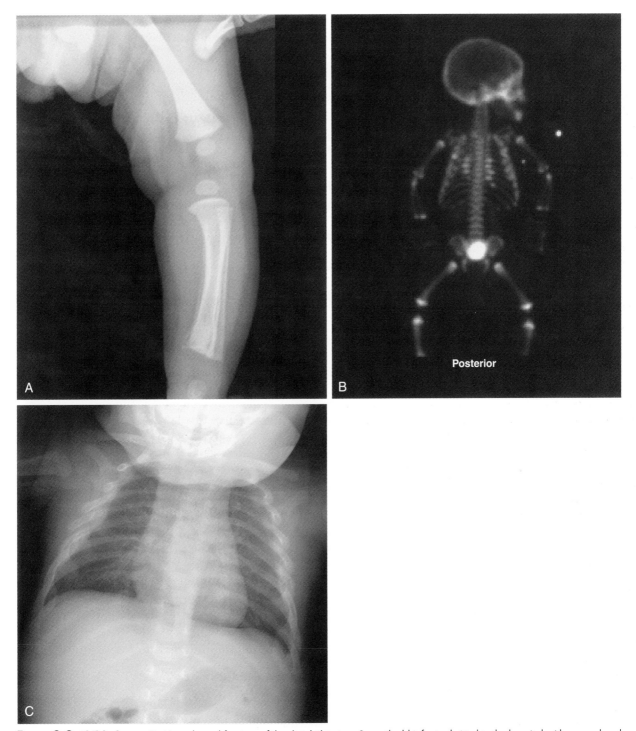

FIGURE 2-2 Child abuse. A, Metaphyseal fracture of the distal tibia in a 3-month-old infant admitted to the hospital with severe head injury. **B,** Bone scan revealed multiple previously unrecognized fractures of the posterior and lateral ribs. **C,** Follow-up radiographs 2 weeks later showed multiple healing rib fractures. This pattern of fracture is highly specific for child abuse. The mechanism of these injuries is usually violent squeezing of the chest. *(From Marcdante K, Kliegman R, Behrman R, Jenson H: Nelson Essentials of Pediatrics, 5th ed. Philadelphia, Saunders, 2005.)*

also are at increased risk for leukemia, duodenal atresia (and other bowel atresia), Hirschsprung disease, celiac disease, hypothyroidism, obstructive sleep apnea, gastroesophageal reflux disease (GERD), upper respiratory tract infections, infertility, visual problems, and early Alzheimer disease.

2. **Edward syndrome (trisomy 18):** more common in females than in males; mental retardation, small size for age, small head, hypoplastic mandible, low-set ears, *clenched fist with index finger overlapping third and fourth fingers* (almost pathognomonic and can be seen on prenatal ultrasound imaging). Early childhood death is typical.

3. **Patau syndrome (trisomy 13):** mental retardation, apnea, deafness, *holoprosencephaly* (fusion of cerebral hemispheres), myelomeningocele, *cleft lip/palate,* cardiovascular abnormalities, rocker-bottom feet. Early pediatric death is typical.

4. **Turner syndrome (females with XO instead of XX):** lymphedema of the neck at birth, short stature, webbed neck, low posterior hairline, widely spaced nipples, amenorrhea, and lack of breast development (due to primary ovarian failure; patients are infertile). Patients are at increased risk for *coarctation of the aorta,* horseshoe kidney, hypothyroidism, diabetes, and *cystic hygroma* (classically of the neck).

5. **Cri-du-chat:** due to a deletion on the short arm of chromosome 5. Look for a high-pitched cry like a cat, along with severe mental retardation.

📁 **CASE SCENARIO:** A 33-year-old man comes to you because he and his wife have been unable to conceive. He is tall and thin. On exam, you note gynecomastia, sparse body hair, and small testicles. What is the patient's most likely karyotype? XXY. Infertility is the classic presentation of Klinefelter syndrome. Patients are tall with microtestes (<2 cm in length), gynecomastia, sterility, and mildly decreased intelligence quotient (IQ).

On the USMLE Step 3 exam, you may see multiple-choice questions regarding genetic counseling or asking you to predict the likelihood of having a second affected child after the first is born with a disease. It is assumed that you know the inheritance pattern for the disease.

Autosomal Dominant

Look for an affected mother or father who passes the disease to 50% of offspring.

○ von Willebrand disease
○ Neurofibromatosis: café-au-lait spots, profuse peripheral nerve tumors, acoustic schwannoma
○ Multiple endocrine neoplasia (MEN) I and II syndromes
○ Achondroplasia (diagnosis from picture of the patient)
○ Marfan syndrome: tall height, arachnodactyly, mitral valve prolapse, aortic dissection, lens dislocation
○ Huntington disease
○ Familial hypercholesterolemia: Look for xanthomas and early coronary artery disease, markedly elevated cholesterol
○ Familial polyposis coli
○ Adult polycystic kidney disease
○ Hereditary spherocytosis
○ Tuberous sclerosis: *facial angiofibromas* (i.e., *adenoma sebaceum*), *seizures, mental retardation* (i.e., classic mnemonic: "zits, fits, and nitwits"), CNS hamartomas, cardiac rhabdomyomas, renal angiomyolipomas, and hypopigmented skin macules
○ Myotonic dystrophy: muscle weakness with *inability to release grip,* balding, cataracts, mental retardation, and cardiac arrhythmias

Autosomal Recessive

Look for family history and unaffected parents who pass the disease to 25% of children.

○ Sphingolipidoses (e.g., Tay-Sachs disease, Gaucher disease; the exception is Fabry disease, which is X-linked)
○ Mucopolysaccharidoses (e.g., Hurler disease; the exception is Hunter disease, which is X-linked)
○ Glycogen storage diseases (e.g., Pompe disease, McArdle disease)
○ Cystic fibrosis
○ Galactosemia: look for congenital cataracts, neonatal sepsis; avoid galactose- and lactose-containing foods
○ Amino acid disorders (e.g., phenylketonuria, alkaptonuria)
○ Sickle cell disease
○ Childhood or infantile polycystic kidney disease
○ Wilson disease
○ Hemochromatosis (usually)
○ Adrenogenital syndrome (e.g., 21-hydroxylase deficiency)

📁 **CASE SCENARIO:** A 45-year-old man is diagnosed with adult polycystic kidney disease. His wife has no kidney disease and no family history of kidney disease. He wants to know the likelihood that his two children may have the disease. What do you tell him? Each child has roughly a 50% chance of having the disease.

▢ **CASE SCENARIO:** An asymptomatic couple has a child with phenylketonuria. What is the chance that their next child will have it? 25%.

X-Linked Recessive
Look for affected fathers, who pass the gene only to their daughters (who become carriers but do not get the disease), and carrier mothers (family history in male relatives), who pass the disease to their sons.
○ Hemophilia
○ Glucose-6-phosphate dehydrogenase (G6PD) deficiency
○ Fabry disease
○ Hunter disease
○ Lesch-Nyhan syndrome: hypoxanthine-guanine phosphoribosyltransferase (HPRT) enzyme deficiency. Look for mental retardation and *self-mutilation* (patients may bite off their own fingers).
○ Duchenne muscular dystrophy
○ Wiscott-Aldrich syndrome
○ Bruton agammaglobulinemia
○ Fragile X syndrome: second most common cause of mental retardation in males (after Down syndrome). Patients have large testes.

▢ **CASE SCENARIO:** A healthy man had a father with hemophilia. He wants to know the likelihood that his sons will have hemophilia. His wife is healthy and has no family history of the condition. What do you tell him? His children's risk is no higher than that for the general population (close to 0%). Fathers cannot pass X-linked conditions on to their sons.

Polygenic Disorders
Relatives are more likely to have disease, but there is no known obvious heritable pattern (yet).
○ Pyloric stenosis
○ Cleft lip/palate
○ Type 2 diabetes
○ Obesity
○ Neural tube defects
○ Schizophrenia
○ Bipolar disorder
○ Ischemic heart disease
○ Alcoholism

▢ **CASE SCENARIO:** Assuming that the parent is an alcoholic, which child has the highest risk for alcoholism—the daughter of an alcoholic father, the son of an alcoholic father, the daughter of an alcoholic mother, or the son of an alcoholic mother? The son of an alcoholic father.

PEDIATRIC SUBSPECIALTIES

Pediatric cardiology
Table 2-5 provides a general description of several congenital heart defects:

TABLE 2-5 Congenital Heart Defects	
DEFECT	**SYMPTOMS, TREATMENT, AND OTHER INFORMATION**
PDA	Constant, machine-like murmur in upper left sternal border; dyspnea and possible CHF; close PDA with indomethacin (surgery is required if this approach fails); keep open with prostaglandin E_1; associated with congenital rubella and high altitudes
VSD	Holosystolic murmur next to sternum; most VSDs resolve on their own; most common congenital heart defect
ASD	Asymptomatic until adulthood; fixed, split S_2 and palpitations; most ASDs do not require correction (unless they are large)
TOF	Consists of 4 anomalies: (1) VSD, (2) right ventricular hypertrophy, (3) pulmonary stenosis, and (4) overriding aorta. Most common cyanotic congenital heart defect; look for "tet" spells (squatting after exertion)

Continued

TABLE 2-5 Congenital Heart Defects—cont'd	
DEFECT	**SYMPTOMS, TREATMENT, AND OTHER INFORMATION**
TGA	Aorta connected to the right ventricle, pulmonary artery connected to the left ventricle—dependent on PDA and/or ASD for survival until surgical correction. Often diagnosed via prenatal ultrasound. Can manifest with cyanosis and dyspnea after birth, or failure to thrive later
C of A	Upper extremity hypertension only, radiofemoral delay, systolic murmur heard over mid- to upper back, rib notching on radiograph; associated with Turner syndrome

ASD, Atrial septal defect; *CHF,* congestive heart failure; *C of A,* coarctation of aorta; *PDA,* patent ductus arteriosus; *TGA,* transposition of the great arteries; *TOF,* tetralogy of Fallot; *VSD,* ventral septal defect.

 Note | *Endocarditis prophylaxis is required for all of the cardiac defects listed in the table except asymptomatic, secundum-type atrial septal defects (80% of ASDs).*

Remember that a heart rate over 100 beats/min may be normal in pediatric patients (up to age 10).

In patients with a ventricular septum defect (VSD), think about the possibility of *fetal alcohol syndrome* (Fig. 2-3), *TORCH syndrome, or Down syndrome.*

📁 **CASE SCENARIO:** A 17-year-old male athlete with a family history of sudden death at an early age collapses suddenly during a basketball game. What condition should you consider? Hypertrophic cardiomyopathy. In living patients, it is diagnosed with echocardiography and/or magnetic resonance imaging (MRI) and treated with β-blockers and a pacemaker. Positive inotropic agents (e.g., digoxin), diuretics, and vasodilators are contraindicated because they make things worse.

Remember that in fetal circulation, oxygen content is highest in the umbilical vein and lowest in the umbilical arteries. In addition, oxygen content is higher in blood going to the upper extremities than in blood going to the lower extremities.

Circulation changes with the transition from intrauterine to extrauterine life. First breaths inflate the lungs and cause decreased pulmonary vascular resistance, which increases blood flow to the pulmonary arteries. This and the clamping of the cord increase left-sided heart pressures, which functionally closes the foramen ovale. Increased oxygen concentration shuts off prostaglandin production in the ductus arteriosus, causing gradual closure.

📁 **CASE SCENARIO:** A child has two episodes of dizziness, dyspnea, or passing out after playing, and then is fine and has no other symptoms. You are shown an electrocardiogram (ECG)

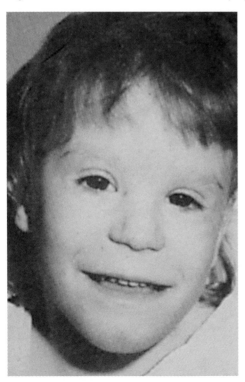

FIGURE 2-3 Classic fetal alcohol syndrome facies with maxillary hypoplasia, shortened palpebral fissures, a flat nasal bridge, and a thin upper lip. Affected children are at increased risk for congenital heart defects, especially ventricular septal defect.

taken while the child has no symptoms. What should you look for on the ECG to make a diagnosis of Wolff-Parkinson-White syndrome? The delta wave (Fig. 2-4). The symptoms were probably caused by transient arrhythmias via accessory pathways.

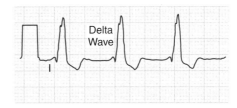

Figure 2-4 Electrocardiogram demonstrating a delta wave, which creates the "double peak" in the QRS complex, as well as a short PR interval and a wide QRS complex, in a patient with Wolff-Parkinson-White syndrome.

Pediatric gastroenterology

Gastrointestinal malformations in children. Each of the following gastrointestinal (GI) conditions (Table 2-6; Fig. 2-5) is generally treated with surgical repair. Other pediatric GI conditions are listed in Table 2-7 (Fig. 2-6).

TABLE 2-6 Gastrointestinal Malformations in Children

NAME	PRESENTING AGE	VOMITUS	FINDINGS/KEY WORDS
Pyloric stenosis	0-2 mo	Nonbilious, projectile	M >> F; palpable olive-shaped mass in epigastrium, low chloride, low potassium, metabolic alkalosis
Duodenal atresia	0-1 wk	Bilious	"Double-bubble" sign, Down syndrome
Tracheoesophageal fistula*	0-2 wk	Food regurgitation	Respiratory compromise with feeding, aspiration pneumonia; cannot thread nasogastric tube past esophagus; stomach distended by air
Hirchsprung disease	0-2 yr	Feculent	Abdominal distention, obstipation, failure or delayed passage of meconium; no ganglia seen on rectal biopsy, M >> F
Anal atresia	0-1 wk	Late, feculent	Detected on initial exam in nursery; M >> F
Choanal atresia	0-1 wk	—	Cyanosis with feeding, relieved by crying; cannot pass nasogastric tube through nose

*Most common variant (85% of cases) has esophageal atresia with a fistula from bronchus to distal esophagus (which explains gastric distention because each breath transmits air to gastrointestinal tract). Be able to recognize a sketch of this most common variant (see figure). A classic chest radiograph shows the nasogastric tube coiled in the esophagus with a large, air-filled stomach.

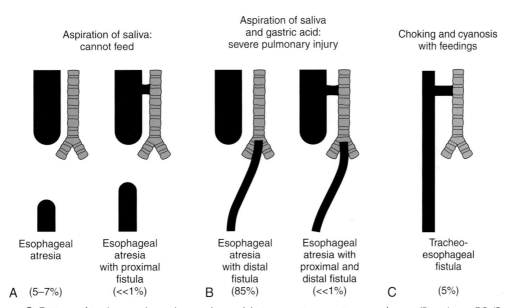

Figure 2-5 Types of tracheoesophageal anomalies and their presenting symptom complexes. *(From James EC, Corry RJ, Perry JF: Principles of Basic Surgical Practice. Philadelphia, Hanley & Belfus, 1987.)*

TABLE 2-7 Pediatric Gastrointestinal Conditions

NAME	PRESENTING AGE	VOMITUS	FINDINGS/KEY WORDS
Intussusception	4 mo–2 yr	Bilious	Currant-jelly stools (blood and mucus); palpable sausage-like mass; treat with air or barium enema (diagnostic and therapeutic), unless there is pneumoperitoneum or evidence of obstruction, then surgery
Necrotizing enterocolitis	0-2 mo	Bilious	Premature infants; fever, rectal bleeding, bowel distention or air in bowel wall on radiographs; treat with NPO status, orogastric tube, intravenous fluids, antibiotics
Meconium ileus	0-2 wk	Feculent, late	Cystic fibrosis manifestation (as is rectal prolapse)
Midgut volvulus	0-2 yr	Bilious	Sudden onset of pain, distention, rectal bleeding, peritonitis, "bird's beak" in small bowel (not large bowel, as in adults) on contrast study; treat with emergent surgery
Meckel diverticulum	0-2 yr	Varies	Rule of 2s,* GI ulceration/bleeding; use Meckel scan to detect; treat with surgery
Strangulated hernia	Any age	Bilious	Physical exam detects bowel loops in the inguinal canal

GI, Gastrointestinal; *NPO,* nothing by mouth.
*Rule of 2s: 2% of population affected (most common GI tract abnormality—remnant of the omphalomesenteric duct), 2 inches long, within 2 feet of ileocolic junction, manifests in the first 2 years of life, twice as likely to occur in males. Meckel diverticulum can cause GI bleeding, intussusception, obstruction, and/or volvulus.

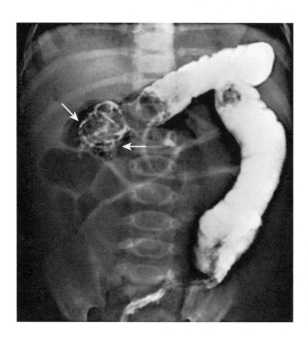

FIGURE 2-6 Intussusception in an infant. The obstruction is evident in the proximal transverse colon. Contrast material between the intussusceptum and the intussuscipiens is responsible for the coiled-spring appearance. *(From Kliegman RM, Stanton BMD, St. Geme J, et al: Nelson Textbook of Pediatrics, 19th ed. Philadelphia, Saunders, 2011.)*

Diaphragmatic hernia is more common on the left side and affects boys more often than girls. Bowel herniates into the thorax, which compresses and impedes lung development (pulmonary hypoplasia results). Patients present with respiratory distress and have bowel sounds in the chest and bowel loops in the thorax on chest radiograph. Treat surgically. Prognosis is related to lung development, not to the hernia.

Omphalocele versus gastroschisis. Omphalocele is in the *midline,* the sac contains multiple abdominal organs, the umbilical ring is absent, and other anomalies are common. Gastroschisis is *to the right of the midline,* only small bowel is exposed (there is no true hernia sac), the umbilical ring is present, and other anomalies are rare.

Henoch-Schönlein purpura may manifest with GI bleeding and abdominal pain. Look for history of upper respiratory or GI infection, *characteristic purpuric rash on lower extremities and buttocks,* swelling in hands and feet, arthritis, and hematuria or proteinuria. Treat supportively.

Children develop nausea, vomiting, and/or diarrhea with *any systemic illness* more commonly than adults. Children can develop inflammatory bowel disease (IBD) or irritable bowel syndrome (IBS) and often have GI complaints with *anxiety* or *psychiatric problems* (e.g., separation anxiety, dislike of school, depression, child abuse).

Neonatal jaundice may be physiologic or pathologic. The first step is to measure total, direct, and indirect bilirubin. The main concern is *kernicterus*, which is due to high levels of unconjugated bilirubin with subsequent deposit into the basal ganglia, causing irreversible damage. Watch for poor feeding, seizures, flaccidity, opisthotonos (muscular spasm that results in spine bending, with body resting on heels and head), and/or apnea to accompany severe jaundice.

1. Physiologic jaundice is seen in 50% of normal infants and is even more common in premature infants. *Symptoms start 1–2 days after birth.* Bilirubin is mostly unconjugated. In full-term infants, bilirubin should be less than 12 mg/dL, peak at day 2–5, and return to normal by 2 weeks. In premature infants, the bilirubin should be less than 15 mg/dL and return to normal by 3 weeks.

2. Pathologic jaundice. Bilirubin levels are higher than normal and continue to rise or fail to decrease appropriately. *Any jaundice present at birth is pathologic.* The differential diagnosis includes the following:

○ Breast milk jaundice is seen in breastfed infants with peak bilirubin levels of 10–20 mg/dL at 2–3 weeks of age. Treat with temporary cessation of breastfeeding (switch to bottle) until jaundice resolves.

○ Illness. Infection or sepsis, hypothyroidism, liver insult, cystic fibrosis, and other illnesses may prolong neonatal jaundice and lower the threshold for kernicterus. The point to remember is that the youngest, sickest infants are at greatest risk for hyperbilirubinemia and kernicterus.

○ Hemolysis due to Rh incompatibility or congenital red cell diseases in the neonatal period. Look for anemia, peripheral smear abnormalities, family history, and higher levels of unconjugated bilirubin.

○ Metabolic. *Criggler–Najjar* disease (rare, with shortened life expectancy) causes severe unconjugated hyperbilirubinemia, and Gilbert disease (common, normal life expectancy) causes mild unconjugated hyperbilirubinemia. *Rotor* and *Dubin-Johnson* syndromes cause conjugated hyperbilirubinemia (benign conditions).

○ Biliary atresia may be seen in full-term infants with *clay-or gray-colored stools* and high conjugated bilirubin. Can diagnose with hepato-iminodiacetic acid (HIDA) scan and treat with surgery.

○ Medications. *Avoid sulfa drugs in neonates;* they displace bilirubin from albumin and may precipitate kernicterus.

The treatment for elevated unconjugated hyperbilirubinemia is *phototherapy* (i.e., ultraviolet [UV] light exposure) to convert the unconjugated bilirubin to a water-soluble form that can be excreted. The indication for phototherapy is based on a nomogram of the bilirubin level and age of patient. The last resort is exchange transfusion. Do not choose this option unless phototherapy has failed and the level of unconjugated bilirubin is high for the patient's age (i.e., >20 mg/dL).

Any infant born to a mother with active hepatitis B should receive the first immunization shot and hepatitis B immune globulin at birth.

Pediatric gynecology

Ambiguous genitalia. Look for adrenogenital syndrome/congenital adrenal hyperplasia (*21-hydroxylase deficiency* in 90% of cases). Patients are usually female; boys with the disease experience precocious sexual development. Neonates with 21-hydroxylase deficiency rapidly develop salt wasting (low sodium), *hyperkalemia, hypotension,* and elevated 17-hydroxyprogesterone. Treat with steroids and intravenous fluids immediately to prevent death. Any child with ambiguous genitalia (Fig. 2-7) should not be assigned a sex until the workup is complete and a karyotype is done.

▢ **CASE SCENARIO:** What does a female child with a "bunch of grapes" (vesicles) protruding from the vagina likely have? Sarcoma botryoides, a malignancy.

Premature/precocious puberty is usually idiopathic but may be caused by a hormone-secreting tumor or CNS disorder, both of which must be ruled out. By definition, the patient must be younger than 8 years (9 years for boys). Treat the underlying cause. If the condition is idiopathic, treat with a *gonadotropin-releasing hormone (GnRH) analog* to prevent premature epiphyseal closure and arrest or reverse puberty until the child reaches an appropriate age.

▢ **CASE SCENARIO:** A mother brings in her 10-year-old daughter and is concerned because the child has just had her first period. What is the correct treatment? Reassurance only, because this is normal.

Vaginitis/discharge. Most cases of vaginitis or discharge are nonspecific or physiologic, but, on the boards, look for foreign body, sexual abuse (especially with sexually transmitted disease in a child), or *Candida* as a presentation of diabetes.

⬜ **CASE SCENARIO:** A mother brings in her 8-year-old daughter because the child has white vaginal discharge. A potassium hydroxide (KOH) prep of the vaginal discharge shows yeast blastospores and pseudohyphae. What laboratory test should be ordered? Blood glucose. *Candida* vulvovaginitis in a healthy young female is unusual. Testing for diabetes mellitus should be performed.

Vaginal bleeding in the neonate is usually physiologic from maternal estrogen withdrawal and resolves spontaneously within a few days.

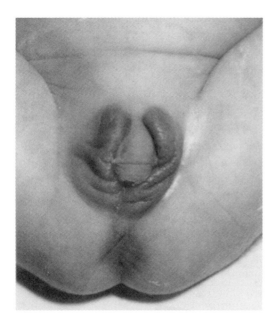

FIGURE 2-7 Ambiguous genitalia in a newborn infant with congenital adrenal hyperplasia. *(From Resnick MJ, Novick AC: Urology Secrets, 2nd ed. Philadelphia, Hanley & Belfus, 1999.)*

Pediatric hematology

The most common cause of nosebleed in children is trauma (often nose picking), but watch for a possible tumor (nasopharyngeal angiofibroma; look for an adolescent boy with no trauma or blood dyscrasia who has recurrent nosebleeds and/or obstruction); leukemia (from pancytopenia, often associated with fever and anemia); and other causes of thrombocytopenia such as idiopathic thrombocytopenic purpura (ITP) and hemolytic uremic syndrome (HUS).

Sickle cell disease (SCD). A blood smear gives it away (Fig. 2-8)—look for a high percentage of reticulocytes. SCD is seen almost always in blacks (8% are heterozygotes in the United States). Watch for the classic manifestations of SCD: aplastic crises due to *parvovirus B19* infection; bone pain due to microinfarcts (often *avascular necrosis* of the femoral head); renal *papillary necrosis*; splenic sequestration crisis;

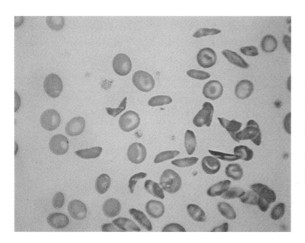

FIGURE 2-8 Sickle cell anemia. A *sickle cell* is a cell with a sickle or crescent shape resulting from the polymerization of hemoglobin S. These cells are seen not only in sickle cell anemia (homozygosity for hemoglobin S) but also in compound heterozygous states such as sickle cell/hemoglobin C disease and sickle cell/β-thalassemia, which also lead to sickle cell disease. This smear also shows target cells and boat-shaped cells, which are the result of a lesser degree of polymerization of hemoglobin S than with a classic sickle cell. *(From Goldman L, Schafer AI: Goldman's Cecil Medicine, 24th ed. Philadelphia, Saunders, 2012.)*

autosplenectomy, often accompanied by increased infections with encapsulated organisms (give pneumococcal vaccine); *acute chest syndrome,* which mimics pneumonia; *pigment* cholelithiasis; priapism; and stroke. Diagnosis is made by hemoglobin electrophoresis. Screening is done at birth, but remember that symptoms usually do not begin until about 6 months of age because of persistent fetal hemoglobin production. Treat with prophylactic penicillin, which is started as soon as the diagnosis is made and continued until age 5 years; proper vaccination including pneumococcal vaccine; folate supplementation; early treatment of infections; and proper hydration.

 A sickle "crisis" is sudden, unheralded, vaso-occlusive event that can have multiple symptoms but most commonly presents as a pain crisis affecting the limbs, lower back, chest, or abdomen. Treat with oxygen, antibiotics and analgesics (including narcotics). If severe, exchange transfusions may be helpful.

CASE SCENARIO: A woman is watching her neighbor's 1-year-old African-American child and brings her in for sudden, symmetric swelling and redness of the hands and feet that develop over a few hours. The child is irritable. The woman thinks that there may be a family history of anemia. The child looks pale. What syndrome does the child probably have? Hand-foot syndrome, or *dactylitis,* a classic manifestation of sickle cell disease in young children.

Classic hematologic/kidney "combo" disorders: see Table 2-8 and Figures 2-9 and 2-10.

TABLE 2-8 Classic Hematology-Kidney Combination Disorders

	HUS	HSP	TTP	ITP
Most common age group	Children	Children	Young adults	Children or adults
Previous infection	Diarrhea (*Escherichia coli*)	URI	None	Viral (especially children)
RBC count	Low	Normal	Low	Normal
Platelet count	Low	Normal	Low	Low
Peripheral smear	Hemolysis	Normal	Hemolysis	Normal
Kidney manifestations	ARF, hematuria	Hematuria	ARF, proteinuria	None
Treatment	Supportive*	Supportive*	Plasmapheresis, NSAIDs Do not give platelets[†]	Steroids[‡], splenectomy if medication fails
Key differential points	Age, diarrhea	Rash, abdominal pain, arthritis, melena	CNS changes, age	Antiplatelet antibodies

ARF, Acute renal failure; *CNS,* central nervous system; *HSP,* Henoch-Schönlein purpura; *HUS,* hemolytic uremic syndrome; *ITP,* idiopathic thrombocytopenic purpura; *NSAIDs,* nonsteroidal anti-inflammatory drugs; *RBC,* red blood cell; *TTP,* thrombotic thrombocytopenic purpura; *URI,* upper respiratory infection.
*In HUS and HSP, patients may need dialysis and transfusions.
[†]Do not give platelet transfusions to patients with TTP because they may form clots.
[‡]Give steroids only if patient is symptomatic (bleeding) or counts fall to dangerous levels (<20,000/µL).

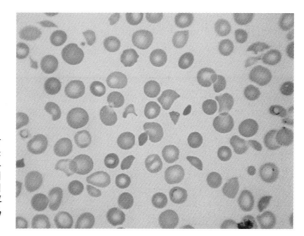

FIGURE 2-9 Schistocytes. *Red cell fragments* or *schistocytes* are seen in microangiopathic hemolytic anemias such as hemolytic uremic syndrome, thrombotic thrombocytopenic purpura, and disseminated intravascular coagulation, as well as in mechanical hemolysis such as artificial heart valves. *(From Goldman L, Schafer AI: Goldman's Cecil Medicine, 24th ed. Philadelphia, Saunders, 2012.)*

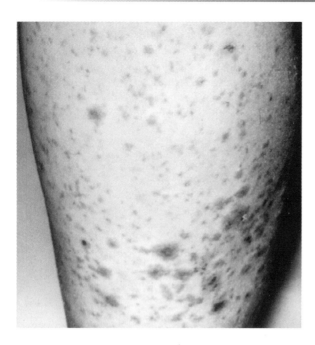

FIGURE 2-10 The anterior leg with raised petechial (<5 mm) and purpuric (>5 mm) skin lesions suggesting vasculitis. This appearance can be seen with Henoch-Schönlein purpura (HSP), in which the rash is generally limited to the buttocks and lower extremities. The platelet count should be normal in HSP.

Pediatric immunology

Primary immunodeficiencies are rare. Your job is simply to recognize the classic case presentations:

1. **IgA deficiency** is the most common primary immunodeficiency. Look for recurrent respiratory and GI infections. IgA levels are low.

📁 **CASE SCENARIO:** What therapy should be avoided in patients with IgA deficiency? *Immunoglobulins*, which may cause anaphylaxis due to anti-IgA antibodies. If a patient develops anaphylaxis after immunoglobulin exposure, consider IgA deficiency.

2. **X-linked agammaglobulinemia** (Bruton agammaglobulinemia) is an X-linked recessive disorder that affects males. It is characterized by low or absent B cells and infections that begin after 6 months when maternal antibodies disappear. Look for recurrent lung or sinus infections with *Streptococcus* and *Haemophilus* spp.

3. **DiGeorge syndrome** is caused by a variable-sized chromosomal deletion. Look for *hypocalcemia* or *tetany* (from absent parathyroids) in the first 24–48 hours of life, facial dysmorphology, along with an absent or hypoplastic thymus (causing variable dysfunctions of cell-mediated immunity). Congenital heart defects are the main cause of morbidity and mortality. Mnemonic: CATCH 22 = **C**ardiac abnormalities (especially tetralogy of Fallot), **A**bnormal facies, **T**hymic aplasia, **C**left palate, **H**ypocalcemia, deletion from chromosome **22.**

4. **Severe combined immunodeficiency** may be autosomal recessive or X-linked. Many cases are due to adenosine deaminase deficiency (autosomal recessive). Patients have B- and T-cell defects and severe infections in the first few months of life. Cutaneous anergy is usually present. The thymus and lymph nodes may be absent or hypoplastic.

5. **Wiskott-Aldrich deficiency** is an X-linked recessive disorder that affects males. Look for the classic triad: *eczema, thrombocytopenia* (bleeding), and *recurrent infections* (usually respiratory).

6. **Chronic granulomatous disease** is usually an X-linked recessive disorder that affects males. Infections with catalase-positive organisms (e.g., *Staphylococcus aureus, Pseudomonas* spp.) are common. The diagnosis is clinched when *deficient nitroblue tetrazolium dye reduction by granulocytes* is confirmed (by a test that measures the respiratory burst, which these patients lack).

7. **Chédiak-Higashi syndrome** is usually autosomal recessive. Look for giant granules in neutrophils (Fig. 2-11), recurrent pyogenic infections, and associated *oculocutaneous albinism*. The syndrome is caused by a defect in microtubule polymerization and subsequently impaired lysis of phagocytosed bacteria.

8. **Complement deficiencies** (factors C5 through C9) cause *recurrent neisserial infections*. Specific complement components are low. Give meningococcal vaccine to affected children.

9. **Chronic mucocutaneous candidiasis** is a cellular immunodeficiency specific for *Candida* Patients have thrush; candidal infections of the scalp, skin, and nails; and anergy to *Candida* organisms with skin testing. The condition is often associated with hypothyroidism; the rest of immune function is intact.

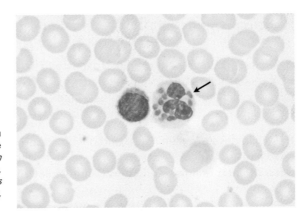

Figure 2-11 Neutrophil and lymphocyte from a patient with Chédiak-Higashi syndrome. Note the large dysmorphic cytoplasmic granules *(arrow).* *(From Mandell GL, Bennett JE, Dolin R: Mandell, Douglas, and Bennett's Principles and Practice of Infectious Diseases, 7th ed. Philadelphia, Churchill Livingstone, 2010.)*

10. **Hyper-IgE syndrome** (Job-Buckley syndrome) is characterized by recurrent staphylococcal infections (especially of the skin). IgA levels are extremely high. Patients commonly have fair skin, red hair, and eczema.

Pediatric infectious disease

Otitis media is most commonly due to *Streptococcus pneumoniae, Haemophilus influenzae,* or *Moraxella catarrhalis.* Manipulation of the auricle produces no pain (in contrast with otitis externa), but the patient has earache, fever, nausea/vomiting, and erythematous and *bulging tympanic membrane* (light reflex and landmarks are difficult to see). Complications include tympanic membrane perforation (bloody or purulent discharge), mastoiditis (fluctuance and inflammation over mastoid process 2 weeks after otitis), labyrinthitis, palsies of cranial nerves VII and VIII, meningitis/cerebral abscess, venous thrombosis, and chronic otitis media. Chronic otitis media may lead to permanent perforation of the eardrum, and patients may develop cholesteatomas with marginal perforations (treat with surgical excision). Treat otitis with antibiotics (amoxicillin or second-generation cephalosporin such as cefuroxime) to avoid these complications.

Recurrent otitis media is a common pediatric clinical problem (as well as prolonged secretory otitis, a result of incompletely resolved otitis) and can cause *hearing loss with resultant developmental problems* (speech, cognitive functions). Treat with prophylactic antibiotics. Tympanostomy tubes are also used but are controversial. Adenoidectomy is thought to help in some cases by preventing blockage of the eustachian tubes.

UTI. In children younger than 6 years of age, UTI is a cause for concern because it may be the presenting manifestation of a *urinary tract malformation.* The most common examples are disordered anatomy leading to vesicoureteral reflux (males and females) and posterior urethral valves (males). The American Academy of Pediatrics (AAP) recommends ordering a renal ultrasound and voiding cystourethrogram (VCUG) after the first febrile UTI in children 2 months to 2 years of age.

Meningitis. The highest incidence of meningitis is seen in neonates; a majority of cases are seen in children younger than 2 years. Younger patients often do not have classic physical findings (Kernig and Brudzinski signs). Look for lethargy, fever or hypothermia, poor muscle tone, *bulging fontanelle,* vomiting, photophobia, *altered consciousness,* and signs of generalized sepsis (hypotension, jaundice, respiratory distress). Seizures may also be seen, but remember simple febrile seizures if the patient is between 5 months and 6 years old and has a fever with temperatures greater than 102°F in the absence of other signs of meningitis. *Do not wait to start treatment* (i.e., antibiotics and IV fluids) if the patient is doing poorly, even if you cannot get an immediate lumbar puncture (treatment is more important than precise diagnosis in this case, which is rare on the boards). If there is clinical evidence of elevated intracranial pressure (e.g., bulging fontanelles, vomiting), do NOT perform lumbar puncture due to risk of uncal herniation.

❍ Mumps and measles are now rare causes of aseptic (nonbacterial or culture-negative) meningitis. The best prevention is immunization.

❍ Watch for herpes encephalitis if the mother has herpes simplex virus (HSV) genital lesions at delivery. In older children and adults, herpes encephalitis is due to HSV-I (vs. HSV-II in neonates), and those affected will have *temporal lobe abnormalities on a head CT scan or MRI.* Give IV acyclovir. Consider TB meningitis in a patient with hydrocephalus and TB risk factors (exposure, immunosuppression, birth in country with high incidence).

See neurology section for cerebrospinal fluid (CSF) findings in meningitis.

▢ **CASE SCENARIO:** A child has high fever, photophobia, vomiting, poor muscle tone, and altered level of consciousness. Vital signs include hypotension and tachycardia. Which should you do first—give antibiotics and IV fluids or perform lumbar puncture? Give antibiotics and IV fluids first. Empirical treatment may save the child's life, and delaying therapy is inappropriate, especially with new direct antigen tests that make CSF culture less important.

CASE SCENARIO: A child recovers from a bout of meningitis after antibiotics. What does the child need as part of routine follow-up? Formal hearing evaluation to check for hearing loss, the most common sequela of meningitis. Other sequelae include vision loss, mental retardation, motor deficits/paresis, epilepsy, and learning/behavioral disorders.

CASE SCENARIO: A child develops meningitis, and antibiotics are given. The direct antigen test is positive for *Neisseria meningitidis*. What do you need to do other than treating the child? Give all the child's close contacts antibiotic prophylaxis (rifampin, ciprofloxacin [in adults], or ceftriaxone usually is given).

Infectious rashes are seen most often in children. Only supportive treatment is necessary unless otherwise specified.

1. **Measles (rubeola).** See whether the patient has been immunized. *Koplik spots* (tiny white spots on buccal mucosa) are seen 3 days after high fever, cough, runny nose, and conjunctivitis/photophobia. On the following day, a maculopapular rash begins on the head and neck and spreads downward to cover the trunk (head-to-toe progression). Complications include pneumonia ("giant cell" pneumonia, especially in very young and immunocompromised patients), otitis media, and encephalitis (either an acute form or *subacute sclerosing panencephalitis,* which usually occurs years later).

2. **Rubella** (German measles) is an important infection in pregnant mothers due to the risk of congenital abnormalities. Screen and immunize any woman of reproductive age before she becomes pregnant. Rubella is milder than measles, with low fever, malaise, and tender swelling of the *suboccipital and postauricular nodes.* Arthralgias also may develop. After a 2- to 3-day prodrome, a faint maculopapular rash starts on the face and neck and spreads to the trunk (head-to-toe progression). Complications include encephalitis, otitis media, and cataracts.

CASE SCENARIO: A pregnant woman says that she was not vaccinated for rubella. She is 6 weeks pregnant. What should you do? Draw a baseline titer and observe. The vaccine is contraindicated during pregnancy. If the woman develops a febrile illness and rash during pregnancy, recheck the titer to see if it has risen to make the diagnosis of rubella.

3. **Roseola infantum** (exanthem subitum). Look for classic progression: high fever (temperature may be >40°C with febrile seizures) with no apparent cause for 4 days, then an abrupt return to normal temperature as a diffuse macular or maculopapular rash appears on the chest and abdomen. Roseola infantum is rare in children older than 3 years. It is caused by the *human herpesvirus type 6* (HHV6).

4. **Erythema infectiosum** (fifth disease). The classic *"slapped-cheek" rash* (confluent erythema over the cheeks) (Fig. 2-12) appears around the same time as mild constitutional symptoms (low fever, malaise). One day later, a maculopapular rash appears on the arms, legs, and trunk. Fifth disease is caused by *parvovirus B19* (the same virus that causes aplastic crisis in sickle cell disease).

5. **Chickenpox** (varicella). The description and progression of the rash should lead to the diagnosis. *Discrete macules (usually on the trunk) turn into papules, which turn into vesicles, which rupture and crust over.* These changes occur within 1 day. The lesions appear in successive crops; therefore the rash is in different stages of progression in different areas. A *Tzanck smear* of tissue from the base of a vesicle shows multinucleated giant cells (rarely required for diagnosis). Varicella-zoster immune globulin is available for prophylaxis in patients with debilitating illness (e.g., leukemia, AIDS) if you see them within 4 days of exposure or for newborns whose mother has chickenpox. Acyclovir can be used in severe cases. Reactivation of the virus later in life can cause *shingles (zoster),* which is characterized by a dermatomal distribution of the rash. Pain and paresthesias often precede the rash. Exposure to a person with active shingles can cause chickenpox in a person who has never been vaccinated or had chickenpox before.

CASE SCENARIO: A 14-year-old boy develops chickenpox, and the mother asks when he will no longer be contagious. What should you tell her? The child is contagious until the last lesion crusts over.

6. **Scarlet fever.** Look for a history of untreated streptococcal pharyngitis (only species that produce *erythrogenic toxin* can cause scarlet fever), followed by a sandpaper-like rash on the abdomen and

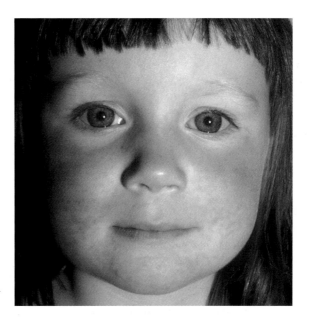

FIGURE 2-12 Erythema infectiosum. Facial erythema "slapped cheek." The red plaque covers the cheek and spares the nasolabial fold and the circumoral region. *(From Habif TP: Clinical Dermatology, 5th ed. Philadelphia, Mosby, 2010.)*

trunk with classic *circumoral pallor* (i.e., area not affected by the rash) and a strawberry tongue. The rash tends to desquamate once the fever subsides. Treat with penicillin to prevent rheumatic fever from developing.

7. **Kawasaki syndrome** (mucocutaneous lymph node syndrome) is a rare disease that usually affects children younger than 5 years. Diagnostic criteria include *fever for longer than 5 days* (mandatory for diagnosis); bilateral *conjunctival injection*; changes in the lips, tongue, or oral mucosa (*strawberry tongue*, fissuring, injection); changes in the extremities (desquamation, edema, erythema); polymorphous *truncal rash* (which usually begins 1 day after the fever starts); and cervical lymphadenopathy. Also look for arthralgia/arthritis. The most feared complications involve the heart (*coronary artery aneurysms*, heart failure, arrhythmias, myocarditis, myocardial infarction). If Kawasaki syndrome is suspected, give *aspirin* and *IV immune globulin* (both reduce cardiac/coronary damage) and follow the patient with echocardiography to detect heart involvement. This is one of the few times that aspirin is given to a pediatric patient.

8. **Infectious mononucleosis** (Epstein-Barr virus [EBV] infection). Look for fatigue, fever, pharyngitis, and lymphadenopathy (similar to streptococcal pharyngitis, but malaise tends to be prolonged and pronounced in EBV infection). To differentiate from streptococcal infection, look for *splenomegaly* (splenic rupture is rare, but patients should avoid contact sports and heavy lifting), hepatomegaly, *atypical lymphocytes* (bizarre forms that may resemble leukemia) with lymphocytosis, anemia/thrombocytopenia, and positive serology (*heterophile antibodies* [e.g., Monospot test] or specific EBV antibodies: viral capsid antigen, Epstein-Barr nuclear antigen). Remember HIV infection in the differential diagnosis. EBV is associated with *nasopharyngeal carcinoma* and *African Burkitt lymphoma*.

📋 **CASE SCENARIO:** A 22-year-old man presents with a sore throat. He is given amoxicillin for presumed streptococcal infection and returns 3 days later with a diffuse maculopapular rash. His sore throat has not improved. Does he have an allergy to amoxicillin? No—he has EBV infection. A rash occurs in roughly 90% of patients with EBV infection who are given ampicillin.

9. **Rocky Mountain spotted fever** (*Rickettsia rickettsii* infection). Look for history of a *tick bite* (especially on the east coast) 1 week before the development of high fever or chills, severe headache, and prostration or severe malaise. The rash appears roughly 4 days after symptoms and *starts on the palms or wrists and soles or ankles, rapidly spreading to the trunk* and face (unique pattern of spread) (Fig. 2-13). Patients are often quite sick (disseminated intravascular coagulation, delirium) and need doxycycline (preferred) or chloramphenicol (in pregnancy) immediately.

10. **Impetigo**. Look for a history of skin break (e.g., previous chickenpox, insect bite, scabies, cut). Rash starts as thin-walled vesicles that rupture and form yellowish crusts. The skin is often described as "weeping." Classically, lesions are seen on the face and tend to be localized. Impetigo

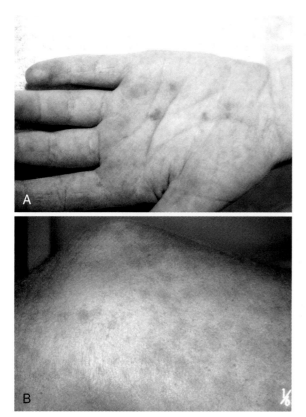

FIGURE 2-13 Rocky Mountain spotted fever rash on the palm and arm. The rash initially appears on the ankles and wrists and the palms and soles. The rash then spreads centripetally to the forearms, arms, legs, thighs, and trunk. *(From Mandell GL, Bennett JE, Dolin R: Mandell, Douglas, and Bennett's Principles and Practice of Infectious Diseases, 7th ed. Philadelphia, Churchill Livingstone, 2010.)*

is infectious; look for sick contacts. Treat with oral antistaphylococcal penicillin (to cover strepto-cocci and staphylococci, the most common causative organisms).

Pediatric respiratory infections. The big three are croup, epiglottitis, and respiratory syncytial virus (RSV) infection.

1. **Croup** (acute laryngotracheitis). Most patients are *1–2 years old*. Croup usually occurs in the fall or winter, and 50%–75% of cases are due to *parainfluenza virus*. The other causative agent is influenza. Patients first develop symptoms of a viral upper respiratory infection (URI) such as rhinorrhea, cough, and fever. Roughly 1–2 days later, patients have a *"barking" cough*, hoarseness, and inspiratory stridor. The *"steeple sign"* (narrowing of the trachea just below the vocal cords due to subglottic edema) is classic on an anteroposterior (AP) radiograph of the neck but is insensitive and nonspecific. Treat supportively with cool *humidified oxygen* (e.g., the "cool mist tent") and corticosteroids (oral dexamethasone preferred). Nebulized *racemic epinephrine* is used in severe cases that do not respond to initial measures.

2. **Epiglottitis**. Most patients are *2–7 years old*. The main cause is *H. influenzae* type b; widespread vaccination has decreased the incidence significantly. *S. pneumoniae* and *S. aureus* are other potential causes. Look for little or no prodrome, with *rapid progression* to high fever, toxic appearance, *drooling*, and respiratory distress. No cough is present. The *"thumb sign"* (i.e., enlarged epiglottis looks like a thumb) is classic on lateral neck radiograph. Do not examine the throat or irritate the child in any way—you may precipitate airway obstruction! When a case of epiglottitis is presented, the first step is to *be prepared to establish an airway* (i.e., intubate or perform a tracheostomy if needed). Treat with antibiotics (e.g., third-generation cephalosporin).

3. **RSV infection/bronchiolitis**. Most patients are *18 months or younger*. Bronchiolitis usually occurs in the fall or winter, and 75% of cases are caused by *respiratory syncytial virus* (RSV). Other causes are parainfluenza and influenza viruses. Initial symptoms of viral URI are followed 1–2 days later by rapid respirations, intercostal retractions, and *expiratory wheezing*. Crackles may be heard on auscultation of the chest. Diffuse hyperinflation of the lungs is classic on radiographs; look for flattened diaphragms. Treat supportively (humidified oxygen, saline nasal drops, bronchodilators, IV fluids). Use *ribavarin* treatment only in patients with severe symptoms and high risk (cyanosis, other health problems). *Palivizumab* prophylaxis (a monoclonal antibody against RSV) can be used in premature children and those with chronic lung disease during RSV season.

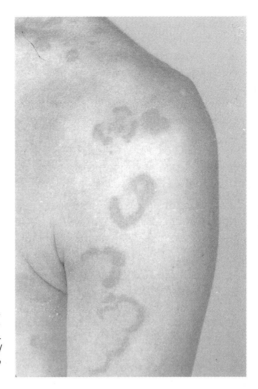

FIGURE 2-14 Erythema marginatum. The rash is classically flat to slightly elevated, erythematous, and annular (ringlike) in appearance. *(From Forbes CD, Jackson WF: Cardiovascular disorders. In Forbes CD, Jackson WF: Atlas and Text of Clinical Medicine. London, Mosby-Wolfe, 1993, pp 209–264.)*

4. **Diphtheria** (*Corynebacterium diphtheriae*) and pertussis (*Bordetella pertussis*). Consider both if the patient has not been immunized. Diphtheria is associated with *grayish pseudomembranes* (necrotic epithelium and inflammatory exudate) on the pharynx, tonsils, and uvula, and myocarditis. Pertussis is associated with severe paroxysmal coughing and a high-pitched, whooping inspiratory noise (classically called *"whooping cough"*). Treat both with antibiotics; for diphtheria, add an antitoxin.

Streptococcus pyogenes (group A streptococcus) causes multiple important infections. The most common is pharyngitis. Look for sore throat with fever, tonsillar exudate, enlarged tender cervical nodes, and leukocytosis. Streptococcal throat culture confirms the diagnosis. The "rapid strep test" is more commonly used because results are available within minutes. Do not treat empirically without a positive test. Elevated titers of antistreptolysin O and anti-DNase can be used retrospectively, as needed (e.g., to diagnose rheumatic fever or poststreptococcal glomerulonephritis). Treat with *penicillin* to avoid rheumatic fever and scarlet fever.

1. **Rheumatic fever.** The diagnosis is based on a history of streptococcal pharyngitis and the Jones criteria: major (migratory polyarthritis, carditis, chorea, erythema marginatum [Fig. 2-14], subcutaneous nodules) and minor (elevated sedimentation rate, elevated levels of C-reactive protein, increased white blood cell (WBC) count, elevated streptococcal antibody titer, prolonged PR interval on ECG, arthralgia). Treat with antiinflammatories and corticosteroids (if needed) for carditis.

2. **Scarlet fever.** Some untreated pharyngitis cases progress to scarlet fever if the streptococcal species produces erythrogenic toxin. Clinical manifestations include a red flush to the skin (which blanches with pressure and classically is associated with *circumoral pallor*), truncal rash, strawberry tongue, and late skin desquamation. Remember *Kawasaki syndrome* as another cause of this set of symptoms.

3. **Poststreptococcal glomerulonephritis** occurs most commonly after a skin infection but may occur after pharyngitis. The patient presents with a history of infection by a nephritogenic streptococcal strain 1–3 weeks earlier and abrupt onset of *hematuria*, proteinuria (mild—not in the nephrotic range), *RBC casts* ("*smoke-colored urine*" is the classic symptom), *hypertension,* edema (especially periorbital), and elevated blood urea nitrogen (BUN)/serum creatinine. Treat supportively. Control blood pressure, and use diuretics for severe edema.

▢ **CASE SCENARIO:** Of the three previously described conditions, which can be prevented by giving antibiotics for strep throat? Rheumatic fever and scarlet fever. Glomerulonephritis cannot be prevented by treating strep throat.

Streptococcus agalactiae (streptococcus group B) is the most common cause of neonatal meningitis and sepsis. The organism is acquired from the maternal birth canal, where it is part of the normal flora. Pregnant mothers are tested and treated (with penicillin or ampicillin) near term to prevent neonatal infection, a measure that has reduced the incidence significantly.

TORCH syndromes. Most TORCH intrauterine fetal infections can cause mental retardation, microcephaly, hydrocephalus, hepatosplenomegaly, jaundice, anemia, low birth weight, and/or IUGR:

1. *Toxoplasma gondii*. Look for *maternal exposure to cats*. Specific defects include intracranial calcifications and chorioretinitis.
2. Other. The "other" agents included under "O" include coxsackievirus, syphilis, varicella-zoster, HIV, and human parvovirus B19. Varicella-zoster infection is associated with limb hypoplasia and *scarring of the skin*, whereas syphilis is associated with rhinitis, saber shins, *Hutchinson teeth*, interstitial keratitis, and skin lesions.
3. Rubella. Some physicians recommend abortion if the mother contracts rubella in the first trimester, when the effects on the fetus are worst. Check maternal antibody status on the first prenatal visit if the immunization history is uncertain. Look for cardiovascular defects (patent ductus, ventricular septal defect), deafness, cataracts, and microphthalmia in the newborn.
4. Cytomegalovirus (CMV) is the most common TORCH infection. Look for deafness, cerebral calcifications, and microphthalmia.
5. Herpes. Look for *vesicular skin lesions* (with positive Tzanck smears) and history of maternal herpes lesions.

 With all in utero infections that cause problems with the fetus, the mother may have a subclinical infection and be asymptomatic. The infant may also be asymptomatic at birth but develop symptoms at a later date.

Pediatric neurology

The "floppy" baby. Two specific concerns in infants with hypotonia/flaccidity are a genetic disorder and infant botulism:

1. **Werdnig-Hoffman disease** is an autosomal recessive degeneration of anterior horn cells in the spinal cord and brainstem (lower motor neurons). Most infants are hypotonic at birth, and all are affected by 6 months. Look for a positive family history. The disease onset and course are *long and slowly progressive;* treatment is supportive.
2. **Infant botulism.** Look for *sudden onset* in a previously normal child and a history of ingestion of *honey* or *home-canned foods*). Diagnosis can be made by finding *Clostridium botulinum* toxin or organisms in the feces. Treatment is given in the hospital, with close monitoring of respiratory status because the child may need intubation for respiratory muscle paralysis. Spontaneous recovery usually occurs within a week.

Muscular dystrophy (most commonly *Duchenne* muscular dystrophy) is an *X-linked* recessive disorder of *dystrophin* that usually manifests in boys aged 3–7 years. Look for muscle weakness, *markedly elevated* creatine kinase (CK), and pseudohypertrophy of the calves (due to fatty and fibrous infiltration of the degenerating muscles). IQ often is less than normal. *Gower sign* is classic (when patients attempt to rise from a prone position, they "walk" their hands and feet toward each other). Muscle biopsy establishes the diagnosis. Treatment is supportive. Most patients die by age 20. Other muscular dystrophies:

1. **Becker muscular dystrophy:** also an X-linked recessive dystrophin problem but milder.
2. **Mitochondrial myopathies:** rare but interesting because they are inherited as mitochondrial defects (passed only from mother to offspring; males cannot transmit). Key phrase is *"ragged red fibers"* in a biopsy specimen. *Ophthalmoplegia* is classically present.
3. **Myotonic dystrophy:** autosomal dominant disorder that manifests between 20 and 30 years of age. Myotonia (inability of muscles to relax) classically manifests as *inability to relax the grip* (e.g., the patient cannot release a handshake). Look for *coexisting mental retardation, baldness,* and testicular or ovarian atrophy. Treatment is supportive and includes genetic counseling. The diagnosis is made on clinical grounds.

Glycogen storage diseases (autosomal recessive) are a rare cause of muscular weakness. *McArdle* disease is characterized by a relatively mild deficiency in glycogen phosphorylase and presents in young patients with weakness *and cramping after exercise.*

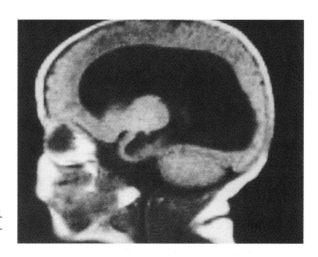

FIGURE 2-15 Hydrocephalus. Sagittal off-midline magnetic resonance image reveals a significantly enlarged lateral ventricle.

Neural tube defects. A triangular patch of hair over the lumbar spine indicates spina bifida occulta, which is asymptomatic and common. More serious defects are usually obvious and occur most commonly in the lumbosacral region (*meningocele* is meninges outside the spinal canal; *myelomengiocele* is CNS tissue plus meninges outside the spinal canal). Most important, giving folate to potential mothers reduces the incidence of neural tube defects.

Hydrocephalus. In children, look for abnormally *increasing head circumference,* increased intracranial pressure, *bulging fontanelle,* scalp vein engorgement, and paralysis of upward gaze. Large ventricles are seen on CT scan or MRI, the confirmatory tests (Fig. 2-15). The most common causes include congenital malformations, tumors, and inflammation (after hemorrhage or meningitis). Treat the underlying cause if possible; otherwise, a surgical shunt is created to decompress the ventricles.

Pediatric oncology

The most common malignancy in children is acute lymphocytic leukemia (ALL). Patients classically present with pancytopenia. Watch for bleeding, signs of anemia, and infection. Patients with *Down syndrome* have a much higher risk than the general population.

Brain tumors in children are usually located in the posterior fossa (e.g., *cerebellum* or *brainstem*). Classic symptoms are due to increased intracranial pressure (vomiting, headaches) and tumor location (seizures, hydrocephalus, ataxia). The most common types are cerebellar *astrocytoma* and *medulloblastoma,* followed by ependymoma.

Wilms tumor versus neuroblastoma. Both manifest as *flank masses* in young children. If the patient is younger than 6 months, neuroblastoma is more likely, but a tissue diagnosis is always necessary for diagnosis. Both have a peak incidence at around the age of 2 years. Wilms tumor is much more common overall. Wilms tumor comes from kidney, whereas neuroblastoma usually derives from the adrenal gland. Rarely, neuroblastomas may regress spontaneously (for unknown reasons). These tumors are the most common primary malignancies of their respective organs in children. Hepatoblastoma is the classic and most common primary liver malignancy in young children.

Retinoblastoma is characterized by *leukocoria* in a young child (red reflex is absent with a penlight) or strabismus (can be exo or eso deviation). Tumor may be bilateral in the inherited form.

Unicameral bone cyst (i.e., simple bone cyst) is an expansile, lucent, well-demarcated lesion usually in the proximal portion of the humerus in children and adolescents (Fig. 2-16). It is benign but may weaken bone enough to cause a pathologic fracture.

Osteosarcoma occurs in 10- to 20-year-olds, usually around the knee (distal femur, proximal tibia) and has a classic "sunburst" appearance of the associated periosteal reaction on x-ray. A mass may be palpable on exam.

Pediatric ophthalmology

Neonatal conjunctivitis is classically due to one of three causes (though typical adult bacterial and viral infections as the cause are also possible during the neonatal period):

1. **Chemical reaction.** Silver nitrate, erythromycin, or tetracycline drops are given prophylactically to newborns to prevent gonorrheal conjunctivitis. The drops may cause a chemical conjunctivitis

(with no purulent discharge), which develops within 6–12 hours of instilling the drops and resolves within 48 hours. *Chemical reaction is* **always** *the answer if conjunctivitis appears in the first 24 hours of life.*

2. **Gonorrhea.** Look for symptoms of gonorrhea in the mother. The infant has an extremely purulent ocular discharge that *starts 2–5 days after birth.* Treatment is topical (erythromycin ointment) plus IV or intramuscular (IM) third-generation cephalosporin (e.g., ceftriaxone). Infants who are given prophylactic drops should not develop gonorrheal conjunctivitis.

3. **Chlamydial infection** (inclusion conjunctivitis). The mother often reports no symptoms. The infant has mild to severe conjunctivitis, which *begins 5–14 days after birth.* Patients must be treated with systemic antibiotics (oral erythromycin is the usual choice) to prevent chlamydial pneumonia, a common complication. Prophylactic eye drops should be used, but alone they do not effectively prevent chlamydial conjunctivitis.

🗀 **CASE SCENARIO:** What is the most important point in the history for neonatal conjunctivitis? The age at presentation (<1 day = chemical, 2–5 days = gonococcal; 5–14 days = chlamydial).

Cataracts in a neonate should make you think of *TORCH infections* or an inherited metabolic disorder (e.g., *galactosemia*), particularly if bilateral.

Strabismus/amblyopia. Any child with a "lazy eye" (strabismus: the eye deviates, usually inward) that persists beyond 3 months of age needs ophthalmologic referral (Fig. 2-17). This condition does not resolve and may cause poor vision (amblyopia) in the affected eye. For this reason, visual screening must be done in all children. The visual system continues to develop until the age of 7 or 8 years. If one eye cannot see well (e.g., cataract, refractive error) or is not straight (can be exotropic or esotropic), the brain cannot fuse the two different images and suppresses the bad eye. Thus the "bad eye" does not develop the proper neural connections and will never see well. Glasses will not correct the problem, which is neural rather than refractive.

Be able to differentiate orbital cellulitis from preorbital cellulitis (i.e., preseptal cellulitis). Both may be associated with swollen lids, fever, chemosis (swollen conjunctiva), and a history of facial laceration, trauma, or insect bite or sinusitis. *Ophthalmoplegia, proptosis, afferent papillary defect, severe eye pain, or decreased visual acuity generally indicates orbital cellulitis* (an emergency). The most common causative

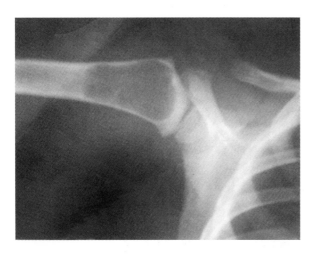

FIGURE 2-16 Unicameral bone cyst. Unicameral (simple) bone cyst. *(From West SG: Rheumatology Secrets. Philadelphia, Hanley & Belfus, 1997.)*

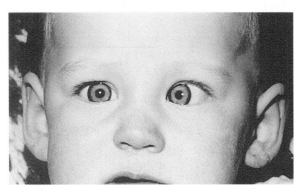

FIGURE 2-17 Strabismus. This child has esotropia (i.e., medial deviation) of the left eye.

agents in both are *Streptococcus pneumoniae, Hemophilus influenzae,* and staphylococci. Complications of orbital cellulitis include extension into the skull, dural sinus thrombosis, and blindness. Treat either condition with blood cultures and administration of broad-spectrum antibiotics until culture results are known. Inpatient IV antibiotics are necessary for orbital cellulitis; surgery may be required for orbital abscess.

Pediatric orthopedic surgery

Pediatric hip problems: see Table 2-9 and Figure 2-18.

TABLE 2-9 Pediatric Hip Problems

NAME	AGE	EPIDEMIOLOGY	SYMPTOMS/SIGNS*	TREATMENT
CHD	At birth	Female, first-born, breech delivery	Barlow and Ortolani signs	Harness
LCP	4-10 yr	Male, short with delayed bone age	Knee, thigh, and groin pain, limp	Orthoses
SCFE	9-13 yr	Overweight, male, adolescent	Knee, thigh, and groin pain, limp	Surgical pinning
TS	2-10 yr	Male	Hip pain, limp, fever after URI	NSAIDs for pain, resolves spontaneously

CHD, Congenital hip dysplasia; *LCP,* Legg-Calvé-Perthes disease; *NSAIDs,* nonsteroidal anti-inflammatory drugs; *SCFE,* slipped capital femoral epiphysis see Figure 2-18; *TS,* toxic/transient synovitis
*Pediatric hip problems are notorious for causing referred pain in the knee, but the knee is not tender, swollen, or otherwise abnormal.

🗀 CASE SCENARIO: How do the hip disorders mentioned in Table 2-9 classically manifest in adults? Early-onset osteoarthritis of the hip. Given the correct history (especially age at onset of symptoms), you may be able to tell which disorder the patient had. Radiographs may be shown, but history can help you guess the answer if you are unsure.

Osgood-Schlatter disease is an osteochondritis of the tibial tubercle that is often bilateral and usually presents between 10 and 15 years of age in males involved in jumping sports with pain, swelling, and tenderness to palpation in the knee. Treat with rest, activity restriction, and nonsteroidal antiinflammatory drugs (NSAIDs). Most cases resolve spontaneously.

Scoliosis usually affects prepubertal girls and is idiopathic. Mild cases are observed. More severe cases are treated with a brace. For deformities that are rapidly progressive or cause respiratory compromise, consider surgery. Check for scoliosis by having the patient touch his or her toes while you look at the spine. An abnormal lateral curvature is seen in patients with scoliosis (Fig. 2-19).

🗀 **CASE SCENARIO:** A 4-year-old girl presents with irritated, red eyes. The mother also mentions that the child has been limping lately and has had a swollen, hot left knee for about 4 weeks. Rheumatoid factor assay is negative. Joint aspiration reveals inflammatory reaction in the joint fluid with no crystals or bacteria, and the culture is negative. What is the likely diagnosis and how should the eye symptoms be managed? The likely diagnosis is juvenile rheumatoid (idiopathic) arthritis, which often has a negative rheumatoid factor assay. The child needs

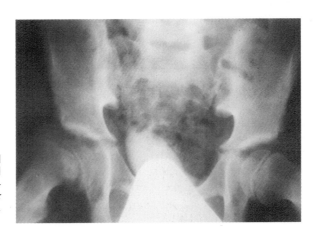

FIGURE 2-18 Slipped capital femoral epiphysis. The right femoral head is displaced medially and posteriorly relative to the right femoral shaft. *(From Katz DS, Math KR, Groskin SA: Radiology Secrets. Philadelphia, Hanley & Belfus, 1998.)*

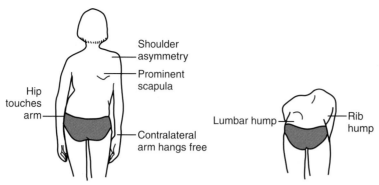

FIGURE 2-19 Scoliosis screening test showing the most important diagnostic features. *(From Staheli LT: Pediatric Orthopedic Secrets. Philadelphia, Hanley & Belfus, 1998.)*

referral to an ophthalmologist (as well as referral to a rheumatologist) for treatment of probable uveitis, which can be confirmed with a slit-lamp exam and requires treatment with steroid drops.

Pediatric psychiatry

Eighty-five percent of cases of intellectual disability (mental retardation [MR]) are mild (IQ range = 55–70), and most are idiopathic. Patients can achieve a reasonable level of independence, with assistance or guidance during periods of stress. Look for *fetal alcohol syndrome,* which is the number-one preventable cause of MR. Down syndrome (number-one overall cause of MR) and *fragile X syndrome* (in boys) are other common causes.

Autism usually starts at a young age. Look for impaired social interaction (e.g., the child is isolated, unaware of surroundings); impaired verbal and nonverbal communication (e.g., strange words, babbling, repetition); and restricted activities and interests (e.g., head banging, strange movements). Autism is usually idiopathic, but look for congenital rubella as a potential cause.

Learning disorder. Math, reading, writing, speech, language, or coordination is impaired, but everything else is normal. No MR is present. ("Johnny just can't do math.")

Conduct disorder. Look for fire-setting, cruelty to animals, lying, stealing, and/or fighting.

▢ **CASE SCENARIO:** A 10-year-old boy repeatedly starts fires, lies, steals, and tortures animals. What disorder will the child likely have when he is an adult? Antisocial personality disorder (in fact, conduct disorder is required in order to make a diagnosis of antisocial personality disorder in adults).

Attention deficit-hyperactivity disorder (ADHD). As the name implies, affected children are hyperactive and have short attention spans. Boys develop the disorder more often than girls. Look for a child with symptoms of hyperactivity, inattentiveness, impulsivity and cannot pay attention but is not cruel. Treat with stimulants (paradoxical calming effect) such as *methylphenidate* (Ritalin), *dextroamphetamine* (Adderall), *modafinil* (Provigil), and *amoxetine,* all of which can cause *insomnia, abdominal pain, decreased appetite, anorexia,* and *weight loss/growth suppression.* ADHD has become a hot topic because of concerns about overdiagnosis and overtreatment. Use "drug holidays" (stop drug for a brief period) to combat side effects.

Oppositional-defiant disorder. Affected children exhibit negative, hostile, and defiant behavior toward authority figures (e.g., parents or teachers). Such children may be a "pain in the butt," but only around adults; they are *normal around peers.* They are not cruel, lying, or criminally inclined.

Separation anxiety disorder. Look for a child who refuses to go to school. Basically, affected children think something will happen to them or their parents if they separate. Patients will do anything, from claiming to have a *stomachache* or *headache* to throwing temper tantrums, to avoid separation.

Anorexia. Look for a female adolescent who is a good athlete, ballerina, and/or student with a perfectionist personality. With a body weight at least 15% below normal, the affected girl exhibits an intense fear of gaining weight, "feels fat" even though she is emaciated, and suffers from *amenorrhea.* All three are required for diagnosis. Death occurs in roughly 10–15% of patients from complications of starvation and/or bulimia (e.g., electrolyte imbalances, cardiac arrhythmias, infections). Patients are sometimes hospitalized against their will for IV nutrition. Up to 50% of patients with anorexia nervosa develop bulimic symptoms, and a smaller percentage of patients who are initially bulimic develop anorexic symptoms.

Bulimia. Although the typical patient is a young, adolescent female, 15% of patients are male and it can occur in older patients as well. Look for someone who is of normal weight or overweight (unless suffering from coexisting anorexia), has binge-eating episodes, then engages in purging behaviors such as *vomiting, using laxatives, exercising,* or *fasting.* Such patients also may require hospitalization for electrolyte disturbances. The classic physical findings in a patient with bulimia are *eroded tooth enamel* from frequent vomiting and/or *eroded skin over the knuckles* from putting fingers in the throat to induce vomiting.

Tourette disorder. Occurs in males 3-4 times more often than females. Look for a patient with *motor tics* (e.g., eye-blinking, grunting, throat clearing, grimacing, barking, or shoulder shrugging) and/or random bouts of swearing (copralalia) that are exacerbated by stress and remit during activity or sleep. Of interest, Tourette disorder can be caused and/or unmasked by the use of stimulants (e.g., for presumed ADHD). Antipsychotics such as haloperidol are used if symptoms are severe. Tourette syndrome symptoms tend to improve in adulthood.

Encopresis/enuresis is not a disorder until after age 4 years (encopresis) or 5 years (enuresis). Rule out physical problems such as Hirschsprung disease and infection, and then treat with *behavioral therapy* (e.g., "gold star for being good" charts, alarms, biofeedback). *Imipramine,* which is not a first-line treatment, is used only for refractory cases of enuresis.

📁 **CASE SCENARIO:** A mother complains about her 2-year-old daughter who still wets her bed, although less often than a year ago. What is the preferred treatment? None, because bed-wetting is normal for a 2-year-old, and symptoms are already abating.

📁 **CASE SCENARIO:** List, in order, the top three causes of death in adolescents. *Accidents, homicide,* and *suicide.* Together, they cause about 75% of teen-age deaths. In black males, homicide is the number-one cause.

Pediatric pulmonology

Respiratory distress syndrome: Due to atelectasis from deficiency of surfactant; almost always in premature babies and/or babies of diabetic mothers. Look for *rapid, labored respirations, substernal retractions, cyanosis, grunting,* and/or *nasal flaring* at birth. Blood gas shows hypoxemia and hypercarbia, radiograph shows diffuse atelectasis. Treat with O_2, intubate if necessary, and give *surfactant.* Complications include intraventricular hemorrhage and pneumothorax/bronchopulmonary dysplasia (acute/chronic mechanical ventilation complications).

📁 **CASE SCENARIO:** What is the predominant presenting symptom in a newborn with a diaphragmatic hernia? Respiratory problems. Bowel herniated into the chest pushes on developing lung, causing lung hypoplasia on the affected side. Look for scaphoid abdomen, and listen for bowel sounds in the chest. Herniated bowel is seen on chest radiograph; 90% of cases are left-sided.

Look for meconium aspiration if an infant is covered with meconium when delivered, which can lead to airway obstruction and/or chemical pneumonitis. Suction secretions first from the mouth (oropharynx) and then from the nose with a bulb syringe or suction catheter immediately after the head is delivered. If intubation is necessary for depressed respiratory status, suctioning through the endotracheal tube is also performed until no more meconium is returned.

The most common type (85%) of tracheoesophageal fistula is an esophagus with a blind pouch proximally and a fistula between a bronchus/carina and the distal esophagus. Look for a neonate with *excessive oral secretions, coughing and cyanosis with attempted feedings,* abdominal distention, and aspiration pneumonia. The diagnosis should be suspected if a nasogastric tube cannot be passed into the stomach; the tube typically becomes *coiled in the esophagus.* An x-ray study using air injected through the nasogastric tube (rarely needed) shows the proximal esophagus only. Treatment is early surgical correction.

Cystic fibrosis: Autosomal recessive inheritance pattern; the most common lethal genetic disease in whites. Cystic fibrosis should be suspected in all children with *rectal prolapse, meconium ileus,* or *esophageal varices;* a "salty-tasting" infant; or any child with recurrent pulmonary infections and/or failure to thrive. The diagnosis can be made by an abnormal increase in the electrolytes of sweat (sodium and

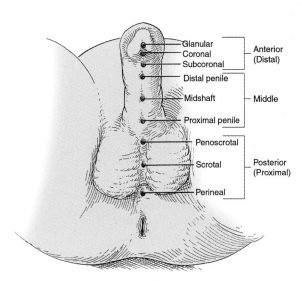

Anterior
(Distal)
- Glanular
- Coronal
- Subcoronal

Distal penile

Midshaft — Middle

Proximal penile

Penoscrotal

Scrotal — Posterior
(Proximal)

Perineal

FIGURE 2-20 Hypospadias. *(From Rakel RE, Rakel D: Textbook of Family Medicine, 8th ed. Philadelphia, Saunders, 2011.)*

chloride) or a DNA probe test. Watch for *pancreatic insufficiency*, which should be treated with pancreatic enzyme replacements and fat-soluble vitamin supplements; *infertility*, which affects 98% of affected males and many affected females; and *cor pulmonale* (right heart failure from lung disease). Look for *Staphylococcus aureus* and *Pseudomonas* spp. to be the cause of the many respiratory infections. Treat with chest physical therapy, vaccinations, fat-soluble vitamin supplements, pancreatic enzyme replacement, and aggressive treatment of infections with antibiotics.

Pediatric urology

Cryptorchidism is arrested descent of the testicle(s) somewhere between the renal area and the scrotum. The more premature the infant, the greater the likelihood of cryptorchidism. Many of the arrested testes eventually descend on their own within the first year of life. After 1 year, surgical intervention (orchiopexy) is warranted in an attempt to preserve fertility and facilitate future testicular exams (because of increased cancer risk). The higher the testicle is found (the farther away from the scrotum), the higher the risk of developing testicular cancer and the lower the likelihood of retaining fertility.

⬛ **CASE SCENARIO:** Does surgical correction of cryptorchidism alter the risk of testicular cancer in the affected testicle? Not definitively (controversial), but may preserve fertility and facilitates testicular exam for early detection of testicular cancer.

Penile anomalies. In hypospadias, the urethra opens on the ventral side (undersurface when the penis is flaccid) of the penis (Fig. 2-20); in epispadias, the urethra opens on the dorsal side (superior surface when the penis is flaccid) of the penis. Treat both surgically.

⬛ **CASE SCENARIO:** Which of the following is associated with exstrophy of the bladder: epispadias or hypospadias? Epispadias.

⬛ **CASE SCENARIO:** Where do the left and right gonadal veins drain? The right testicular/ovarian vein usually drains into the inferior vena cava (a lower-pressure system), whereas the left gonadal vein drains into the left renal vein. Isolated left varicoceles are common secondary to increased pressure in the left renal vein. An isolated right varicocele should raise suspicion for compression of the right testicular vein secondary to retroperitoneal malignancy/lymphadenopathy.

Potter syndrome. Bilateral renal agenesis causes oligohydramnios in utero (the fetus swallows fluid but cannot excrete it), limb deformities, abnormal facies, and hypoplasia of the lungs. Potter syndrome is incompatible with life.

3 INTERNAL MEDICINE AND MEDICAL SUBSPECIALTIES

GENERAL INTERNAL MEDICINE

Smoking

Smoking is the *single most significant source of preventable morbidity and premature death* in the United States. Whenever you are not sure which risk factor is most responsible for death, gloom, or doom, smoking is a safe guess on the boards.

☐ **CASE SCENARIO:** In a 58-year-old male smoker with no exercise, high stress, high cholesterol, and a drinking problem, what is the best way to reduce risk of death? Quit smoking.

Smoking is the best risk factor to eliminate to prevent deaths due to *heart disease* (responsible for 30–45% of coronary heart disease deaths). The risk is decreased by 50% within 1 year after quitting compared with continuing smokers, and the risk decreases to that of people who have never smoked 15 years after quitting smoking.

Smoking increases the risk for the following cancers: *lung* (causes 85–90% of cases); *oral cavity* (traditionally 90% of cases, though human papillomavirus [HPV] is rising as a cause); *esophagus* (70–80% of cases); *larynx, pharynx, bladder* (30–50% of cases); *kidney* (20–30% of cases); *pancreas* (20–25%); *cervix; vulva; penis; anus;* and *stomach.* It may also increase the risk of *acute myeloid leukemia* (AML).

Emphysema and *chronic bronchitis* (i.e., chronic obstructive pulmonary disease [COPD]) are almost always due to smoking. Although the changes associated with emphysema are irreversible, the risk of death still decreases after quitting smoking.

Smoking retards healing of the lesions of *peptic ulcer disease.*

Smoking by a pregnant woman increases the risk of *low birth weight, prematurity, spontaneous abortion, stillbirth,* and *infant mortality.*

☐ **CASE SCENARIO:** A 27-year-old woman has smoked five cigarettes per day for the past 2 years and now has emphysema. What is the cause? α_1-Antitrypsin deficiency. The patient has not smoked enough cigarettes to be the primary cause of emphysema (usually need at least 5–10 pack years).

☐ **CASE SCENARIO:** A 3-year-old child has asthma and recurrent otitis media. Both parents smoke. What is the best initial treatment? Persuade the parents to quit smoking.

☐ **CASE SCENARIO:** A 29-year-old man who is a heavy smoker gets painful red fingers and cold toes. What is the diagnosis? The patient has *Buerger disease (thromboangiitis obliterans).* Findings on angiography are diagnostic. If he stops smoking, the disease should resolve.

☐ **CASE SCENARIO:** Is it acceptable for a 36-year-old female smoker to take birth control pills? No. Oral contraceptives are contraindicated in women older than age 35 who smoke.

☐ **CASE SCENARIO:** Is it acceptable for a 58-year-old female smoker to take estrogen replacement therapy? Yes.

Alcohol

Health maintenance: Alcohol abuse is more common in men. Roughly 10–15% of people abuse alcohol. Alcoholism has a heritable component and is especially passed from *fathers to sons.*

Alcohol increases the risk for the following cancers: *oral, larynx, pharynx, esophagus,* and *liver.* It may increase the risk for gastric, pancreatic, colorectal, and *breast* cancer as well.

Alcohol is the most common cause of cirrhosis and esophageal varices and is involved in motor vehicle collisions, drowning, suicides, homicides, divorce, violent crime, child abuse, unemployment, and disruption of the family.

Patient management issues:

1. **Alcohol withdrawal** can be fatal and should be treated on an inpatient basis (Table 3-1).

TABLE 3-1 Manifestations of Alcohol Withdrawal

SIGNS/SYMPTOMS	TIME TO ONSET
Acute withdrawal syndrome: insomnia, tremors, mild anxiety, gastrointestinal upset, headache, sweating, anorexia	6-12 hr
Alcohol hallucinations: visual, auditory, or tactile. Withdrawal seizures: generalized tonic-clonic type, the so-called "rum fits"	12-48 hr
Delirium tremens: hallucinations (predominantly visual), disorientation, tachycardia, hypertension, low-grade fever, agitation, diaphoresis	2-5 days

Treatment of alcohol withdrawal involves:

❍ Supportive care: quiet room; soft lighting; intravenous (IV) fluids; electrolyte corrections (alcoholics typically have decreased potassium, glucose, and magnesium); and folic acid supplementation

❍ Thiamine supplementation to prevent Wernicke-Korsakoff syndrome

❍ Benzodiazepines reduce the severity of withdrawal symptoms

❍ For seizures, hallucinations, or agitation, use a benzodiazepine

❍ For tachycardia, use β-blockers

CASE SCENARIO: About 24 hours after surgery, a middle-aged patient becomes delirious and shaky. He has no hypoxia, no obvious infection, and no abnormal electrolytes. He is taking no medications, has never taken corticosteroids, and is on a regular surgery floor (not the intensive care unit). Why is he delirious? The patient is most likely a closet alcoholic going into withdrawal.

2. **Know the stigmata of chronic liver disease and cirrhosis in alcoholics:** varices, hemorrhoids, caput medusae, jaundice, ascites, palmar erythema, spider angiomas, gynecomastia, testicular atrophy, encephalopathy, *asterixis,* prolonged prothrombin time, hyperbilirubinemia, spontaneous bacterial peritonitis, hypoalbuminemia, and anemia.

3. **Know the various diseases associated with alcohol:** gastritis, Mallory-Weiss tears, pancreatitis (acute and chronic), peripheral neuropathy, dilated cardiomyopathy, fatty change in the liver, hepatitis, cerebellar degeneration/ataxia, and rhabdomyolysis (acute and chronic).

CASE SCENARIO: In a patient with hepatitis, the aspartate aminotransferase (AST) level is 250 units and the alanine aminotransferase (ALT) level is 110. What is the likely cause of the hepatitis? Alcohol (AST ≥2 times the ALT value typically indicates alcohol abuse, versus a 1:1 ratio or higher ALT with viral and other forms of hepatitis).

CASE SCENARIO: What is the best treatment for alcoholics who want to quit? Alcoholics Anonymous or a support group that offers cognitive and behavioral therapy.

4. Alcohol is a teratogen and can cause **fetal alcohol syndrome.** Findings in affected infants include mental retardation, microcephaly, microphthalmia, short palpebral fissures, midfacial hypoplasia, and cardiac defects. Generally, alcohol should be avoided during pregnancy. An estimated 1 in 3000 births are affected by fetal alcohol syndrome.

CASE SCENARIO: What is the most common cause of preventable mental retardation? Maternal alcohol consumption.

CASE SCENARIO: A homeless alcoholic is combative and found to have a low glucose level. He is given glucose and starts acting confused and ataxic and cannot move his eyes. What happened? Wernicke encephalopathy was precipitated by giving glucose before thiamine. Always give thiamine first, then glucose (or in the same IV bag) for alcoholics.

📖 **CASE SCENARIO:** A chronic alcoholic patient cannot form new memories and makes up stories. Why? Chronic thiamine deficency has led to Korsakoff syndrome, which is chronic and irreversible.

5. Watch for **aspiration pneumonia** with enteric organisms such as *Klebsiella* spp. (currant jelly sputum), anaerobes, *Escherichia coli*, streptococci, and staphylococci.
6. Alcoholics can have just about any **vitamin or mineral deficiency** but are especially prone to deficiencies of folate, magnesium, and thiamine.

📖 **CASE SCENARIO:** A known alcoholic with jaundice, ascites, and caput medusae vomits large quantities of blood. What should you do? First, stabilize the patient with IV fluids and blood and assess baseline lab values. Most frequently, upper endoscopy and sclerotherapy are performed with cauterization, banding, or vasopressin administration if esophageal varices are the cause. The mortality rate with varices is high, and rebleeding is common, especially early after the initial episode. *Placement of a transjugular intrahepatic portosystemic shunt* (TIPS) is another treatment option for variceal bleeding if it is life-threatening or recurrent after sclerotherapy. A TIPS procedure can also be performed to prolong life after variceal bleeding is stabilized, which is used instead of open surgical portocaval shunting (splenorenal shunt is the most physiologic type of standard surgically created shunt).

Obesity

Body mass index formula: (weight in kilograms)/(height in meters)^2
○ Overweight: body mass index (BMI) of 25–29.9 kg/m^2
○ Obesity: BMI of ≥30 kg/m^2
○ Morbid (also called severe or extreme) obesity: BMI ≥ 40 kg/m^2

Obesity increases the risk of the following problems:
1. Overall mortality (at every age)
2. Insulin resistance and diabetes mellitus (roughly 80–90% of cases of type 2 diabetes, or 70–80% of all cases of diabetes in the United States due to obesity)
3. Hypertension (HTN) (roughly two-thirds to three-fourths of cases caused or aggravated by obesity)
4. Dyslipidemia—hypertriglyceridemia is classic, but obesity can also increase low-density lipoprotein (LDL) and lower high-density lipoprotein (HDL)
5. Heart disease and coronary artery disease (CAD), including congestive heart failure (CHF) and myocardial infarction (MI)
6. Stroke
7. Gallstones (cholesterol stones)
8. Hypoventilation, Pickwickian syndrome, and sleep apnea
9. Osteoarthritis
10. Cancer—especially endometrial cancer, but also cancers of the breast, colon, and esophagus
11. Thromboembolism
12. Varicose veins
13. Polycystic ovary syndrome
14. Gastroesophageal reflux disease (GERD)
15. Depression

Treatment is multifactorial (Table 3-2). Starvation/drastic diets should be avoided and have potentially dangerous side effects. Slow progress that can be maintained for life is better than drastic improvement that cannot be maintained. Bariatric surgery (i.e., weight reduction procedures such as gastric bypass, gastric stapling, or sleeve procedures) is used with short-term success in persons with morbid obesity that is refractory to other treatments, who demonstrate an ability and willingness to comply with follow-up regimens, and accept the risks (including death) of the procedure.

TABLE 3-2 Weight-Loss Treatment Guidelines

TREATMENT	BMI				
	25-26.9	27-29.9	30-34.9	35-39.9	>40
Diet, physical activity, behavioral therapy, or all three	Yes	Yes	Yes	Yes	Yes
Pharmacotherapy Orlistat: blocks digestion and absorption of fat Phentermine: amphetamine derivative causing appetite suppression		In patients with obesity-related diseases	Yes	Yes	Yes
Surgery				In patients with obesity-related diseases	Yes

Data are from www.nhlbi.nih.gov/guidelines/obesity/ob_home.htm. These guidelines are generally consistent with those from the American Heart Association, the American Medical Association, the American Diabetic Association, the Obesity Society (Practical Guide), the American Diabetes Association, the American Academy of Family Physicians, the American College of Sports Medicine, and the American Cancer Society.
BMI, Body mass index.

Acid-base disorders
Common formulas in acid-base analysis (Fig. 3-1):
○ $pH = 6.1 + \log([HCO_3^-]/0.03 \times PCO_2)$
○ Anion gap $= [Na^+] - ([Cl^-] + [HCO_3^-])$
○ Urine anion gap $= U_{Na} + U_K - U_{Cl}$
○ Calculated osmolarity $= 2[Na] + [Glucose]/18 +$ blood urea nitrogen $[BUN]/2.8 + [Ethanol]/4.6$

▢ **CASE SCENARIO:** What is the primary disturbance in the following settings?
1. pH high, carbon dioxide high: Metabolic alkalosis (with respiratory compensation).
2. pH high, bicarbonate low: Respiratory alkalosis (with metabolic compensation).

▢ **CASE SCENARIO:** A patient takes "a handful of pills" and has tinnitus, near-normal pH, low carbon dioxide, and low bicarbonate. What did she take? Aspirin, which causes both a primary metabolic acidosis and a primary respiratory alkalosis. Alkalinization of the urine (with bicarbonate) speeds excretion.

▢ **CASE SCENARIO:** A patient with an acute asthma exacerbation has hyperventilation and respiratory alkalosis on arterial blood gas analysis. If the pH changes to normal, the patient

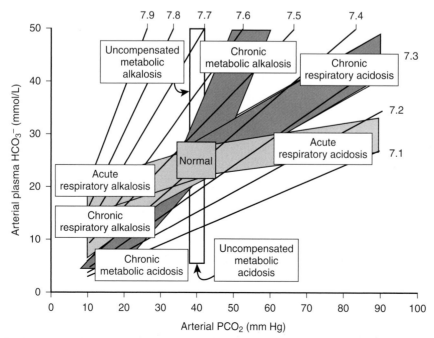

FIGURE 3-1 The relationship of PCO_2, HCO_3, and pH in acid-base disorders. *(From Mason RJ, Broaddus VC, Martin T, et al: Murray and Nadel's Textbook of Respiratory Medicine, 5th ed. Philadelphia, Saunders, 2010.)*

becomes sleepy, and carbon dioxide starts to rise, what should you do? Prepare to intubate! There is no time for metabolic compensation in an acute asthma exacerbation. The patient is developing fatigue due to the work of breathing and is about to "crash."

◻ **CASE SCENARIO:** A 68-year-old woman with emphysema who takes 2 L/min of oxygen by nasal cannula 24 hours per day at home presents with increased shortness of breath. She is given 6 L/min via nasal cannula to maintain oxygen saturation above 93%, but carbon dioxide starts to rise and the pH falls on repeat blood gas analysis. What should you do? Turn down the oxygen. High oxygen levels may shut down the respiratory drive of patients with severe chronic obstructive pulmonary disease.

◻ **CASE SCENARIO:** What do you expect the blood gas analysis to show in patients with a heroin overdose? Respiratory acidosis with high carbon dioxide, low pH, and near-normal bicarbonate (due to lack of time for metabolic compensation).

◻ **CASE SCENARIO:** A 32-year-old woman presents with severe dyspnea and anxiety, 100% oxygen saturation, high pH, low carbon dioxide, normal bicarbonate, and a normal chest radiograph and electrocardiogram (ECG). She is also afebrile and has no wheezing. What is happening? Probably a *panic attack* causing primary respiratory alkalosis.

◻ **CASE SCENARIO:** In an obese, fatigued 36-year-old man whose wife says that he snores a lot, why does the blood gas analysis show high pH, high bicarbonate, and normal carbon dioxide during an office visit? The patient has sleep apnea. Chronic respiratory acidosis during sleep causes chronic metabolic compensation. During the day, the patient is awake and blows off enough carbon dioxide. Alkalosis develops because the bicarbonate is still high (i.e., the compensation becomes the primary disturbance).

◻ **CASE SCENARIO:** In a 37-year-old woman with new-onset HTN, the chemistry panel shows hypokalemia and high bicarbonate. Why? Aldosterone-secreting adenoma *(Conn syndrome).*

◻ **CASE SCENARIO:** What is the difference between the acid-base disturbances caused by diarrhea and by vomiting? Diarrhea usually results in metabolic acidosis, whereas vomiting usually results in metabolic alkalosis (and hypokalemia).

 Avoid using bicarbonate to treat low pH unless the pH is <7.0 and other measures have failed. First try to correct the underlying problem and/or give normal saline.

Hyponatremia: Watch for confusion, lethargy, mental status changes, anorexia, *seizures*, disorientation, cramps, and coma.

The first step in determining the cause of hyponatremia is to ensure that the patient does not have "false" hyponatremia due to *hyperglycemia*. The most important next step is to check the volume status (Table 3-3).

Table 3-3 Causes and Treatment of Hyponatremia

	CAUSES	TREATMENT
Hypovolemic hyponatremia	Dehydration, diuretics, diabetes, Addison disease, hypoaldosteronism	Normal saline
Isovolemic hyponatremia	SIADH psychologic polydipsia, oxytocin use	SIADH: Fluid restriction, demeclocycline. If acute and symptomatic: hypertonic saline
Hypervolemic hyponatremia	CHF nephritic syndrome, cirrhosis, toxemia, renal failure	Sodium and water restriction. Captopril and furosemide if due to CHF

CHF, Congestive heart failure; *SIADH,* syndrome of inappropriate antidiuretic hormone.

The syndrome of inappropriate antidiuretic hormone (SIADH) commonly results from head trauma, surgery, meningitis, *small cell cancer of the lung,* postoperative or other painful states, pulmonary infections (pneumonia or tuberculosis [TB]), opioids, or chlorpropamide.

◻ **CASE SCENARIO:** A patient with small cell lung cancer develops severe hyponatremia. Water restriction does not help. What drug can you try? *Demeclocycline,* which causes nephrogenic diabetes insipidus and counteracts the SIADH.

📁 **CASE SCENARIO:** A patient with a history of severe asthma undergoes an uncomplicated appendectomy and develops hypotension turning into shock, as well as hyponatremia and hyperkalemia that does not respond to IV fluids. What should you do? Give IV corticosteroids. The patient probably has acute adrenal insufficiency from taking steroids in the past.

📁 **CASE SCENARIO:** A nursing home patient taking furosemide presents with marked tenting of skin, hyponatremia, and hypokalemia. What should you do? Give normal saline—the treatment for hypovolemic hyponatremia. Do not give hypertonic saline!

📁 **CASE SCENARIO:** An alcoholic patient who presents with very low sodium is given hypertonic saline, and the sodium becomes normal within 12 hours. The patient goes into a coma. What happened? Brainstem damage *(central pontine myelinolysis)*. Hypertonic saline should be avoided on the boards (used only when a patient has seizures from hyponatremia and even then only briefly and cautiously). Normal saline is a better choice 99 times out of 100 for board purposes.

📁 **CASE SCENARIO:** A 27-year-old woman (G1P0) is in labor and is given *oxytocin* for failure to progress. After a few hours, she has a seizure. The sodium level is low. What should you do first? Stop the oxytocin, which can cause hyponatremia.

Note ✎ *In a surgical patient, the most common cause of hyponatremia is inappropriate or excessive fluid administration.*

Hypernatremia: Signs and symptoms are similar to those of hyponatremia: confusion, mental status changes, hyperreflexia, seizures, and coma (Table 3-4).

TABLE 3-4 Causes and Treatment of Hypernatremia

	CAUSES	TREATMENT
Hypovolemic hypernatremia	Renal losses (diuretics), dehydration, gastrointestinal or respiratory loss, adrenal deficiency	Normal saline
Isovolemic hypernatremia	Diabetes Insipidus, skin loss	Thiazide diuretic, D_5W IV fluid
Hypervolemic hypernatremia	Iatrogenic, Cushing syndrome, Conn syndrome, salt ingestion	Loop diuretic, D_5W IV fluid

📁 **CASE SCENARIO:** A demented patient is found unconscious at home. He has marked tenting of the skin. The sodium level is extremely high. What should you do? Give normal saline because the patient is dehydrated. Do not give ½ normal saline or D5W. The patient needs volume.

📁 **CASE SCENARIO:** Pituitary versus nephrogenic diabetes insipidus. In a patient with diabetes insipidus, how do you know if the cause is nephrogenic or pituitary? Give vasopressin and measure the urine concentration before and after giving it. Pituitary diabetes insipidus respond appropriately (i.e., urine becomes more concentrated); nephrogenic diabetes insipidus does not.

📁 **CASE SCENARIO:** A manic-depressive patient taking lithium has fatigue and polyuria. The serum sodium level is very high, and glucose is normal. What is the problem? Nephrogenic diabetes insipidus due to lithium.

📁 **CASE SCENARIO:** What drug can be used to treat a patient with nephrogenic diabetes insipidus? A *thiazide diuretic* (paradoxical effect decreases urine formation).

📁 **CASE SCENARIO:** A 29-year-old woman has severe postpartum hemorrhage and goes into shock. She recovers after aggressive resuscitation. Later she cannot breast-feed and produces 20 L/day of urine. What happened? The patient developed Sheehan syndrome (pituitary infarction), which may result in central diabetes insipidus and other endocrine problems (e.g., in this case, lack of prolactin; thus, she cannot breast-feed).

Hypokalemia: Look for *muscular weakness,* which can lead to paralysis and ventilatory failure. Hypokalemia also affects the smooth muscles; the patient may have an adynamic *ileus* and/or hypotension.

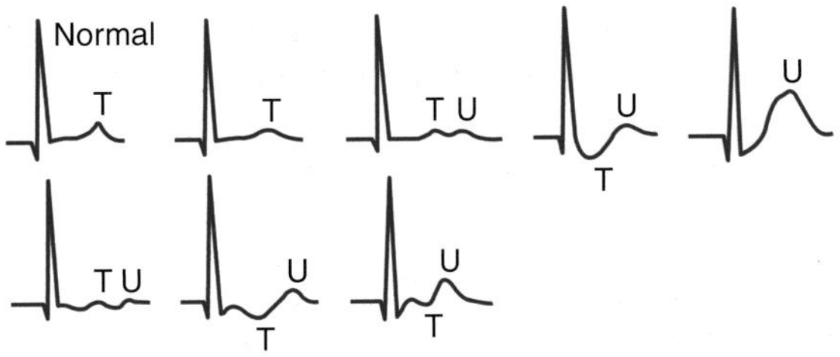

FIGURE 3-2 Variable electrocardiogram patterns can be seen with hypokalemia, ranging from slight T wave flattening to the appearance of prominent U waves, sometimes with ST depressions or T wave inversions. *(From Ferri FF: Practical Guide to the Care of the Medical Patient, 8th ed. Philadelphia, Mosby, 2011.)*

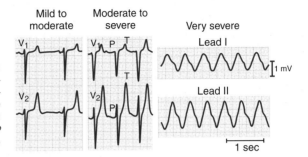

FIGURE 3-3 The earliest change with hyperkalemia is peaking ("tenting") of the T waves. With progressive increases in serum potassium, the QRS complexes widen, the P waves decrease in amplitude and may disappear, and finally, a sine wave pattern leads to asystole. *(From Ferri FF: Practical Guide to the Care of the Medical Patient, 8th ed. Philadelphia, Mosby, 2011.)*

📁 **CASE SCENARIO:** A 58-year-old woman taking furosemide develops palpitations. The ECG shows loss of T waves, the presence of U waves, and multiple premature ventricular contractions (Fig. 3-2). Cardiac enzymes are normal. What is the problem? Hypokalemia.

📁 **CASE SCENARIO:** A 22-year-old man presents with diabetic ketoacidosis and has severe acidosis with a normal potassium level. Why should you give potassium? Because acidosis causes hyperkalemia. Thus the "normal" potassium level will become low once you start treating the acidosis with fluids and insulin. To make matters worse, insulin drives potassium from the extracellular space and plasma into the intracellular space. The end result is that if you do not start potassium replacement now, you will probably get into trouble with hypokalemia later.

The heart is particularly sensitive to hypokalemia when *digitalis* is present.

Always check magnesium levels. If low, replace with IV or oral magnesium.

Do not replace potassium too quickly. The best replacement route is oral, but if potassium is given IV, use ECG monitoring and do not exceed 20 mEq/hr.

Hyperkalemia: The classic symptom of hyperkalemia is *weakness* or paralysis.

ECG changes (in order of increasing potassium value) include *tall, peaked T waves* (Fig. 3-3); widening of QRS; PR interval prolongation; loss of P waves; and a sine-wave pattern. Arrhythmias include asystole and ventricular fibrillation.

Common causes of hyperkalemia are *renal failure* (acute or chronic) and *medications* (potassium-sparing diuretics, nonsteroidal antiinflammatory drugs [NSAIDs], and angiotensin-converting enzyme [ACE] inhibitors). Other causes include severe tissue destruction, hypoaldosteronism (watch for hyporeninemic hypoaldosteronism in diabetes), and adrenal insufficiency (patients also have low sodium levels and low blood pressure).

📁 **CASE SCENARIO:** A patient has a high potassium level but is asymptomatic and has a normal ECG. What is the best treatment? Oral sodium polystyrene resin (Kayexalate).

📁 **CASE SCENARIO:** What should you give to a severely hyperkalemic patient with ECG changes? First, give *calcium gluconate* (cardioprotective), then *sodium bicarbonate* (alkalosis causes potassium to shift inside cells). Also consider giving IV glucose with insulin (also forces potassium inside cells). Dialysis can be used in an emergency or in patients with renal failure.

Hypocalcemia: The classic sign of hypocalcemia is *tetany*, which can be elicited by tapping on the facial nerve to elicit contraction of the facial muscles *(Chvostek sign)*. Other symptoms and signs include depression, encephalopathy, dementia, laryngospasm, and convulsions. The ECG shows *QT interval prolongation.*

🖵 **CASE SCENARIO:** When a nurse checks a patient's blood pressure, the patient's hand goes into spasm. She tries the other arm, and the same thing happens. What does the patient have? Hypocalcemia. This is a *Trousseau sign.*

🖵 **CASE SCENARIO:** A neonate born with low-set ears, cleft palate, and ventricular septal defect demonstrates irritability and facial muscle contractions when the face is touched. The child then goes into convulsions. What rare syndrome might the child have? *DiGeorge syndrome.*

🖵 **CASE SCENARIO:** What surgery classically results in iatrogenic hypocalcemia? Thyroidectomy, when all four parathyroids are accidentally removed.

Other causes of hypocalcemia include *renal failure* (remember the kidney's role in vitamin D metabolism); vitamin D deficiency; pseudohypoparathyroidism (short fingers, short stature, mental retardation, and normal levels of parathyroid hormone with end-organ unresponsiveness to parathyroid hormone); and acute pancreatitis (hypocalcemia is one of Ranson's criteria for poor outcome).

🖵 **CASE SCENARIO:** When a patient has a low calcium level, what other lab test do you have to check to interpret the low calcium level? An albumin level. *Hypoalbuminemia* of any etiology can cause hypocalcemia because the protein-bound fraction of calcium is decreased. In this instance, however, the patient is asymptomatic because the ionized/unbound, biologically active fraction of calcium is unchanged.

Rickets and osteomalacia are the skeletal effects of vitamin D deficiency in children and adults, respectively.

Alkalosis can cause symptoms similar to hypocalcemia because of its effects on the ionized fraction of calcium. Treat by correcting the pH.

Remember that phosphorus and calcium levels usually go in opposite directions. Derangements in one can cause problems with the other. In patients with renal failure, you must try to not only raise calcium but also restrict phosphorus (Table 3-5).

TABLE 3-5 Approach to Various Causes of Hypocalcemia

CAUSE	TREATMENT
Acute, severe hypocalcemia due to hypoparathyroidism or vitamin D deficiency	Intravenous calcium gluconate
Chronic hypocalcemia due to hypoparathyroidism or vitamin D deficiency	Oral calcium carbonate, vitamin D replacement (calcitriol)
Chronic hypocalcemia due to renal failure	Phosphate-binding antacids, calcium carbonate, vitamin D (calcitriol)
Hypoalbuminemia	Diet and nutrition improvement. Free calcium levels are normal, so no treatment of calcium levels is indicated
Hypomagnesemia	Magnesium sulfate

Hypercalcemia: Hypercalcemia is usually asymptomatic and discovered on routine lab tests. When symptoms are present, remember *"bones, stones, groans, and psychiatric overtones"* ("bones" = bone changes such as osteopenia and pathologic fractures; "stones" = kidney stones and polyuria; "groans" = abdominal pain, anorexia, constipation, ileus, nausea, and vomiting; and "psychiatric overtones" = depression, psychosis, delirium, confusion).

The ECG shows QT interval shortening.

🖵 **CASE SCENARIO:** Hypercalcemia is discovered on routine lab tests in an outpatient. What is the most likely cause? Hyperparathyroidism.

Other causes of hypercalcemia include *malignancy,* vitamin A or D intoxication, sarcoidosis, thiazide diuretics, familial hypocalciuric hypercalcemia (look for low urinary calcium, which is rare with hypercalcemia), and immobilization.

Hyperproteinemia of any cause can lead to hypercalcemia because of an increase in the protein-bound fraction of calcium, but the patient will be asymptomatic, because the ionized/unbound, active fraction is unchanged (and no treatment is necessary).

Severe prolonged hypercalcemia can cause *nephrocalcinosis* and *renal failure* from calcium salt deposits in the kidney.

📋 **CASE SCENARIO:** A patient has severe hypercalcemia. What is the first step in treatment? IV normal saline. After the patient is well hydrated, *furosemide* may be of benefit as the next step in treatment to cause a calcium diuresis.

Other possible hypercalcemia treatments include oral phosphorus administration (IV phosphorus is rarely used because it is dangerous), calcitonin, bisphosphonates (e.g., etidronate in Paget disease), plicamycin, and prednisone (for malignancy-induced hypercalcemia).

Other Electrolyte Disturbances: Hypomagnesemia is often seen in alcoholics. The signs and symptoms (including ECG changes and tetany) are similar to those of hypocalcemia. Hypomagnesemia is notorious because it *makes hypokalemia and hypocalcemia difficult to correct.* Treat with oral or IV replacement.

Hypermagnesemia is common in patients with renal failure.

📋 **CASE SCENARIO:** A woman treated with magnesium sulfate for severe preeclampsia develops low blood pressure and trouble with breathing. Deep tendon reflexes are markedly decreased bilaterally. What should you do first? Stop the magnesium, because the patient has developed hypermagnesemia.

Hypophosphatemia is seen primarily in patients with diabetic ketoacidosis and in alcoholics. Signs and symptoms include neuromuscular disturbances (encephalopathy, weakness), rhabdomyolysis, and anemia.

Hyperphosphatemia is usually seen in patients with renal failure. Treat with phosphate restriction, dialysis, and phosphate-binding resins (e.g., calcium carbonate or sevelamer).

📋 **CASE SCENARIO:** In a hypotensive trauma patient, what is the IV fluid of choice? Ringer's lactate. The second choice is normal saline.

In hypovolemic patients, normal saline or Ringer's lactate is often the best choice for IV fluid, regardless of other electrolyte problems.

📋 **CASE SCENARIO:** What is the best choice of maintenance fluid in patients who are not allowed to eat? D5 ½ normal saline. In younger pediatric patients, use D5 ¼ normal saline or D5 1⅓ normal saline because of renal differences. Do not forget to monitor potassium levels (and replace as needed) if the patient is not going to be eating.

Geriatrics

The most rapid increase in the U.S. population (percentage-wise) is in people older than 65. Within this subgroup, the older-than-85 group is increasing most rapidly. About 15% of the population is older than age 65.

At age 80, elderly patients have half the lean body mass of a 30-year-old. Because the basal metabolic rate depends on lean body mass, the elderly need fewer calories.

Normal changes in elderly people: Slightly impaired immune response; visual *(presbyopia)* and hearing *(presbyacusis)* impairment; decreased muscle mass; increased fat deposits; osteoporosis; brain changes (decreased weight, enlarged ventricles, and dilated sulci); and slightly decreased ability to learn new material.

Normal sexual function changes in men: Longer time to get an erection; increased refractory period (after ejaculation, it takes longer before the patient can have another erection); and delayed ejaculation (the patient may ejaculate only one of every three times he has sex). *Impotence and lack of sexual desire are not normal* and should be investigated. Look for psychiatric (depression) and physical causes. Medications, especially antihypertensives, are notorious culprits.

Normal sexual function changes in women: Decreased lubrication may require use of a water-soluble lubricant; atrophy of the clitoris, labia, and vaginal tissues may cause dyspareunia (treat with estrogen cream); and orgasm may be delayed. *Lack of sexual desire is not normal* and should be investigated (psychiatric or physical causes).

Sleep changes in elderly people: The elderly sleep less deeply, wake up more frequently during the night, and awaken earlier in the morning. They take longer to fall asleep (longer sleep latency) and have less stage 3, 4, and rapid eye movement (REM) sleep.

Depression in the elderly can manifest as dementia (known as *pseudodementia*). Look for a history that would trigger depression (e.g., loss of a spouse, terminal or debilitating disease).

Dementia affects 15% of people older than age 65. The most common causes of dementia are (in decreasing order) *Alzheimer disease* (gradually progressive, neurofibrillary tangles); *multiple cerebral infarcts* (stepwise, risk factors for stroke); and others (e.g., human immunodeficiency virus [HIV], Pick disease).

Only 5% of people older than the age of 65 live in nursing homes.

More than 90% of hip fractures are associated with falls. Most occur in patients older than 70. Decrease the risk of falls in the elderly with mobility problems by "fall-proofing" the home (e.g., repair broken hand rails or steps and slippery floors, remove items that can be tripped over) and by watching for medications that decrease the patient's sense of balance (the classic offenders are sedatives and anticholinergic drugs).

CARDIOLOGY

Cholesterol

Health maintenance: Screen all people by obtaining a fasting lipoprotein profile (total cholesterol, LDL, HDL, and triglycerides) every 5 years (unless abnormal) starting at age 20. Consider earlier and more aggressive screening for a strong family history and/or obesity. Screen all first-degree relatives of a patient with familial hyperlipidemia. Total cholesterol goal is <200 mg/dL, with >240 considered high; normal triglyceride levels are <150 mg/dL, with >200 considered high; LDL is usually the main player for treatment decisions (see later).

Cholesterol is important mainly because it is a risk factor for atherosclerosis. To keep the importance in perspective, atherosclerosis is involved in about half of all deaths in the United States and one-third of deaths in people between ages 35 and 65. Atherosclerosis is the most important cause of permanent disability and accounts for more hospital days than any other illness.

New patient management issues: Look for *xanthelasma, xanthomas* (Fig. 3-4), and *corneal arcus* in younger people, as well as lipemic-looking serum and obesity (markers of possible familial hypercholesterolemia). Also look for pancreatitis with no risk factors (e.g., no alcohol use or gallstones) as a marker for familial hypertriglyceridemia.

Lipoprotein analysis involves measuring total cholesterol, HDL, and triglycerides. LDL cholesterol can be calculated from the formula LDL = total cholesterol − HDL − (triglycerides/5).

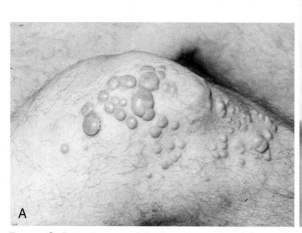
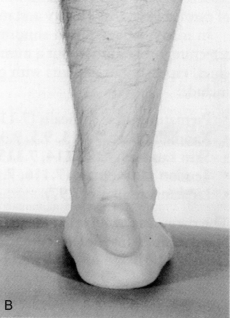

FIGURE 3-4 Xanthomata of the knee **(A)** and Achilles tendon **(B)**, two classic and common locations. Most are located along tendons and extensor surfaces of joints. *(From Forbes CD, Jackson WF: Endocrine, metabolic, and nutritional disorders. In Forbes CD, Jackson WF [eds]: Color Atlas and Text of Clinical Medicine. St. Louis, Mosby, 1993, pp 303-352.)*

Standard management guide for cholesterol levels (mg/dL)—ATPIII Guidelines: see Table 3-6.

TABLE 3-6 LDL Cholesterol Levels and Interventions Based on Risk

RISK CATEGORY	LDL GOAL	LDL LEVEL TO RECOMMEND LIFESTYLE CHANGES	LDL LEVEL TO CONSIDER DRUG THERAPY
CAD, or CAD risk equivalents† (10-yr risk >20%)	≤100 mg/dL	≥100 mg/dL	≥130 mg/dL (100-129 mg/dL: drug optional)
2+ risk factors* (10-yr risk ≤20%)	≤130 mg/dL	≥130 mg/dL	≥130 mg/dL if 10-yr risk 10-20% ≥160 mg/dL if 10-yr risk <10%
0-1 risk factor*	≤160 mg/dL	≥160 mg/dL	≥190 mg/dL (160-189 mg/dL: drug optional)

CAD, Coronary artery disease; *LDL,* low-density lipoprotein.
*Risk factors for CAD are listed in the text.
†CAD equivalents include diabetes mellitus, peripheral arterial atherosclerotic disease, symptomatic carotid artery disease, and abdominal aortic aneurysm.

Risk factors for CAD:
1. Age (men ≥45, women ≥55, or women with premature menopause and no hormone replacement therapy)
2. Family history of premature CAD (defined as definite MI or sudden death in first-degree male relative <55 years old or first-degree female relative <65 years old)
3. Current cigarette smoking (>10 cigarettes per day)
4. Hypertension (BP ≥140/90 mm Hg or taking antihypertensive medications)
5. Low HDL (<40 mg/dL). Note, however, that HDL ≥60 mg/dL is considered to be protective and negates one risk factor.

"Softer" risk factors and other information:
○ Obesity, stress, physical inactivity, and "type A" personality are not independent risk factors for board purposes. However, watch for these clues in a clinical case scenario describing CAD.
○ *Male sex* is a risk factor for CAD because men develop CAD earlier than women. Postmenopausal women quickly catch up to age-matched men, however. If you give a man one risk factor for male gender, do not give him a second risk factor for age.
○ *High LDL* and *total cholesterol* are risk factors for CAD, but do not count them when deciding to treat or not treat hyperlipidemia using the table. *Hypertriglyceridemia* alone is not considered a risk factor, but in association with high cholesterol it causes more CAD than high cholesterol alone.

▭ **CASE SCENARIO:** A 59-year-old man taking amlodipine and with no family cardiac history or other health problems has an LDL of 170 mg/dL on multiple visits over 1 year, even after dietary changes. He quit smoking 3 months ago. What should you do? Prescribe lipid-lowering medication such as HMG-CoA reductase inhibitor (statin) due to the presence of two risk factors (age and taking HTN medications).

General management issues: Give lower-risk patients 3 to 6 months to try lifestyle modifications (exercise, a diet lower in calories, cholesterol, saturated fats, less alcohol consumption, and smoking cessation) before intiating drug therapy. If the patient has CAD or a CAD disease equivalent (e.g., diabetes, peripheral vascular disease) and the LDL is ≥100, medication therapy is indicated.

First-line agents are HMG-CoA reductase inhibitors (statins). Second-line agents include niacin ezetimibe and bile acid-binding resins (e.g., cholestyramine).

Order baseline liver function tests for patients taking statins and periodically *monitor liver enzymes* in people taking these agents due to potential hepatotoxicity. Statins should not be used in patients with liver disease and can also cause muscle damage (watch for sore muscles and/or elevated creatine kinase [CK] levels).

Gemfibrozil lowers only triglycerides.

HDL is protective against atherosclerosis and is increased by *moderate (not high) alcohol consumption* (1–2 drinks/day), *exercise,* and *estrogens.* HDL is decreased by smoking, androgens, progesterone, and hypertriglyceridemia.

Secondary causes of hyperlipidemia include diabetes, hypothyroidism, uremia, nephrotic syndrome, obstructive liver disease, excessive alcohol intake (increases triglycerides), and medications (birth control pills, glucocorticoids, thiazides, and β-blockers). If the underlying problem is corrected in such cases, no other treatment may be necessary.

Hypertension

Health maintenance: Screening for HTN should be done roughly every 1–2 years starting at the age of 18, although blood pressure is typically measured routinely during any health encounter.

    Patient management issues: Hypertension is diagnosed when the blood pressure from two separate measurements is >140 mm Hg systolic or >90 mm Hg diastolic (values lower in children; typically the 95th percentile for age is used in pediatric patients) (Table 3-7).

TABLE 3-7 Hypertension Classification and Management in People 18 Years of Age and Older (2003 Joint National Committee Guidelines):

SYSTOLIC BP* (mm Hg)	DIASTOLIC BP* (mm Hg)	CLASSIFICATION	INITIAL DRUG TREATMENT (ALL PATIENTS SHOULD MAKE LIFESTYLE MODIFICATIONS)
<120	<80	Normal	None
120-139	80-89	Prehypertension	None unless compelling indications†
140-159	90-99	Stage I hypertension	Thiazides preferred. Use other agents for co-morbid conditions or combination treatment
≥160	≥100	Stage II hypertension	Thiazide plus at least one other agent (if tolerated) typically needed

*Classification is based on the worst number (e.g., 168/60 mm Hg is considered stage II hypertension even though diastolic pressure is normal).
†Compelling indications are *diabetes, chronic kidney disease, heart failure, prior myocardial infarction,* and *prior stroke.*

After the first abnormal blood pressure measurement, prescribe lifestyle modifications as appropriate: *weight reduction, exercise, low-salt and low-cholesterol diet, moderation of alcohol intake,* and *smoking cessation.* If these measures fail after a 1- to 2-month observation period, start medications. Lifestyle modifications should continue to be prescribed once drug therapy is initiated.

    Basic studies and evaluation in a new hypertensive patient include *urinalysis, basic blood chemistry panel* (i.e., basic metabolic profile [BMP] or Chem-7 panel), *ECG, complete blood count* (CBC), and a *fasting lipid profile.* These tests, along with the history, help to screen for secondary causes of HTN and check for end-organ damage and associated cardiovascular risk factors.

    General management issues: The goal of treatment is to *maintain a blood pressure <140/90 mm Hg.* There are five primary first-line agents for the treatment of HTN: *thiazide diuretics* (preferred agent in patients without additional comorbid conditions/indications), *β-blockers, ACE inhibitors, angiotensin receptor blockers (ARBs),* and *calcium channel blockers.* The choice is often made because of coexisting conditions (Table 3-8).

TABLE 3-8 Hypertension Management

DRUG CLASS	USE IN PATIENTS WITH:	AVOID IN PATIENTS WITH:
Thiazides	Heart failure, diabetes, high risk for coronary artery disease or stroke, osteoporosis	Gout, electrolyte disturbances (e.g., hyponatremia), pregnancy, sulfa allergy
β-Blockers	Stable angina, acute coronary syndrome/unstable angina, acute or prior myocardial infarction, high risk for coronary artery disease, atrial tachycardia/fibrillation, thyrotoxicosis (short-term), essential tremor, migraines	Asthma, chronic obstructive pulmonary disease, heart block, sick sinus syndrome
ACE inhibitors	Heart failure, diabetes, acute coronary syndrome/unstable angina, acute or prior myocardial infarction, high risk for coronary artery disease or stroke, chronic kidney disease	Pregnancy, angioedema, renovascular hypertension (may cause renal failure)
ARBs (e.g., losartan, irbesartan)	Heart failure, diabetes, chronic kidney disease	Pregnancy, renovascular hypertension (may cause renal failure)
Calcium channel blockers	Raynaud syndrome, atrial tachyarrhythmias	Heart block, sick sinus syndrome, congestive heart failure (all related to central-acting agents), pregnancy
Aldosterone receptor blockers (e.g., spironolactone)	Heart failure, prior myocardial infarction	Hyperkalemia, pregnancy

ACE, Angiotensin-converting enzyme; *ARBs,* angiotensin receptor blockers.

🗀 **CASE SCENARIO:** What antihypertensive agents are appropriate for pregnant patients? Use hydralazine, β-blockers (typically labetolol), or α-methyldopa. Remember that in preeclamptic patients, *magnesium sulfate* (used for seizure prophylaxis) lowers blood pressure.

🗀 **CASE SCENARIO:** Which agent is the best for a 32-year-old woman with hypertension? Any agent that is not teratogenic! Especially avoid ACE inhibitors and ARBs. Do not forget to counsel women of reproductive age about the risks of pregnancy. Always do a pregnancy test before starting a standard antihypertensive agent (or any other possible teratogen).

🗀 **CASE SCENARIO:** What antihypertensive agent may be a good choice for men with coexisting benign prostatic hypertrophy (BPH)? α-Adrenergic antagonists (e.g., prazosin, doxazosin).

Secondary HTN: Clues are onset before age 30 or after age 55, very high or hard-to-control blood pressure, lab values showing renal disease, or presence of abdominal bruit.
1. Drugs (NSAIDs, oral contraceptives, corticosteroids): Birth control pills are the most common secondary cause in young women. Discontinue their use to see if HTN resolves.
2. Renovascular HTN: may be due to *fibromuscular dysplasia* in young women or *atherosclerosis* in elderly persons. Watch for a renal bruit or renal failure after taking an ACE inhibitor. Consider ultrasonography, computed tomography (CT) or magnetic resonance angiogram, or conventional arteriogram to diagnose. Treatment is typically angioplasty.
3. Excessive alcohol intake: a common cause, especially in young men.
4. Pheochromocytoma: Watch for *intermittent severe HTN, dizziness,* and *diaphoresis.* Check plasma fractionated metanephrines or 24-hour urinary catecholamines (e.g., vanillylmandelic acid, metanephrine) as a screening test.
5. Polycystic kidney disease: flank mass(es), family history, renal insufficiency.
6. Cushing disease: Patient taking steroids or with Cushingoid appearance. Use 24-hour urine cortisol level or dexamethasone suppression test as screening tool.
7. Conn syndrome: Aldosterone-secreting adrenal adenoma causes high aldosterone, low renin, and hypokalemia.
8. Coarctation of the aorta: upper extremity hypertension only, unequal pulses, radiofemoral delay, associated with *Turner syndrome,* rib notching on radiograph.

Hypertensive urgency and emergency: A systolic BP >200 mm Hg and/or diastolic BP >120 mm Hg is generally defined as a hypertensive urgency if the patient is *asymptomatic* and an emergency if there is evidence of *acute end-organ damage.* Signs of end-organ damage include acute left ventricular failure/pulmonary edema; unstable angina; MI encephalopathy (i.e., headaches, mental status changes, vomiting, blurry vision, dizziness, and/or papilledema); stroke; life-threatening arterial bleeding; aortic dissection; optic disc swelling; or acute renal insufficiency/failure. Admit affected patients and treat with IV *nitroprusside, nitroglycerin, nicardipine,* or *labetalol* emergently.

Epidemiology facts
1. Lowering HTN lowers the risk for stroke (hypertension is the most important risk factor), congestive heart failure, MI renal failure, atherosclerosis, and aortic dissection.
2. CAD is the most common cause of death among untreated hypertensive patients.
3. The risk of cardiovascular disease doubles with each blood pressure increment of 20/10 mm Hg starting at 115/75 mm Hg.

Myocardial infarction
With *acute chest pain*, the main/first question is whether the pain is related to the heart. Always order a *chest radiograph, ECG,* and *troponin* at a minimum.

Use *pretest probability* to help you through the process. A 30-year-old patient with no risk factors for atherosclerosis who develops chest pain after eating a spicy meal does not have ischemic cardiac pain. By contrast, "chest pain" in a 65-year-old heavy smoker with high cholesterol, hypertension, diabetes, and a strong family history of heart disease is cardiac pain until you prove otherwise (even if his complaint is throat tightness!).

Look for key clues to suggest an MI:
1. ECG: After an MI, you should see flipped or flattened T waves, ST-segment elevation, and/or Q waves in a segmental distribution. The leads in which ST-segment elevation is seen help determine the location of the infarct (Table 3-9).

TABLE 3-9 Electrocardiogram after Myocardial Infarction (MI)

LOCATION	LEADS	ST-SEGMENT CHANGE
Anterior wall MI	V1 through V4	Elevation
Lateral wall MI	I, aVL, V5, and V6	Elevation
Inferior wall MI	II, III, and aVF	Elevation
Right ventricular wall MI	aVR	Elevation
Posterior wall MI	V8 and V9	Elevation
	V1 through V3	Depression

2. Pain characteristics: Pain is usually described as crushing, poorly localized substernal pain that may *radiate to the shoulder, arm,* or *jaw;* it is not reproducible on palpation. Pain usually does not resolve with nitroglycerin (as it often does with angina) and usually lasts at least 15–30 minutes.

3. Lab tests: Assays for troponin I or T are usually performed every 8 hours times 3 before MI is ruled out. CK (the MB isoenzyme) is now less commonly used but can also be positive. Chest radiograph may show cardiomegaly, pulmonary vascular congestion, and/or congestive heart failure; echocardiography may show ventricular wall motion abnormalities.

4. Physical exam: Bilateral pulmonary rales in the absence of other pneumonia-like symptoms, distended neck veins, S_3 or S_4, new murmurs, hypotension, and/or shock should make you think along the lines of an MI. Patients are classically *diaphoretic, tachycardic* (unless the conduction system has been damaged), and *pale;* nausea and vomiting may be present.

5. History: Patients with MI often have a history of angina or previous chest pain, murmurs, arrhythmias, and/or risk factors for CAD. They may also be taking heart medications (digoxin, furosemide, hypertension or cholesterol medications).

Treatment for MI: Treatment for an MI involves hospital admission to the intensive care or cardiac care unit with adherence to several basic principles:

1. Morphine (pain control and helps with pulmonary edema)
2. Oxygen (maintain O_2 saturation >90%)
3. Nitroglycerin (causes venodilation, decreased preload)
4. Aspirin
5. Clopidogrel if the patient is post–percutaneous coronary intervention (PCI) or has unstable angina or non–ST-elevation MI
6. β-Blocker (if no contraindication such as bradycardia or heart block; reduces oxygen demand and decreases mortality)
7. ACE inhibitor or ARB within 24 hours, even in patients with CHF
8. Unfractionated or low-molecular-weight heparin
9. Heparin should be started if unstable angina is diagnosed, if the patient has a cardiac thrombus, a larger area of dyskinetic ventricle, or if severe CHF is seen on echocardiogram
10. Lipid profile within 24 hours with initiation of statin therapy (goal LDL <70 units)
11. ECG monitoring—to monitor for arrhythmias such as ventricular fibrillation. If ventricular tachycardia develops, use amiodarone.
12. Reperfusion therapy with PCI or thrombolysis. Coronary artery bypass grafting (CABG) may be required if thrombolysis is contraindicated (or in combination with it). If PCI is planned, administer clopidogrel and unfractionated heparin before PCI.
13. Thrombolytic therapy (tissue plasminogen activator [tPA], tenecteplase) can be used up to 12 hours from pain onset, though early thrombolysis (less than 4–6 hours) is preferred to try to salvage myocardium. Contraindications to thrombolytic therapy include hemorrhagic stroke and serious bleeding. Hemoccult positive stool with no active bleeding is not a contraindication. Heparin therapy should also be given.

 Note *Remember that patients can experience reinfarction on the same hospital visit even with good medical management.*

Complications of MI:

1. Left ventricular dysfunction and heart failure: causes pulmonary edema. Treat with oxygen, diuretics, ACE inhibitor.
2. Ventricular rupture or pseudoaneurysm: occurs 2–7 days after MI. High mortality. Emergency cardiac surgery.
3. Mitral regurgitation: most common after inferoposterior MI. Listen for pansystolic murmur.
4. Right ventricular failure: seen with inferoposterior MI. Look for hypotension, jugular vein distention with clear lungs, and no dyspnea. Treat with IV fluids and inotropes such as dobutamine to increase preload and cardiac output.
5. Arrythmias: Ventricular tachycardia and ventricular fibrillation can cause sudden death. Treat with defibrillation, epinephrine, and amiodarone. For atrioventricular (AV) block and bradycardia, treat with atropine and pacing.
6. Thrombosis: Deep venous thrombosis (DVT) and pulmonary embolism (PE) are now relatively uncommon due to standard use of anticoagulants.
7. Pericarditis: generally after anterior infarction, occurs 1–4 days after MI. ECG shows ST-segment elevation in all leads. Treat with NSAIDs. Dressler syndrome is pericarditis 2–4 weeks after MI often with pleural and pericardial effusions. It is thought to be autoimmune and treated with NSAIDs.
8. Depression occurs in 20% of post-MI patients.

Other causes of chest pain and clues to diagnosis:

1. Reflux or peptic ulcer disease: related to certain foods (spicy, chocolate); smoking; caffeine; or lying down flat; relieved by antacids or acid-reducing medications. Patients with ulcers often test positive for *Helicobacter pylori*.
2. Stable angina: Pain begins with exertion or stress and remits with rest or calming down; pain is relieved by nitroglycerin. The ECG shows *ST-segment depression* with the pain and then reverts to normal when the pain stops. Pain lasts <20 minutes.
3. Chest wall pain (costochondritis, bruised or broken ribs): pain reproducible on palpation and localized.
4. Esophageal problems (achalasia, nutcracker esophagus, or esophageal spasm): difficult differential. The question will probably give you a negative workup for MI; look for barium swallow with *bird beak tapering* distally (achalasia) or esophageal manometry abnormalities. Treat achalasia with pneumatic dilatation or botulinum toxin injection; treat nutcracker/esophageal spasm with calcium channel blockers. Surgical myotomy can be used if other treatments are ineffective.
5. Pericarditis: Look for viral upper respiratory infection prodrome. The ECG shows *diffuse ST-segment elevation*. Other clues include elevated sedimentation rate and low-grade fever. The most common cause is viral (coxsackievirus); others include uremia, TB, malignancy, and lupus or other autoimmune diseases.
6. Pneumonia: Chest pain is due to pleuritis. Patients also have cough, fever, and/or sputum production. Look for possible sick contacts.
7. Aortic dissection: Do not forget the "other" cardiovascular emergency! Watch for severe pain *radiating to the back, hypertension,* difference in blood pressure between the arms, and widened mediastinum on chest radiograph. Get a CT scan with intravenous contrast to rule out or confirm this diagnosis. If the ascending aorta or proximal arch is involved in the dissection, prompt surgery is indicated (i.e., Stanford type A dissection).

Unstable angina is defined as a change in pattern of chest pain. Signs of unstable angina are chest pain at rest, a marked increase in the frequency of attacks, discomfort that occurs with minimal activity, and new-onset angina of increased severity. As in ST-segment elevation and non–ST-segment elevation MI, ECG changes may be seen, but cardiac biomarkers are typically negative. Treatment is similar to that for non–ST-segment elevation MI and includes oxygen, morphine, nitroglycerin, aspirin, β-blocker, clopidogrel, heparin (unfractionated or low molecular weight), and glycoprotein IIb/IIIa receptor inhibitor. An ACE inhibitor or ARB should be given as well. Consider emergent PCI if the pain does not resolve.

Variant (Prinzmetal) angina is rare and associated with anginal pain at rest with *ST-segment elevation* (cardiac enzymes, however, are normal). The cause is coronary artery spasm. Variant angina responds to nitroglycerin and is usually treated over the long term with *calcium channel blockers.*

Twenty-five percent of MIs are "silent." They manifest without chest pain (especially in *diabetics,* who have neuropathy). Patients present with heart failure, shock, or confusion and delirium (especially elderly patients).

Valvular heart disease

Murmur characteristics: see Table 3-10.

Table 3-10 Summary of Murmur Characteristics

VALVE PROBLEM	PHYSICAL CHARACTERISTICS (BEST HEARD HERE)	OTHER FINDINGS
Mitral stenosis	Late diastolic blowing murmur (at apex)	Opening snap, loud S1, atrial fibrillation, LAE, PH
Mitral regurgitation	Holosystolic murmur (radiates to axilla)	Soft S_1, LAE, PH, LVH
Aortic stenosis	Harsh systolic ejection murmur (aortic area, radiates to carotids)	Slow pulse upstroke, S_3/S_4, ejection click, LVD, cardiomegaly; syncope, angina, CHF
Aortic regurgitation	Early diastolic descrescendo murmur (apex)	Widened pulse pressure, LVH, LV dilation, S_3
Mitral prolapse	Mid-systolic click/late systolic murmur	Panic disorder

LAE, Left atrial enlargement; *PH,* pulmonary hypertension; *LVH,* left ventricular hypertrophy; *CHF,* congestive heart failure.

Endocarditis prophylaxis: Cardiac conditions for which antibiotic prophylaxis before dental procedures is recommended include:

○ Prosthetic cardiac valve
○ Previous infectious endocarditis
○ Congenital heart disease
○ Valvulopathy developing in cardiac transplant recipients

An antibiotic for prophylaxis should be administered in a single dose before the procedure. Amoxicillin is the preferred choice for oral therapy. Cephalexin, clindamycin, azithromycin, or clarithromycin may be used in patients with penicillin allergy. IV ampicillin, cefazolin, ceftriaxone, or clindamycin may be used for patients unable to take oral medication.

Congestive heart failure

Health maintenance: Most cases of congestive heart failure (CHF) are due to atherosclerosis and its effects on the adult heart. Aggressive management of risk factors for atherosclerosis is the key to prevention.

▭ **CASE SCENARIO:** In a 54-year-old man with sudden-onset signs and symptoms of CHF, what condition should you rule out first? An MI.

Symptoms and signs of CHF: see Table 3-11.

Table 3-11 Symptoms and Signs of Congestive Heart Failure

LEFT-SIDED FAILURE	RIGHT-SIDED FAILURE
Fatigue, dyspnea, cardiomegaly	Fatigue, dyspnea, cardiomegaly
Left-sided S_3/S_4	Right-sided S_3/S_4
Orthopnea	Peripheral edema
Paroxysmal nocturnal dyspnea	Jugular venous distention
Pulmonary congestion/rales	Hepatomegaly/ascites

Note: Patients will often have signs and symptoms of biventricular failure, particularly given that the most common cause of right-sided heart failure is left sided heart failure.

Patient management issues:

1. First make sure that the patient is stable (ABCs).
2. Check an ECG and cardiac enzymes to rule out MI or arrhythmia.
3. Check chest radiograph to look for pulmonary edema, cardiomegaly, or chronic obstructive pulmonary disease (which may cause right-sided failure/cor pulmonale).
4. Check brain natriuretic peptide (BNP) level to clinch the diagnosis in many cases. If the level is <100 pg/mL, heart failure is highly unlikely. If between 100 and 500, the results are uncertain but suspicious, and if >500, heart failure (or another acute and serious cardiovascular disorder) is highly likely. False positives for a CHF diagnosis using BNP levels include other diseases that cause right or left ventricular stretching, pulmonary embolism, pulmonary hypertension, cor pulmonale, renal failure, acute coronary syndrome, and cirrhosis.

5. Check a CBC to rule out anemia as a CHF cause or aggravating factor.
6. Check levels of thyroid-stimulating hormone (TSH) to rule out hyperthyroidism as a CHF cause or aggravating factor.
7. Echocardiography is used to estimate ejection fraction, check for valvular dysfunction, and rule out pericardial effusion or tamponade.

Treat patients with sodium restriction and an *ACE inhibitor* (first-line agent proven to reduce mortality in CHF); add a *β-blocker* once the patient is stable. Diuretics, usually *furosemide,* may help to reduce symptoms but have no effect on mortality rates.

❍ Digoxin and vasodilators (arterial and venous) are second-line agents.
❍ IV sympathomimetics (dobutamine, dopamine, amrinone) or nesiritide (recombinant brain-natriuretic peptide) plus furosemide and oxygen can be used for inpatients with severe CHF.

🗀 **CASE SCENARIO:** A 25-year-old man has an upper respiratory infection. Ten days later he develops chest pain and then CHF. What condition does he probably have? Myocarditis, usually from a virus (e.g., coxsackievirus). Treatment is supportive with NSAIDs for pain (and possibly corticosteroids to reduce inflammation).

Cor pulmonale: right ventricular enlargement, hypertrophy, or failure due to primary lung disease. Watch for tachypnea, *cyanosis, clubbing, parasternal heave,* loud P_2, and right-sided S_4 in addition to signs and symptoms of pulmonary disease. The most common cause is chronic obstructive pulmonary disease. Chronic sleep apnea can also cause cor pulmonale.

🗀 **CASE SCENARIO:** What conditions should you worry about if signs and symptoms of right-sided heart failure develop suddenly in a younger patient without a cardiac history or risk factors? Pulmonary embolus and cardiac tamponade.

🗀 **CASE SCENARIO:** A 28-year-old woman with gradually worsening dyspnea over a few months develops peripheral edema, clubbing, hypoxia, and a right-sided S_4. She takes no medications and has no risk factors for heart disease. CT pulmonary angiogram is negative for pulmonary embolism. What condition does she probably have? Primary pulmonary hypertension. Treat with pulmonary vasodilators such as prostacyclins (parenteral epoprostenol), antiendothelins (bosentan), and/or calcium channel blockers while awaiting heart-lung transplantation.

Dilated cardiomyopathy: classically due to *alcohol, myocarditis,* or *doxorubicin* because, by definition, ischemia is not considered a cardiomyopathy (although CAD/ischemia is the most common cause of a dilated, poorly functioning heart). The heart is enlarged, with thin, "flabby" walls. Diagnosis is made with echocardiography after excluding CAD as the etiology for dilated heart. Manage like regular CHF.

Restrictive cardiomyopathy usually results from amyloidosis, sarcoidosis, hemochromatosis, or myocardial fibroelastosis (ventricular biopsy is abnormal in all of these conditions). Constrictive pericarditis acts similarly clinically but has a pericardial knock on exam, calcification of the pericardium, and a normal ventricular biopsy and can be treated by removing the pericardium. CT or MRI of the heart can usually distinguish between restrictive cardiomyopathy and constrictive pericarditis, allowing treatment without the need for ventricular biopsy in patients with constrictive pericarditis.

Arrythmias
Atrial fibrillation and flutter:
❍ With atrial fibrillation, consider hyperthyroidism (check TSH) as the cause. Alcohol is another classic cause; tell the patient to stop drinking.
❍ If the patient is asymptomatic, no specific treatment is necessary acutely. Consider anticoagulation on the basis of CHADS2 score (Tables 3-12 and 3-13).

TABLE 3-12 CHADS2 Score

	CONDITION	POINTS
C	Congestive heart failure	1
H	Hypertension	1
A	Age 75 or older	1
D	Diabetes mellitus	1
S2	Prior stroke or transient ischemic attack	2

TABLE 3-13 Anticoagulation for Atrial Fibrillation Based on CHADS2 Score

SCORE	RISK	ANTICOAGULATION
0	Low	Aspirin
1	Moderate	Aspirin or warfarin
≥2	High	Warfarin

❍ If the patient is symptomatic but stable, slow the ventricular rate with medication such as verapamil, diltiazem, β-blocker, or digoxin.

❍ If the patient is symptomatic and unstable (i.e., decreased blood pressure, chest pain, hypoxia), use direct current cardioversion.

Be able to recognize the ECG abnormalities shown in Table 3-14 and know their treatments. Always check for ischemia and electrolyte disturbances as the cause.

TABLE 3-14 Arrhythmias

ARRHYTHMIA	TREATMENT AND WARNINGS
Heart block	
First-degree	No treatment, but avoid β-blockers and central calcium channel blockers (both slow conduction) (Fig. 3-5)
Second-degree	Use pacemaker or atropine only if symptomatic in Mobitz type 1. Pacing usually indicated for the more dangerous Mobitz type 2 (Figs. 3-6 and 3-7)
Third-degree	Pacemaker (Fig. 3-8)
WPW syndrome	Use procainamide or quinidine; avoid medications that affect the atrioventricular node such as digoxin, verapamil, adenosine, and metoprolol
V-Tach	If pulseless, treat with immediate defibrillation followed by epinephrine, vasopressin, amiodarone, lidocaine. If a pulse is present, treat with amiodarone or lidocaine and synchronized cardioversion (Fig. 3-9)
V-Fib	Immediate defibrillation
PVCs	Usually not treated; if severe and symptomatic, consider β-blocker or amiodarone
Sinus bradycardia	Usually not treated; use atropine if severe and symptomatic (post MI). Avoid β-blockers, calcium channel blockers, and other conduction slowers
Sinus tachycardia	Usually none; correct underlying cause; use β-blocker if symptomatic

PVCs, Premature ventricular contractions; *VFib,* ventricular fibrillation; *VTach,* ventricular tachycardia; *WPW,* Wolff-Parkinson-White syndrome.
Note: Sinus tachycardia and atrial fibrillation are common presentations for hyperthyroidism. Check TSH.

Deep venous thrombosis and pulmonary embolus

Virchow triad *(endothelial damage, stasis,* and *hypercoagulable state)* is a clue to the presence of DVT.

Common causes or situations in which DVT occurs: Surgery (especially orthopedic, pelvic, or abdominal), neoplasms, trauma, immobilization, pregnancy, birth control pills, lupus anticoagulant/

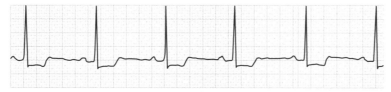

FIGURE 3-5 First-degree block (PR interval = 0.26 second). *(From Seelig CB: Simplified EKG Analysis. Philadelphia, Hanley & Belfus, 1992.)*

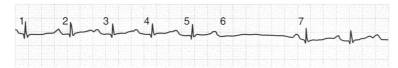

FIGURE 3-6 Mobitz type 1 second-degree atrioventricular block (Wenckebach). Note the gradual prolongation of the PR interval (1-5), the missing QRS complex after the sixth P wave, and the return of the PR interval to its shortest duration (7). *(From Seelig CB: Simplified EKG Analysis. Philadelphia, Hanley & Belfus, 1992.)*

antiphospholipid syndrome, prothrombin G20210A gene mutation, hyperhomocysteinemia, factor V Leyden, thrombin variant, and/or deficiency of antithrombin III, protein C, or protein S.

The classic symptoms are unilateral leg swelling, pain and tenderness, and/or *Homan sign* (present in 30% of patients and unreliable, but classic).

The best way to diagnose DVT is compression ultrasonography; CT venography is an option and allows simultaneous CT chest angiography, giving a whole body assessment for thromboembolic disease. Impedance plethysmography and invasive conventional venography are no longer used. A *negative D-dimer* test helps exclude DVT in patients with low pretest probability with a fairly high degree of accuracy, but a positive D-dimer test is less specific (does not necessarily indicate thrombosis).

Superficial thrombophlebitis (erythema, tenderness, edema, and a palpable clot in a superficial vein) is not a risk factor for pulmonary embolism and is generally considered a benign condition. Treat with NSAIDs or aspirin. Antibiotics may be used for outpatient treatment of mild cases (dicloxacillin or cephalexin) and for septic thrombophlebitis (IV nafcillin + genatmicin or cefotaxime)

If a patient has DVT, systemic anticoagulation is necessary. Use low-molecular-weight heparin (or regular heparin), followed by gradual crossover to oral warfarin. Patients are maintained on warfarin for at least 3–6 months and possibly permanently if they have more than one episode of clotting.

DVT prophylaxis for surgery: early ambulation postoperatively for low-risk patients. Low-molecular-weight heparin, low-dose unfractionated heparin, or fondaparinux is recommended for patients at moderate risk. High-risk patients should be given low-molecular-weight heparin, fondaparinux, or an oral vitamin K antagonist. Pneumatic compression stockings should be used instead if the patient is moderate risk or higher and is at high risk of bleeding.

Pulmonary embolus (PE) follows DVT, delivery (amniotic fluid embolus), or fractures (fat emboli). Symptoms include *tachypnea, dyspnea, chest pain, hemoptysis* (with lung infarct), and hypotension,

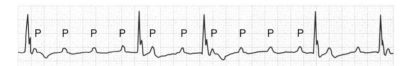

FIGURE 3-7 Mobitz type 2 second-degree atrioventricular block. Note that when beats are conducted, the PR interval is unvarying. *(From Seelig CB: Simplified EKG Analysis. Philadelphia, Hanley & Belfus, 1992.)*

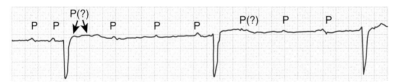

FIGURE 3-8 Third-degree atrioventricular block with a ventricular escape rhythm at 32 beats/minute. P-wave activity is somewhat irregular. *(From Seelig CB: Simplified EKG Analysis. Philadelphia, Hanley & Belfus, 1992.)*

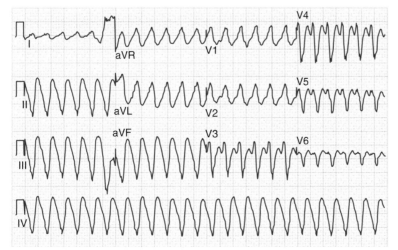

FIGURE 3-9 Electrocardiogram showing ventricular tachycardia. *(From Carabello BA, Gazes PC: Cardiology Pearls, 2nd ed. Philadelphia, Hanley & Belfus, 2000.)*

syncope, or death in severe cases. Rarely, on a chest radiograph you may see a wedge-shaped defect due to a pulmonary infarct.

Left-sided heart clots (from atrial fibrillation, ventricular wall aneurysm, severe CHF, or endocarditis) that embolize cause arterial-sided infarcts (stroke; renal, gastrointestinal [GI], or extremity infarcts), *not* PEs. Right-sided clots (DVTs) that embolize cause PEs, not arterial infarcts. The exception is a "paradoxical embolus" that occurs due to abnormal cardiovascular shunts such as a patent foramen ovale/atrial septal defect, which may allow a DVT to embolize and cause a systemic arterial infarct.

🔲 **CASE SCENARIO:** A 58-year-old woman with rate-controlled atrial fibrillation presents with sudden onset of a cold, swollen, painful right leg. What probably happened? An intracardiac thrombus embolized to the leg.

CT angiography is now considered the first-line test to evaluate for PE (or ventilation-perfusion nuclear scan if intravenous contrast is contraindicated) because it is safe and noninvasive. If the scan is positive, PE is diagnosed and treated. If the CT is of poor quality, or the ventilation-perfusion scan indeterminate, and there is a high clinical suspicion for PE, a conventional pulmonary angiogram can be performed for definitive diagnosis. If the scan is negative or indicates a low probability of PE, it is unlikely that the patient has a clinically significant PE and another diagnosis should be sought.

Treat PE with IV heparin or low-molecular-weight heparin to prevent further clots and emboli and then gradually switch to oral warfarin, which the patient should take for at least 3–6 months.

🔲 **CASE SCENARIO:** A woman has DVT with PE. She is put on heparin/warfarin and 1 month later develops a second DVT and PE. What should you do? Place an inferior vena cava (IVC) filter (e.g., Greenfield filter) to prevent further PE.

🔲 **CASE SCENARIO:** Four days after a patient is put on heparin, his platelet count is very low. What should you do? Stop the heparin, which can cause thrombocytopenia (heparin-induced thrombocytopenia) and even arterial thrombosis in some patients.

Heparin is followed by determination of the *partial thromboplastin time* (PTT) (internal pathway) and *warfarin* by determination of the *prothrombin time* (PT) (external pathway). In emergencies, reverse heparin with protamine; reverse warfarin with fresh frozen plasma and/or vitamin K; and reverse aspirin with platelet transfusion.

🔲 **CASE SCENARIO:** In a patient receiving enoxaparin, how often should you check the PTT? You should not. Low-molecular-weight heparin does not affect the PT, PTT, or bleeding time. Its effects are not monitored with lab values; in fact, one of the reasons for its popularity is that no monitoring is required. In rare cases when monitoring is necessary, an *anti-factor Xa* assay can be used to measure the effects.

Other conditions may affect coagulation tests: see Table 3-15.

TABLE 3-15 Conditions Affecting Coagulation Tests

DISEASE	PROLONGS THIS TEST	OTHER AIDS TO DIAGNOSIS
Hemophilia A	PTT	Low levels of factor 8; normal PT; X-linked
Hemophilia B	PTT	Low levels of factor 9; normal PT; X-linked
VWF disease	PTT	Normal or low levels of factor 8 depending on type; normal PT; autosomal dominant; low ristocetin cofactor or VWF antigen
Disseminated intravascular coagulation	PT, PTT	Positive D-dimer or FDPs; postpartum, infections, malignancy; schistocytes/fragmented cells of peripheral smear
Liver disease	PT	PTT normal or prolonged; vitamin K dependent factors are low—2, 7, 9, 10—but other factors 5, 8 are normal; stigmata of liver disease; no correction with vitamin K
Vitamin K deficiency	PT, PTT (slight)	Low levels of factors 2, 7, 9, and 10, proteins C and S; look for neonate (who did not receive prophylactic vitamin K), malabsorption, alcoholism, or prolonged use of antibiotics (which kill vitamin K–producing bowel flora)

FDPs, Fibrin degradation products; *PT,* prothrombin time; *PTT,* partial thromboplastin time; *VWF,* von Willebrand factor.

Uremia causes a qualitative platelet defect, and vitamin C deficiency or chronic corticosteroid therapy can cause a petechial-type bleeding tendency with normal coagulation tests.

DERMATOLOGY (See Table 3-16)

TABLE 3-16 Common Terms to Describe Skin Findings

PRIMARY LESION	DEFINITION	MORPHOLOGY	EXAMPLES
Macule	Flat, circumscribed skin discoloration that lacks surface elevation or depression	Macule	Café-au-lait, vitiligo, freckle, junctional nevus, ink tattoo
Papule	Elevated solid lesion <0.5 cm in diameter	Papule	Acrocordon (skin tag), basal cell carcinoma, molluscum contagiosum, intradermal nevi, lichen planus
Plaque	Elevated, solid "confluence of papules" (>0.5 cm in diameter) that lacks a deep component	Plaque	Bowens disease, mycosis fungoides, psoriasis, eczema, tinea corporis
Patch	Flat, circumscribed skin discoloration; a large macule >1 cm in diameter	Patch	Nevus flammeus, vitiligo
Nodule	Elevated, solid lesion >0.5 cm in diameter; a larger, deeper papule	Nodule	Rheumatoid nodule, tendon xanthoma, erythema nodosum, lipoma, metastatic carcinoma
Wheal	Firm, edematous plaque that is evanescent and pruritic; a hive	Wheal	Urticaria, dermographism, urticaria pigmentosa

Continued

TABLE 3-16 Common Terms to Describe Skin Findings—cont'd

PRIMARY LESION	DEFINITION	MORPHOLOGY	EXAMPLES
Vesicle	Papule that contains clear fluid; a blister	Vesicle	Herpes simplex, herpes zoster, dyshidrotic eczema, contact dermatitis
Bulla	Localized fluid collection >0.5 cm in diameter; a large vesicle	Bulla	Pemphigus vulgaris, bullous pemphigoid, bullous impetigo
Pustule	Papule that contains purulent material	Pustule	Folliculitis, impetigo, acne, pustular psoriasis
Cyst	Nodule that contains fluid or semisolid material	Cyst	Acne, epidermoid cyst, pilar cyst

General Dermatology

Vitiligo: Depigmentation of unknown etiology, but probably autoimmune (Fig. 3-10). Associated with other autoimmune conditions such as *pernicious anemia,* hypothyroidism, Addison disease, and diabetes. Patients often have antibodies to melanin, parietal cells, and/or the thyroid gland.

Pruritus: May be a clue to a diagnosis of *obstructive biliary disease* (classically primary biliary cirrhosis), *uremia, polycythemia rubra vera* (classically after a warm shower or bath), contact or *atopic dermatitis,* scabies, and lichen planus.

Contact dermatitis: Often due to a type 4 hypersensitivity reaction; also may be due to an irritating or toxic substance. Look for the question to mention new exposure to a classic offending agent (e.g., poison ivy, nickel earrings, deodorant) (Fig. 3-11). The rash is well circumscribed and found only in the area of exposure. The skin is *red and itchy* and often has *vesicles* and *bullae.* Avoidance of the agent is required. Patch testing can be done, if necessary, to determine the antigen.

Atopic dermatitis: Look for family and personal history of *allergies* (e.g., hay fever) or *asthma.* This is a chronic condition that begins in the first year of life with *red, itchy, weeping skin* on the head and upper extremities and sometimes around the diaper area. The major problem is pruritus and resultant scratching, which leads to skin breaks and possible bacterial infection. Treatment involves avoidance of hot water, drying soaps, hydration using creams and ointments, and the use of *antihistamines* and *topical corticosteroids.*

Seborrheic dermatitis: Causes the common conditions known as cradle cap and *dandruff,* as well as *blepharitis* (eyelid inflammation). Look for scaling skin on the scalp and eyelids. Treat with dandruff shampoo (i.e., selenium sulfide).

Acne: Know the medical description of acne: *comedones (whiteheads/blackheads), papules, pustules, inflamed nodules,* and *superficial pus-filled cysts* with possible inflammatory skin changes.

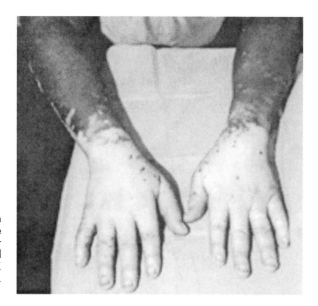

Figure 3-10 Vitiligo in an African-American man. Note the complete loss of pigmentation in the hands and wrists. Although usually not required for diagnosis, a biopsy of affected skin would reveal an absence of melanocytes. *(From Fitzpatrick JE, Aeling JL [eds]: Dermatology Secrets. Philadelphia, 1996, Hanley & Belfus, p. 122.)*

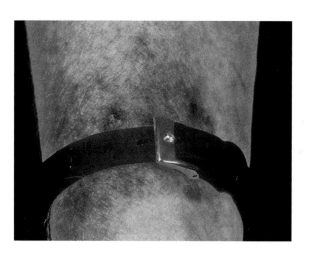

Figure 3-11 Allergic contact dermatitis from nickel. *(From Lim EKS, Loke YK, Thompson AM: Medicine and Surgery. Philadelphia, Churchill Livingstone, 2010.)*

Propionibacterium acnes is thought to be partially involved in the pathogenesis of acne, as is blockage of pilosebaceous glands. Acne has not been proved to be related to food, but if the patient makes such a relation, you can try discontinuance of the presumably offending food. Acne is not related to exercise, sex, or masturbation, but cosmetics may aggravate it. Treatment options are multiple. Start with *topical benzoyl peroxide;* then try *topical antibiotics or topical retinoids,* oral tetracycline, or oral erythromycin (for *Propionibacterium acnes* eradication). The last resort is *oral isotretinoin.* Isotretinoin is highly effective but *teratogenic* (pregnancy testing before and during therapy is mandatory) and can cause *dry skin and mucosae, muscle and joint pain,* and *abnormal liver function tests.*

Rosacea: Looks like acne but starts in middle age. Look for *rhinophyma* (bulbous red nose) and coexisting blepharitis. Treat with topical metronidazole or oral tetracycline. The pathogenesis is unknown, but it is not related to diet or caused by alcohol (though alcohol can aggravate it).

Hirsutism: Most commonly idiopathic, but look for other signs of *virilization* (deepening voice, clitoromegaly, frontal balding) to represent an androgen-secreting ovarian tumor. Other causes include *corticosteroid administration, Cushing syndrome, polycystic ovary disease,* and drugs (*minoxidil* and *phenytoin*).

Baldness: Watch for exotic causes of irregular, patchy baldness such as *trichotillomania,* a psychiatric disorder in which patients pull out their own hair, and *alopecia areata,* which is idiopathic and associated with antimicrosomal and other autoantibodies. Alopecia areata is also seen in patients with lupus or syphilis and after chemotherapy. Male-pattern baldness is benign and considered to be a genetic disorder that requires androgens to be expressed.

Psoriasis: Classic lesions are *dry, not pruritic, well-circumscribed, silvery, scaling papules, and plaques* found on the *extensor surfaces of the elbows and knees* or on the *scalp* (Fig. 3-12). The family history is often positive. Psoriasis occurs mostly in whites with onset in early adulthood. Patients may have *pitting of the nails* and an

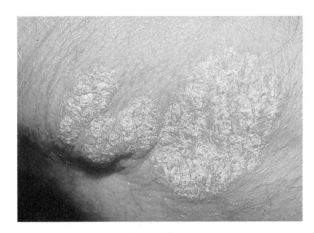

FIGURE 3-12 Psoriasis. Elbow involvement in psoriasis vulgaris, demonstrating typical well-demarcated, red plaques with silvery scale. *(From Fitzpatrick JE, Aeling JL: Dermatology Secrets. Philadelphia, Hanley & Belfus, 1998.)*

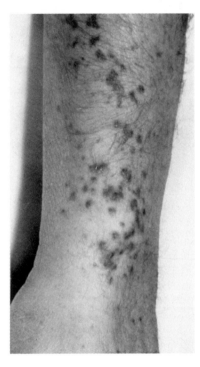

FIGURE 3-13 Drug reaction resulting in palpable purpura due to vasculitis. This type of rash is also classically seen in Henoch-Schonlein purpura, meningococcal meningitis/sepsis, and other autoimmune/vasculitis disorders. *(From Silver RM, Smith EA: Rheumatology Pearls. Philadelphia, Hanley & Belfus, 1997.)*

arthritis that resembles rheumatoid arthritis but is rheumatoid factor negative. Diagnosis is made by appearance, but biopsy can be used if there is doubt. Treatment is complex. For mild cases, recommend sunbathing and avoiding triggers. For more severe cases, use exposure to *ultraviolet light,* lubricants, topical corticosteroids, vitamin D analogues (calcipotriene), tar products, and keratolytics (salicylic acid, anthralin). Antibody therapy (e.g., etanercept, efalizumab) can be useful in patients with refractory disease.

Pityriasis rosea: Usually seen in older children and young adults; idiopathic. Look for a *"herald patch"* (scaly, slightly erythematous, ring-shaped or oval patch classically seen on the trunk), followed 1 week later by many similar lesions that tend to *itch.* Look for lesions on the back with a long axis that *parallels the Langerhans' skin cleavage lines,* typically in a *"Christmas tree"* pattern. The disease usually remits spontaneously in 1–3 months. Syphilis and tinea-type infections should be included in the differential diagnosis (biopsy/scrapings may be necessary if the diagnosis is in doubt). Treat with reassurance.

Lichen planus: Look for oral mucosal lesions *(patches of fine white lines and dots)* and the four Ps: **p**ruritic, **p**urple, **p**olygonal **p**apules, classically on the *wrists* and/or *ankles.* The condition is usually self-limiting and goes away within a few years and only symptomatic treatment (i.e., to relieve itching) is typically necessary.

Drug reactions and skin (Fig. 3-13): Penicillin, cephalosporins, and sulfa drugs commonly cause rashes; tetracyclines and phenothiazines commonly cause *photosensitivity.*

Erythema multiforme (Fig. 3-14): Look for classic *target* (also known as *iris*) lesions. This condition is usually caused by drugs or infections (e.g., herpes virus). The severe form, which may be fatal, is known as Stevens-Johnson syndrome (eye and oral mucosal involvement); treat supportively.

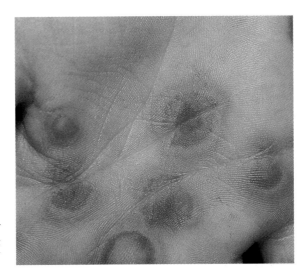

Figure 3-14 Erythema multiforme. Classic palmar involvement with target lesions. *(From Bolognia JL, Jorizzo JL, Rapini RP, et al: Dermatology, 2nd ed. Philadelphia, Mosby, 2008.)*

Erythema nodosum: Inflammation of the subcutaneous tissue and skin, classically over the shins (pretibial). Tender, red nodules are present. Look for exotic diseases such as *sarcoidosis, coccidioidomycosis*, and *ulcerative colitis* to be the cause, although more commonly the cause is unknown or a streptococcal infection.

Pemphigus vulgaris: An autoimmune disease of middle-aged and elderly people that manifests with *multiple bullae*, starting in the *oral mucosa* and spreading to the skin of the rest of the body, with subsequent sloughing of the blisters that leaves raw, denuded skin. Biopsy tissue can be stained for the desmoglein antibody and shows a *lacelike or fishnet immunofluorescence pattern* (versus a *linear pattern in bullous pemphigoid*, a similar but milder condition). Non-Hodgkin lymphoma or other malignancy can sometimes trigger this disorder. Treat with corticosteroids or rituximab. Death can occur from skin infection or fluid losses without successful treatment.

Dermatitis herpetiformis: Should alert you to the presence of *gluten-sensitivity* (i.e., *celiac disease*). Look for coexisting diarrhea and weight loss. The skin has *immunoglobulin A (IgA) deposits* even in unaffected areas. Patients present with intensely *pruritic vesicles, papules, and wheals on the extensor aspects of the elbows and knees* (sometimes on the face and neck). Treat with a gluten-free diet.

Decubitus ulcers (bedsore or pressure sore): Due to prolonged pressure against the skin. Cleanliness and dryness help to prevent this condition, and periodic skin inspection makes sure that you catch the problem early. When missed, the lesions can ulcerate down to the bone and become infected, possibly leading to sepsis and death. Treat major skin breaks with aggressive surgical debridement; use antibiotics if the patient has signs of infection.

▢ **CASE SCENARIO:** What is the best way to prevent bedsores? Periodic turning of paralyzed, bedridden, or debilitated patients (those at highest risk). Special air mattresses also change areas of pressure continuously and can help in prevention.

▢ **CASE SCENARIO:** What are the classic causes for new onset of excessive perspiration? Hyperthyroidism, pheochromocytoma, and hypoglycemia (the latter two usually have more intermittent perspiration symptoms).

Skin Infections

Fungal skin infections include dermatophyte infections, tinea versicolor, and candidiasis.

Dermatophyte infections include the following:

1. **Tinea corporis** (body and trunk): look for red, ring-shaped lesions that have raised borders and tend to clear centrally while they expand peripherally.
2. **Tinea pedis** (athlete's foot): look for macerated, scaling web spaces between the toes that often itch, as well as associated thickened, distorted toenails (onychomycosis). Good foot hygiene is part of the treatment.
3. **Tinea unguium** (nails; also known as *onychomycosis*): thickened, distorted nails with debris under the nail edges.
4. **Tinea capitis** (scalp): mainly affects children (highly contagious), who have scaly patches of hair loss. Those affected may have an inflamed, boggy granuloma of the scalp known as a *kerion* (previous

board exams have shown a picture of this finding), which usually resolves with antifungal treatment (griseofulvin) and is not a tumor/malignancy.

5. **Tinea cruris** (jock itch): more common in obese males; usually seen in the crural folds of the upper, inner thighs.

Most of these fungal skin infections are due to *Trichophyton* spp.

○ Diagnosis of any of these infections can be confirmed by scraping the lesion and using a potassium hydroxide (KOH) preparation to visualize the fungus or by doing a culture.

○ Oral agents (e.g., *terbinafine, fluconazole*) must be used to treat tinea capitis and onychomycosis; the others can be treated with topical antifungals (imidazoles such as miconazole, clotrimazole, keto-conazole) or oral agents for resistant/more severe disease.

○ In tinea capitis, if the hair *fluoresces under the Wood's lamp, Microsporum* spp. is the causative agent; if the hair does not fluoresce, the probable causative agent is *Trichophyton* spp.

Candidiasis: Thrush (creamy white patches on the tongue or buccal mucosa that can be scraped off) may be seen in normal children, and candidal vulvovaginitis is seen in normal women, especially during pregnancy or after taking antibiotics. However, at other times and in different patients, candidal infections may be a sign of *diabetes* or *immunodeficiency.* For example, thrush in an adult man should raise the possibility of *HIV/acquired immunodeficiency syndrome (AIDS).* Treat with local/topical nystatin or imidazole (e.g., miconazole, clotrimazole) for uncomplicated cases and oral fluconazole or itracon-azole if recurrent or the patient is HIV-positive.

Tinea versicolor: Caused by a fungal infection of the genus Malassezia, formerly known as Pityros-porum, which presents most commonly in young adults with *multiple patches of various size and color (brown, tan, and white) on the torso.* Often the lesions become noticeable in the summer because the affected areas fail to tan and thus look white. Diagnose from lesion scrapings (KOH preparation). Treat with oral or topical imidazoles or use selenium sulfide shampoo.

Scabies: Caused by the mite *Sarcoptes scabei,* which tunnels into the skin and leaves *visible "burrows"* on the skin, classically in the *finger web spaces* and *flexor surface of the wrists.* Watch for severe pruritus and itching, which can lead to secondary bacterial infection. Diagnosis is made by scraping the mite out of a burrow and seeing it under a microscope. Treat with topical permethrin cream. Remember to treat all contacts (e.g., the whole family, nursing care residents).

📁 **CASE SCENARIO:** What is the preferred treatment for scabies? *Permethrin* cream applied to the whole body. Do not use lindane unless permethrin is not a choice. Lindane used to be the treatment of choice but can cause neurotoxicity, especially in young children.

Lice (pediculosis): Lice can infect the head (*Pediculus capitis*; common in school children), body (*Pediculus corporis*; unusual in people with good hygiene), or pubic area (*Phthirus pubis,* also known as "crabs" and transmitted sexually). Infected areas tend to itch, and diagnosis is made by *seeing the lice on hair shafts.* Treat with *permethrin* cream (preferred over lindane due to lindane's neurotoxicity) and decontaminate sources of reinfection (wash and sterilize combs, hats, bed sheets, and clothing).

Warts: Caused by *HPV.* Warts are infectious and most commonly seen in older children, often on the hands. There are multiple treatment options that include salicylic acid, liquid nitrogen, and curet-tage. Genital warts are also caused by HPV, and HPV plays a causative role in cervical, vulvar, vagi-nal, penile, anal, and oral cancers.

Molluscum contagiosum: A *poxvirus* infection that is common in children but also may be trans-mitted sexually. A child who has genital molluscum may or may not have contracted the disease from sexual contact; autoinnoculation is possible. Do not automatically assume child abuse, although it must be ruled out. The diagnosis is made by the characteristic appearance of the lesions (*skin-colored, smooth, waxy papules with a central depression* [umbilicated] that are roughly 0.5 cm) or by looking at the con-tents of the lesion, which include cells with characteristic *inclusion bodies.* Molluscum contagiosum is usually treated with freezing or curettage and is self-limited.

Skin growths and cancers

Moles: Common and benign, but malignant transformation is possible. Excise any mole (or do a biopsy if the lesion is large) if it *enlarges suddenly, develops irregular borders, darkens or becomes inflamed, changes color* (even if only one small area of the mole changes color), *begins to bleed, begins to itch,* or *becomes painful.* Dysplastic nevus syndrome is a genetic condition (watch for family history) with mul-tiple dysplastic-appearing nevi (usually >100). Treat with careful follow-up and excision/biopsy of any suspicious-looking lesions, as well as sun avoidance and sunscreen use.

Keratoacanthoma: Considered a benign variant of squamous cell carcinoma. Look for a flesh-colored lesion with a central crater that contains keratinous material, classically on the face. The lesion involutes spontaneously in a few months and requires no treatment. Kertoacanthoma is often difficult to differentiate from squamous cell carcinoma, so if you are unsure, the best step is a biopsy and treatment as for a squamous cell carcinoma.

Keloid: An overgrowth of scar tissue after an injury, most frequently seen in *Blacks*. The lesion is usually slightly pink and classically found on the upper back, chest, and deltoid area. Also look for keloids to develop after ear piercing. Surgery alone is associated with recurrence. Surgery with intralesional steroids is the preferred treatment.

Basal cell carcinoma: The most common of all skin neoplasms. Begins as a shiny papule and slowly enlarges and develops an *umbilicated center*, which later may *ulcerate*, with *peripheral telangiectasias* (Fig. 3-15). Almost never metastasizes. As with all skin cancer, *sunlight exposure* increases the risk and it is more common in light-skinned people. Found on exposed areas, classically the (lower) eyelid, nose. Treat with excision. Biopsy any suspicious skin lesion in elderly patients.

Squamous cell cancer: Look for preexisting *actinic keratoses* (hard, sharp, red, often scaly lesions in sun-exposed areas) or burn scars that become nodular, warty, or ulcerated. Do a biopsy if this happens. Squamous cell cancer in situ is known as *Bowen disease*. Treatment is excision, which is usually curative. Radiation used for cases with difficult surgical planes, locally advanced disease, and/or recurrence. Metastases are uncommon but can occur.

Malignant melanoma: *Superficial spreading melanoma* (Fig. 3-16), which tends to stay superficial, has the best prognosis, whereas *nodular melanoma* has the worst prognosis because it tends to grow downward (i.e., vertical spread) first. Although uncommon in Blacks, melanoma tends to be of the *acrolentiginous* type; look for black dots on the *palms* or *soles* or *under the fingernail* (i.e., subungual). Treat with surgery. If melanoma is <2 mm thickness, excise with 2-cm margins; if ≥2 mm in thickness, excise with 3-cm margins. Adjunctive therapies for locally advanced or metastatic disease include interferon alfa-2b, temozolomide, dacarbazine, and interleukin-2.

▭ **CASE SCENARIO:** What characteristic of the primary lesion is most closely related to prognosis in melanoma? The depth of vertical invasion.

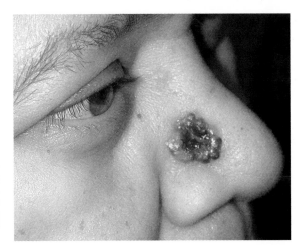

FIGURE 3-15 Basal cell carcinoma, the most common skin cancer of the face. There is a pearly papule or nodule with raised edges and central ulceration. Typically, the lesion is painless but bleeds, forms a scab, and fails to heal. *(From Bolognia JL, Jorizzo JL, Rapini RP, et al: Dermatology, 2nd ed. Philadelphia, Mosby, 2008.)*

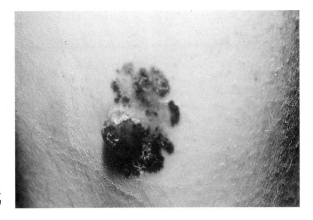

FIGURE 3-16 Superficial spreading malignant melanoma that has developed a nodular melanoma. *(From Fitzpatrick JE, Aeling JL: Dermatology Secrets. Philadelphia, Hanley & Belfus, 1996.)*

Kaposi sarcoma: Classically seen in patients with AIDS. Look for classic mucosal lesions (e.g., inside the mouth) or an expanding, strange rash or skin lesion that does not respond to multiple treatments. Excision is often adequate treatment for single lesions; use chemotherapy for more advanced lesions.

Paget disease of the nipple: Watch out for a *unilateral red, oozing/crusting nipple* in an adult woman. You must rule out an underlying breast carcinoma with extension to the skin. Excision of the nipple with radiation is indicated if no underlying carcinoma is found, and conservation breast treatment or mastectomy is indicated if underlying carcinoma is present.

🗂 **CASE SCENARIO:** What is the classic nutritional cause of stomatitis? Deficiencies of B complex vitamins (riboflavin, niacin, pyridoxine). Vitamin C deficiency may also cause stomatitis.

ENDOCRINOLOGY

Diabetes mellitus

Screening: Universal screening is generally not recommended. Screening is recommended in patients who are overweight, are older than 45 years, are members of certain subgroups (Black, Native American, Hispanics) or have diabetes risk factors such as family history in a first-degree relative, habitual inactivity, gestational diabetes, hypertension, or dyslipidemia is more accepted, but not uniformly.

Diagnosis: the diagnosis is made when:
○ fasting plasma glucose is ≥126 mg/dL (after an 8-hour fast)
○ random glucose is ≥200 mg/dL with symptoms of hyperglycemia
○ Hemoglobin A_{1c} ≥6.5%
○ 75 g oral glucose tolerance test ≥200 mg/dL at 2 hours (glucose tolerance test is commonly used in pregnancy but otherwise is rarely used for the diagnosis of diabetes)

If the patient has classic symptoms, one measurement is enough to confirm a diagnosis, but in an asymptomatic patient, repeat the test.

Classic differences between type 1 and type 2 diabetes mellitus (though overlap exists): see Table 3-17

TABLE 3-17 Type 1 versus Type 2 Diabetes Mellitus

FEATURE	TYPE 1	TYPE 2
Age at onset	Most commonly <30 yr	Most commonly >30 yr*
Associated body habitus	Thin	Obese
Develop ketoacidosis	Yes	No
Develop hyperosmolar state	No	Yes
Level of endogenous insulin	Low to none	Low to high (insulin resistance)
Twin concurrence	<50%	>50%
HLA association	Yes	No
Response to oral hypoglycemics	No	Yes
Antibodies to insulin	Yes (at diagnosis)	No
Risk of diabetic complications	Yes	Yes
Islet cell pathology	Insulitis	Normal number, but with amyloid deposits

*Be aware, however, of the "epidemic" of type 2 diabetes in those younger than 30 years including children and adolescents, which is due in part to the obesity epidemic.
HLA, Human leukocyte antigen.

Patient management issues: Classic symptoms of diabetes mellitus (DM) are *polydipsia, polyuria, polyphagia,* and unexplained *weight loss.* Patients also may have a classic infection such as *candidiasis* and sometimes complain of near-sightedness or report improved vision if far-sightedness is due to osmotic lens swelling (goes away with treatment).

Routine health maintenance issues in diabetic patients:
1. Measure *urine microalbumin* and creatinine level annually to monitor for early renal disease. Consider ACE inhibitor in all diabetics to delay nephropathy.
2. Schedule annual visit to ophthalmologist to monitor for diabetic retinopathy and vision problems (ophthalmologist may space visits out if normal exam). Start exams immediately after diagnosis of type 2 diabetes, or 5 years after the diagnosis of type 1 diabetes.
3. Do a formal foot exam and assess for *neuropathy* with monofilament and/or tuning fork roughly every 12 months. Patients with neuropathy should wash and inspect their own feet daily; wear comfortable, properly fitting shoes; and undergo a clinical foot exam every 6 months.

4. Patients should self-monitor their blood glucose levels on a daily basis, preferably three times per day if on insulin and at least once per day if on oral medications only. Follow compliance with a *hemoglobin A1c level* quarterly initially and twice per year in stable compliant patients who are meeting therapy goals. The goal is generally a level <7. This parameter is an accurate measure of overall control for the previous 3 months. To get a crude estimate of average glucose level, multiply the hemoglobin A_{1c} level by 20.
5. Screen for and treat coexisting modifiable risk factors for atherosclerosis (e.g., HTN, lipid profile) yearly.
6. Screen for thyroid dysfunction (TSH), vitamin B_{12} deficiency, and celiac disease in type 1 diabetes due to increased frequency of coexisting autoimmune diseases.

General management issues: The goal of treatment is to keep postprandial glucose <180 units, fasting glucose <130 units, and hemoglobin A_{1C} <7% in most patients. The goal hemoglobin A_{1C} may be stricter in those with CAD, significant CAD risk factors, or long-standing diabetes. Principles of management include the following:
○ Diet: limit calories, salt intake, and alcohol intake
○ Exercise: increases glucose uptake by increasing the number of cell receptors
○ Education regarding diabetes self-management
○ Monitoring of complications—nephropathy, retinopathy, neuropathy
○ Medications: insulin in type 1, oral medications and/or insulin in type 2

For the "typical" type 2 diabetes mellitus patient, remember that the cheapest and most effective treatment is a combination of dietary changes, exercise, and weight loss. In the real world, however, this does not often work, so use oral medications.

Oral medications for diabetes mellitus:
○ **Biguanides** (e.g., metformin): Decrease hepatic glucose output. Do not cause hypoglycemia when used for monotherapy, therefore often used as first-line therapy. Useful in patients with dyslipidemia because they reduce LDL and triglycerides. Contraindicated in patients with severe renal and liver disease due to risk of lactic acidosis.
○ **Sulfonylureas** (e.g., glyburide, glipizide): Increase postprandial insulin secretion from the pancreas, therefore work best before meals. May cause hypoglycemia. Contraindicated in patients allergic to sulfa.
○ **α-Glucosidase inhibitors** (e.g., acarbose): Inhibit intestinal glucosidase and pancreatic amylase reducing GI absorption of glucose. Useful in patients with postprandial hyperglycemia, therefore work best when taken with meal. Not often used because of side effects of diarrhea, flatulence, abdominal cramps.
○ **Thiazolidinediones** (e.g., pioglitazone, rosiglitazone): Reduce peripheral insulin resistance. Now falling out of favor due to potential cardiac effects. Used as a second agent in combination with another agent. Useful in patients with dyslipidemia. Contraindicated in patients with liver disease. Some studies show possible increase rates of MI, heart failure, and bladder cancer.
○ **Dipeptidyl peptidase-4 inhibitors** (e.g., sitagliptin, saxagliptin): DPP-4 inhibitors potentiate insulin synthesis and release, as well as decrease glucagon production. Used as second agent.
○ **Incretin mimetic** (e.g., exenatide): stimulates pancreatic beta cells to secrete insulin, therefore taken before meals. Useful as second agent. Contraindicated in patients with type 1 DM and renal failure.
○ **Amylin analogues** (e.g., pramlintide): Hormones secreted by beta cells of the pancreas that aid glucose absorption by slowing gastric emptying, promote satiety, and inhibit inappropriate secretion of glucagon. Used as an adjunctive treatment for patients who inject insulin at mealtimes.

Insulin therapy: Know how to use different preparations of insulin, especially lispro, regular, and neutral protamine Hagedorn (NPH) insulin (Table 3-18). Type 1 diabetics generally require 0.5–1 unit/kg of body weight per day of insulin, though initial requirements are often less due to a small amount of residual endogenous insulin production. For those with type 2 diabetes, save insulin for inpatients and those who fail oral preparations. Requirements may be greater than 1 unit/kg/day due to resistance.

TABLE 3-18 Insulin Preparations and Use

INSULIN PREPARATION	ONSET (hr)	PEAK (hr)	DURATION (hr)	WHEN TO USE
Ultra Rapid Acting				
Insulin aspart	<0.25	1-3	3-5	Right before meals
Insulin lispro	0.25-0.5	0.5-2.5	3-5	Right before meals

Continued

TABLE 3-18 Insulin Preparations and Use—cont'd

INSULIN PREPARATION	ONSET (hr)	PEAK (hr)	DURATION (hr)	WHEN TO USE
Rapid Acting				
Regular insulin	0.5-1	2-4	5-8	Inpatients (can be given IV), 0.5-1 hr before a meal for outpatients
Intermediate to Long Acting				
NPH insulin	1-2	4-12	12-24	Generally part of standard regimens that mix with shorter-acting insulin (e.g., 70/30 or 50/50 of NPH/regular)
Ultra Long Acting				
Insulin glargine	1.5-4	None	24+	Provide basal insulin level; supplement with short-acting insulin
Insulin detemir	3-4	3-9	Dose dependent; 6-23 hours	Provides basal insulin level

IV, Intravenous; *NPH,* neutral protamine Hagedorn.

📁 **CASE SCENARIO:** How should doses of lispro/aspart, regular, or neutral protamine Hagedorn (NPH) insulin be adjusted in the following cases?
1. Patient has high (low) 7 AM glucose? Increase (decrease) NPH insulin at dinner the night before.
2. Patient has high (low) noon glucose? Increase (decrease) morning dose of regular or increase (decrease) before-breakfast lispro or aspart insulin.
3. Patient has high (low) 5 PM glucose? Increase (decrease) morning dose of NPH or increase (decrease) before-lunch dose of aspart or lispro insulin.
4. Patient has high (low) 9 PM glucose? Increase (decrease) dinner-time dose of regular insulin or increase (decrease) before-dinner dose of aspart or lispro insulin.

📁 **CASE SCENARIO:** Somogyi effect versus dawn phenomenon. How do you treat a 52-year-old man with 7 AM glucose of 220? Measure the 3 AM glucose. If it is 40, the patient has the Somogyi effect due to hypoglycemia. You should decrease the PM dose of NPH. If the 3 AM glucose is 160, the patient has the dawn phenomenon due to normal morning surge of growth hormone and cortisol. You should increase the PM dose of NPH.

📁 **CASE SCENARIO:** What is the best insulin regimen on the day of elective surgery? Because patients do not eat before surgery, give one-third to one-half of the normal insulin dose. The glucose should be monitored throughout surgery and postoperatively; typically, 5% dextrose in water (D5W) and IV regular insulin are used to maintain glucose control.

📁 **CASE SCENARIO:** A 47-year-old diabetic woman takes metoprolol for prior heart attack and hypertension. She keeps passing out without warning. What should you do? Have the patient check the glucose level after the next attack. If it is low, decrease the amount of diabetes medications. Do not stop the β-blocker if you can avoid doing so because it has been shown to prolong survival after an infarct. Counsel the patient that a β-blocker can eliminate the warning signs of hypoglycemia.

📁 **CASE SCENARIO:** A 59-year-old diabetic man taking metformin gets a CT scan with contrast and subsequently develops lactic acidosis. How could this complication have been prevented? Stop metformin in high-risk patients for 48 hours before the contrast is given and restart it 48 hours later if creatinine level is stable. Also, consider aggressive intravenous hydration and acetylcysteine before and after giving IV contrast in patients with diabetes and/or renal disease (recommendations vary).

Stricter control may result in too many episodes of hypoglycemia.

📁 **CASE SCENARIO:** A 42-year-old woman who takes three insulin injections daily and is compliant complains of episodes of sweating and palpitations with confusion. What is the cause? Episodes of hypoglycemia from overaggressive glucose control.

📁 **CASE SCENARIO:** A 31-year-old male nurse who is histrionic has episodes of severe hypoglycemia. What lab value should you measure? *C-peptide level.* If the C-peptide level is low immediately after an episode, the patient has factitious disorder and is secretly taking insulin. If C-peptide is high, the patient has an insulinoma.

Acute complications of DM:

○ **Diabetic ketoacidosis:** primarily seen in type 1 diabetics. Patients have hyperglycemia, hyperketonemia with ketonuria, and metabolic acidosis. Give fluids and IV regular insulin, closely monitor electrolytes and glucose level, and give potassium and phosphorus replacement. Do not give bicarbonate unless the pH is <6.9 because it can worsen hypokalemia. Remember to search for the cause, which is often infection or noncompliance. Can be fatal.

○ **Nonketotic hyperglycemic hyperosmolar state:** seen in type 2 diabetics. Patients have *hyperglycemia* and *hyperosmolarity* without ketonemia. Treatment involves aggressive IV fluids, IV insulin, and electrolyte replacement. Can be fatal.

Long-term complications of DM:

1. **Atherosclerosis** including CAD and peripheral vascular disease with their associated risks and complications.
2. **Retinopathy:** DM is one of the leading causes of acquired blindness. Retinal findings include microaneurysms, hemorrhages, cotton wool spots, and macular edema.
3. **Nephropathy:** Use ACE inhibitors to help prevent renal complications. DM causes 30% of end-stage renal disease.
4. **Neuropathy:** The classic example is sensory neuropathy leading to numb feet, infection, *gangrene,* and/or *Charcot joints.* In addition, diabetics can have "silent" heart attacks (i.e., no chest pain) due to sensory loss. Autonomic peripheral neuropathy can lead to *gastroparesis* (early satiety and nausea), constipation and/or diarrhea, resting tachycardia, orthostatic hypotension, and *impotence.* Gastroparesis can be diagnosed with a nuclear medicine gastric emptying study and treated with dietary modifications (e.g., smaller more frequent meals) and *metoclopramide* for severe cases.
5. **Increased risk of infections:** Hyperglycemia interferes with neutrophil function. Vascular disease and neuropathy contribute to infection and delayed patient detection.

▭ **CASE SCENARIO:** What is the treatment for proliferative diabetic retinopathy? Panretinal laser photocoagulation helps to prevent progression to blindness. The laser is used to make multiple burns in the peripheral retina.

Hypothyroidism

Classic symptoms: fatigue, bradycardia, depression, menstrual disturbances (usually menorrhagia), slow speech, cold intolerance, constipation, carpal tunnel syndrome, decreased reflexes, anemia of chronic disease, and/or coarse hair. Hypothyroidism may cause hypercholesterolemia, which resolves with treatment. Check thyroid function labs (TSH, free thyroxine [T_4]). Usually TSH is high and free T_4 is low (i.e., primary gland disturbance). TSH may be normal in secondary or tertiary hypothyroidism or concurrent use of dopamine or corticosteroids. Treat with *thyroxine* (T_4). Doses can be changed every 6–8 weeks. Pregnant women may need higher doses.

Causes of hypothyroidism:

1. **Hashimoto thyroiditis:** most common cause of hypothyroidism in the United States; autoimmune disease. Remember the association with other autoimmune diseases (e.g., pernicious anemia, vitiligo, lupus). Look for positive *antimicrosomal antibodies.* Histology shows lymphocyte infiltration of the gland.
2. **Subacute thyroiditis:** acute viral inflammation with fever and an enlarged, *tender* thyroid gland. A history of upper respiratory infection is common. Give NSAIDs for symptom relief. Patients often recover without treatment.
3. **Hypothyroidism due to treatment of hyperthyroidism** (iodine-131 for Graves disease): second most common cause of hypothyroidism in the United States.
4. **Sick euthyroid syndrome:** can be caused by any illness. Treatment is necessary only for the underlying disorder because the condition is self-limiting.
5. **"Central" cause** (i.e., pituitary or hypothalamic cause—thyroid gland is normal and not the problem): TSH will be low along with T_4. This is a rare/exotic cause of hypothyroidism. Think tumor (e.g., pituitary macroadenoma) or Sheehan syndrome. Order an MRI of the brain and pituitary gland.

▭ **CASE SCENARIO:** A 52-year-old man is hospitalized for 2 weeks with pneumonia. He feels tired 2 days after leaving the hospital. Triiodothyronine (T_3) and T_4 levels are slightly low. What lab value will confirm sick euthyroid syndrome? TSH, which should be near normal.

▭ **CASE SCENARIO:** A 29-year-old woman has a goiter. Is she hyperthyroid or hypothyroid? You cannot know until you have a more detailed history and check the lab tests. She may be hypothyroid, hyperthyroid, or euthyroid. A goiter simply means the thyroid gland is enlarged and can be due to many different conditions (Fig. 3-17). Significant thyroid enlargement can cause dysphagia or respiratory symptoms due to local mass effect.

Hyperthyroidism

Classic symptoms: Nervousness, anxiety, insomnia, tachycardia, palpitations, *atrial fibrillation*, heat intolerance, weight loss, diarrhea, menstrual irregularities (hypomenorrhea), increased appetite and proptosis or "thyroid stare." Usually TSH is low and T_4 is high (i.e., primary gland disturbance).

    Causes of hyperthyroidism:

1. **Graves disease** (Fig. 3-18): By far the most common cause. *Exophthalmos* and *pretibial myxedema* are common. Patients have positive *thyroid-stimulating immunoglobulins* and *antibodies*, which activate the TSH receptor. They also have a nontender, diffuse goiter. The whole gland takes up excessive radioactive iodine (RAI) on a thyroid nuclear scan.
2. Plummer disease/toxic multinodular goiter: Hyperfunctioning nodules cause a lumpy goiter without positive antibodies or exophthalmos/pretibial myxedema. RAI uptake is high in nodules but decreased in the rest of the gland.

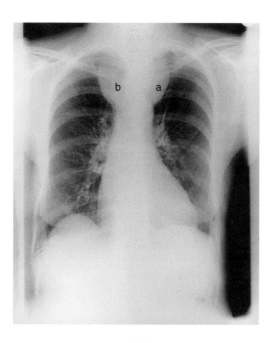

FIGURE 3-17 Large substernal goiter *(a)* deviating the trachea *(b)* to the patient's right. Ectopic thyroid that arises in the mediastinum does not cause this deviation. *(From James EC, Corry RJ, Perry JF: Principles of Basic Surgical Practice. Philadelphia, Hanley & Belfus, 1987.)*

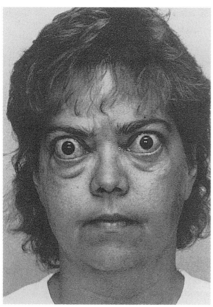

FIGURE 3-18 Graves disease: Note the thyroid stare, asymmetry, proptosis, and periorbital edema. *(From Ferri FF: Ferri's Clinical Advisor 2012. Philadelphia, Mosby, 2012.)*

3. Toxic adenoma: One nodule is palpable and has high RAI uptake; the rest of the gland has decreased uptake (thyroid cancer is almost never hyperfunctional).
4. Thyroiditis: Hashimoto or subacute thyroiditis may have a transient hyperthyroidism from inflammation before converting to hypothyroidism.
5. "Central" cause (i.e., pituitary or hypothalamus dysfunction—the thyroid gland is normal and is not the problem): Quite rare. TSH will be high along with T_4. Order an MRI of the brain and pituitary gland (probably a hyperfunctional TSH-secreting pituitary adenoma).

Treatment of hyperthyroidism: You can start with antithyroid drugs (*propylthiouracil* or *methimazole*), but these do not fix the underlying problem. Use propylthiouracil in pregnant patients due to the risk of fetal anomalies with methimazole. For patients older than 21 whose hyperthyroidism not controlled with meds for 1 year, radioactive iodine is usually the treatment of choice. Do not use in pregnant and lactating patients. Surgery is considered for young patients and pregnant women (i.e., avoid radiation to fetus) but is not used often. Propranolol (or another β-blocker) is used for *thyroid storm* (when patients decompensate, physically and mentally, from high thyroid hormone levels) and symptomatic tachycardia, palpitations, or arrhythmias.

🗀 **CASE SCENARIO:** A 29-year-old woman feels anxious about her pregnancy. Total T_4 is high, but other thyroid tests are normal. What type of hyperthyroidism does she probably have? None. Pregnancy and other factors (birth control pills, estrogens, infections) can cause elevation of thyroid-binding globulin, which causes elevation of total thyroid hormone levels. However, free (active) thyroid levels are not elevated and the TSH is normal. The free (unbound) T_4 can be checked to confirm, but no treatment is warranted!

Hypoadrenalism

Primary hypoadrenalism (also known as *Addison disease* or primary adrenal insufficiency) is usually autoimmune in nature or due to TB. Look for *increased skin pigmentation,* weight loss, dehydration, anorexia, nausea and vomiting, dizziness and syncope, hyponatremia, and hyperkalemia. Diagnosis is with rapid adrenocorticotropic hormone (ACTH) test (give IV ACTH; measure cortisol at 1, 30, and 60 min). Treat with dexamethasone, hydrocortisone, and/or fludrocortisone for mineralocortocoid replacement. Under metabolic stress (e.g., infection, surgery), patients may have an adrenal crisis characterized by abdominal pain, hypotension or cardiovascular collapse, renal shutdown, and death. Give hydrocortisone and IV fluids to avoid this complication.

The diagnosis of hypoadrenalism can be made by administering ACTH and determining whether there is an appropriate increase in plasma cortisol over baseline. Do not delay giving steroids to do this test if the patient is crashing—he or she may die while you are waiting for the results.

Secondary adrenal insufficiency is more common (and more commonly tested). ACTH levels are low compared with primary adrenal insufficiency, and no hyperpigmentation is seen. It is due most often to previous administration of steroids. Once patients take steroids for more than a few weeks, they may not be able to mount an appropriate increase in ACTH during stress for *up to 1 year!* The classic example is a surgery patient with a history of severe asthma (implied use of steroids) who develops hypotension and electrolyte disturbances after surgery. Give corticosteroids. Other secondary causes of adrenal insufficiency are *Sheehan syndrome* (i.e., pituitary infarction, history of postpartum hypotension, inability to breast-feed, and other endocrine insufficiencies typically present) and neoplasms (e.g., pituitary tumor).

In secondary hypoadrenalism, mineralocorticoid (aldosterone) secretion is not affected because it is not directly under pituitary control. Thus electrolyte disturbances are not as severe.

🗀 **CASE SCENARIO:** What physical finding may help to differentiate between primary and secondary hypoadrenalism? Skin hyperpigmentation, which is seen only in primary cases. This symptom is thought to be due to excessive melanocyte-stimulating hormone, which is secreted with ACTH. In secondary cases, ACTH is decreased.

Hyperadrenalism

Hyperadrenalism (Cushing syndrome) is usually due to administration of steroids (Fig. 3-19) but may also be due to adrenal neplasms or ectopic ACTH production in tumors. Look for moon facies, truncal obesity, "buffalo hump," striae, poor wound healing, hypertension, osteoporosis, secondary diabetes or glucose intolerance, proximal muscle weakness, menstrual abnormalities, and psychiatric disturbances

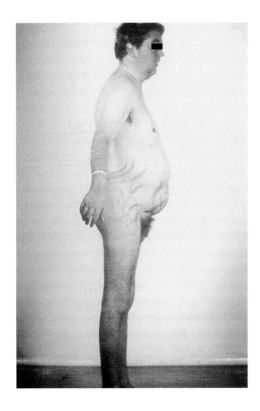

FIGURE 3-19 Cushing syndrome. Note the rash on the face and obese torso with prominent striae. *(From du Vivier A: The skin and systemic disease. In du Vivier A [ed]: Atlas of Clinical Dermatology, 3rd ed. New York, Churchill Livingstone, 2002, pp 509-561.)*

(depression, psychosis). *Cushing disease* is Cushing syndrome caused by pituitary overproduction of ACTH (i.e., pituitary adenoma). Order an MRI study of the pituitary gland/brain if the patient has no history of taking steroids and reports headaches or visual disturbances.

📁 **CASE SCENARIO:** A patient presents with fatigue, moon facies, and abdominal striae. What screening test should you order for hyperadrenalism? A 24-hour urine collection for assessment of free cortisol. Plasma cortisol level is not a good test because of wide interpatient and intrapatient fluctuation. The second choice is a dexamethasone suppression test.

Watch for side effects of steroids in patients on long-term therapy. Classic step 3 questions ask about *secondary diabetes,* hypertension, *osteoporosis,* psychiatric disturbances, and *proximal extremity muscle weakness.*

Miscellaneous Topics

Primary versus secondary endocrine disorders: Remember basic physiology!

❍ In primary endocrine disorders, the gland itself is the problem and the pituitary gland and hypothalamus react normally. For example, TSH is low in Graves disease because the gland is overproducing thyroid hormone. The appropriate response is for the pituitary to secrete less TSH because of feedback inhibition.

❍ In secondary and tertiary endocrine disturbances, the gland is normal but the pituitary or hypothalamus is malfunctioning. For example, if the pituitary secretes low levels of TSH or the hypothalamus secretes low levels of TRH, hypothyroidism occurs even though the thyroid gland is normal.

📁 **CASE SCENARIO:** What gland is the problem in the following conditions?

1. Low TRH, high TSH, high free T_4: Pituitary gland (probable adenoma).
2. Low corticotropin-releasing hormone, low ACTH, high free cortisol: Adrenal gland (or iatrogenic).
3. Low gonadotropin-releasing hormone, low follicle-stimulating hormone and luteinizing hormone, low testosterone: Hypothalamus.

Primary hyperaldosteronism is known as *Conn syndrome* and is due to an adrenal adenoma. Look for hypertension, hypernatremia, hypokalemia, and *low renin* levels. Order a CT scan of the abdomen. Secondary hyperaldosteronism is much more common and is often related to renovascular hypertension (i.e., renal artery stenosis) and edematous disorders (e.g., heart failure, cirrhosis, nephrotic syndrome). Look for the underlying cause and *high renin* levels. Treat the underlying cause.

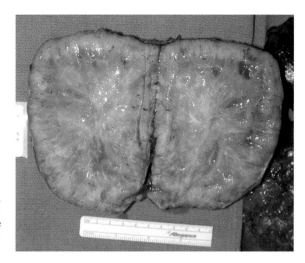

FIGURE 3-20 Pheochromocytoma: gross appearance of tumor in the medulla of the enlarged adrenal gland. *(From Townsend CM, Beauchamp RD, Evers M, and Mattox KL: Sabiston Textbook of Surgery, 18th ed. Philadelphia, Saunders, 2008.)*

Pheochromocytoma (Fig. 3-20): Look for intermittent severe hypertension and wild swings in blood pressure, tachycardia, postural hypotension, headaches, sweating, dizziness, mental status changes, and/or feeling of impending doom. Patients may also have glucose intolerance due to high catecholamines. If pheochromocytoma is suspected, first screen with plasma free metanephrines. If the screen is positive, order abdominal CT or MRI to confirm adrenal mass (usual location). MRI is most sensitive. Treat with surgery after stabilizing the patient with both α- and β-blockers (if only a β-blocker is used, unopposed alpha agonism may cause potentially severe hypertension). Screen all patients for multiple endocrine neoplasia type 2 (MEN type 2) and von Hippel-Lindau disease.

Diabetes insipidus (DI): Patients have severe *polydipsia* and *polyuria* (urinary volume may be 25 L/ day!). DI has no relation to blood sugar; therefore, suspect DI if urine glucose is negative. When access to water is restricted, patients rapidly develop dehydration and hypernatremia, which can cause death. Labs show decreased urine osmolarity and increased serum osmolality. Administration of antidiuretic hormone (ADH) determines whether the cause is central or nephrogenic. Central DI responds to ADH (i.e., urine osmolarity increases when ADH given); nephrogenic DI does not.
1. Nephrogenic DI: Look for medications as the cause (e.g., *lithium*, methoxyflurane, demeclocycline). Treat with removal of causative medication, adequate hydration, low-sodium diet, and *thiazide diuretics* (paradoxical effect); ADH does not help!
2. Central DI: Look for trauma, neoplasm, or sarcoidosis, although central DI is often idiopathic. Treat with 1-deamino-8-D-arginine vasopressin (DDAVP)/vasopressin, and treat the underlying cause, if possible.

📁 **CASE SCENARIO:** What is the relationship of serum to urine osmolarity when DI is present? Serum osmolarity is high, and urine osmolarity is inappropriately low (due to lack of ADH or its effects).

SIADH causes hyponatremia and low levels of every other electrolyte (and lab value) because of dilution from excessive water retention. Look for neoplasm, pulmonary disorders, and medications (e.g., morphine), and watch for a pregnant patient (oxytocin effect). Other causes include small cell lung cancer, postoperative status (watch for all electrolytes to fall after surgery), trauma, lung infections, and pain. Treat with *water restriction*. For board purposes, avoid hypertonic saline (unless seizures or coma are present) and do not attempt aggressive or quick correction of hyponatremia (which may cause central pontine myelinolysis).

📁 **CASE SCENARIO:** What drug can be given in SIADH if conservative treatment (water restriction) fails? Demeclocycline, which at controlled doses induces mild nephrogenic DI to counteract the SIADH.

GASTROENTEROLOGY

Gastroesophageal reflux disease
High-yield pearls:
○ Due to inappropriate, intermittent lower esophageal sphincter (LES) relaxation.
○ Incidence increased in patients with a sliding hiatal hernia and with obesity and pregnancy.

❍ Classically manifests as "heartburn," often related to eating and lying supine. However, it also may manifest as chest pain, regurgitation, cough, asthma, sore throat, dysphagia, laryngitis and hoarseness, or recurrent pneumonia. Testing or treating for *Helicobacter pylori* is generally not effective in GERD.

❍ The initial treatment is to elevate the head of the bed and avoid coffee, alcohol, tobacco, chocolate, spicy and fatty foods, and medications with anticholinergic properties. Weight loss should be encouraged in overweight individuals. If this approach fails, proton pump inhibitors (omeprazole) are most effective, but antacids or histamine H_2 receptor blockers can be tried; often they are started empirically at the initial presentation (and often by the patient before presenting for medical attention).

❍ Surgery is reserved for severe and resistant cases (Nissen fundoplication or similar procedure).

❍ Sequelae include esophagitis, esophageal stricture (which may mimic esophageal cancer), esophageal ulcer, hemorrhage, *Barrett metaplasia,* and *esophageal adenocarcinoma.*

❍ In cases that are atypical or do not respond to medical therapy, consider endoscopy. The gold standard for diagnosis is 24-hour esophageal pH monitoring (a probe is inserted into the esophagus).

Hiatal hernia, as the term is commonly used, implies a *sliding* hiatal hernia. The entire gastroesophageal junction moves above the diaphragm, pulling the stomach with it—a common and benign finding associated with GERD. In a *paraesophageal* hiatal hernia, the gastroesophageal junction stays below the diaphragm but the stomach herniates through the diaphragm into the thorax. This uncommon, serious type of hernia can become strangulated and should be repaired surgically if detected.

Peptic ulcer disease

Peptic ulcer disease (PUD) classically manifests with chronic, intermittent, epigastric burning, gnawing, or aching pain that is localized and often relieved by antacids or milk. Look for epigastric tenderness. PUD can also cause atypical chest pain. Patients may have occult blood in the stool, nausea, and vomiting. PUD is more common in men. There are two types: gastric and duodenal (Table 3-19).

TABLE 3-19 Types of Peptic Ulcer Disease

FEATURE	DUODENAL	GASTRIC
Percentage of cases	75	25
Acid secretion	Normal to high	Normal to low
Main cause	*Helicobacter pylori*	Use of nonsteroidal antiinflammatory drugs
Peak age	40s	50s
Blood type	O	A
Eating food	Pain gets better, then worse 2-3 hr later	Pain often not relieved or made worse

Other pearls:

❍ Endoscopy is the preferred initial study because it also allows biopsy and *H. pylori* testing. Urea breath test is >90% sensitive and specific. Serologic testing for *H. pylori* is inexpensive, however, antibodies may be seen with previous infection but not necessarily current infection. Histologic evaluation of the endoscopic biopsy specimen is the gold standard for *H. pylori.* Stool antigen testing is useful for testing 8 weeks after therapy for eradication of *H. pylori.*

❍ Biopsy all gastric ulcers to exclude malignancy if given the option. Always worry about gastric cancer if a stomach ulcer fails to heal after 2 months of treatment. Duodenal ulcers are almost never malignant and do not need biopsy.

❍ The classic complication is perforation. Look for peritoneal signs, history of PUD, and free air under the diaphragm on upright abdominal radiograph. Treat with antibiotics and laparotomy with repair of perforation.

❍ If duodenal ulcers are severe, atypical (e.g., located in distal duodenum), or nonhealing, think about *Zollinger-Ellison syndrome* and check the gastrin level.

❍ Diet changes (e.g., avoidance of spicy foods) do not help to heal ulcers, but reduced usage of alcohol and tobacco does. Avoid NSAIDs and foods that aggravate symptoms.

❍ For initial treatment, use H_2 blockers or proton pump inhibitors. Use antibiotics to eliminate *H. pylori* if positive. Three- or four-drug therapy is commonly used, with many possible regimens. A classic regimen consists of a proton pump inhibitor with two other antibiotics such as amoxicillin and clarithromycin. In patients with penicillin allergy, substitute metronidazole for amoxicillin. Misoprostol is useful for prevention of NSAID-induced gastric ulcers.

❍ Patients with recurrent ulcers should be treated for 8 additional weeks and placed on maintenance H_2 blockers or PPIs. Surgical options are considered after failure of medication or development of complications (perforation, bleeding). Antrectomy, vagotomy, or Billroth I or II procedures may be performed. After surgery (especially with Billroth procedures), watch for dumping syndrome (weakness, dizziness, sweating, nausea and vomiting after eating). Patients with dumping syndrome also develop hypoglycemia 2–3 hours after the meal, which causes the same symptoms to recur. Also watch for afferent loop syndrome (bilious vomiting after a meal relieves abdominal pain), bacterial overgrowth, and vitamin deficiencies (B_{12} and/or iron deficiency, which causes anemia).

Gastrointestinal Bleeding

GI bleeds may originate in the upper or the lower tract : see Table 3-20.

Table 3-20 Upper versus Lower Gastrointestinal (GI) Bleeds

	UPPER GI	LOWER GI
Location	Proximal to ligament of Treitz	Distal to ligament of Treitz
Common causes	Gastritis, peptic ulcer disease, varices	Vascular ecstasia, diverticulosis, colon cancer, colitis, inflammatory bowel disease, hemorrhoids
Stool	Tarry, black stool (melena)	Red blood seen in stool (hematochezia)
Nasogastric tube aspirate	Positive for blood	Negative for blood

Management issues:

❍ The first step is to make sure that the patient is stable. Check vital signs and hemoglobin level (and recheck frequently). Remember the ABCs, and give IV fluid or blood, if necessary. Then get a diagnosis once the patient is stabilized. Monitor the patient and obtain blood counts every 4–8 hours on an inpatient basis until hemoglobin is stable for at least 24 hours.

❍ Endoscopy is the first test performed (upper and/or lower, depending on symptoms). Endoscopically treatable lesions include polyps, vascular ectasias, and varices.

❍ Radionuclide (i.e., nuclear medicine) scans can detect slow or intermittent bleeds if the source cannot be found with endoscopy. Angiography can detect more rapid bleeds and allows embolization of bleeding vessels.

❍ Surgery is reserved for severe or resistant bleeds and usually involves resection of affected bowel (usually colon).

❍ *A lower GI bleed (or just a positive occult blood test of the stool) in an adult older than age 40 is colon cancer until proved otherwise.* A complete workup is required.

Diverticulosis is extremely common, and the incidence increases with age (present in roughly 50% of people older than age 60). It is thought to be caused in part by a low-fiber, high-fat (i.e., Western) diet. Complications are *GI bleeding* (common cause of lower GI bleeds) and diverticulitis (inflammation of a diverticulum). In patients with *diverticulitis,* look for lower left quadrant pain and tenderness, fever, diarrhea/constipation, and an elevated white blood cell (WBC) count. Confirm the diagnosis with a CT scan with IV contrast (endoscopy is avoided in the setting of suspected diverticulitis or colitis due to increased risk of causing bowel perforation). Right-sided diverticulitis is less common but can occur in young patients, especially of Asian ethnicity. Treat mild cases with broad-spectrum antibiotics (ciprofloxacin); severe cases with IV antibiotics (ampicillin-sulbactam, cefoxitin); and life-threatening cases with imipenem. Surgery should be considered in patients with >2 episodes of diverticulitis, poor response to medical therapy, peritonitis, abscess, or fistula.

Diarrhea

Diarrhea can have multiple causes and is best broken down into the following categories:

1. **Systemic:** any illness can cause diarrhea as a systemic symptom (e.g., hyperthyroidism, flu), especially in children.

2. **Osmotic:** nonabsorbable solutes remain in the bowel, where they retain water (e.g., lactose or other sugar intolerances). When the person stops eating the offending substance (e.g., no more milk or a trial of NPO status [nothing by mouth]), the diarrhea stops.

3. **Secretory:** Bowel secretes fluid because of bacterial toxins (cholera, some strains of *E. coli*), VIPoma (pancreatic islet cell tumor), or bile acids (after ileal resection). Diarrhea continues with NPO status.
4. **Malabsorption** (e.g., celiac sprue, Crohn disease). In patients with celiac sprue, look for *dermatitis herpetiformis*, and stop gluten in the diet. Diarrhea stops with NPO status.
5. **Infectious:** Look for fever, recent history of travel (Montezuma's revenge caused by *E. coli*), and WBCs in the stool (not present with toxigenic bacteria; only with invasive bacteria such as *Shigella*, *Salmonella*, *Yersinia*, and *Campylobacter* spp.).

📁 **CASE SCENARIO:** An avid hiker presents with steatorrhea (fatty, greasy, malodorous stools that float) and crampy abdominal pain. What should you look for in the stool? *Giardia lamblia* (Fig. 3-21). Steatorrhea is due primarily to small bowel involvement. Treat with metronidazole.

6. **Exudative:** Inflammation in bowel mucosa causes seepage of fluid; classically due to inflammatory bowel disease or cancer.
7. **Altered intestinal transit:** after bowel resections or medications that interfere with bowel function.

   Management issues:
   ❍ Watch for dehydration and check for electrolyte disturbances (metabolic acidosis, hypokalemia), which are a common and preventable cause of death in underdeveloped areas.
   ❍ Do a rectal exam, check for occult blood in stool, and examine stool for bacteria, ova, parasites, fat content (steatorrhea), and WBCs.
   ❍ If the cause is not obvious, a trial of NPO status is helpful to see if the diarrhea stops.
   ❍ If the patient has a history of antibiotic usage, think of *Clostridium difficile* and test the stool for toxin. If the test is positive, treat with oral metronidazole; if metronidazole fails or is not a choice, use vancomycin.
   ❍ Remember diabetes mellitus (diabetic diarrhea), factitious diarrhea (secret laxative abuse, usually by medical personnel), hyperthyroidism, and colorectal cancer as causes of diarrhea.
   ❍ After bacterial diarrhea (especially if due to *E. coli* or *Shigella* spp.) in children, watch for *hemolytic uremic syndrome* (HUS). Symptoms include thrombocytopenia; hemolytic anemia (schistocytes, helmet cells, fragmented red blood cells); and acute renal failure. Treat supportively. Patients may need dialysis and/or transfusions.

   Irritable bowel syndrome (IBS) is a common cause of GI complaints. Classic patients are anxious or neurotic and have a history of *symptoms aggravated by stress*, often *alternating between diarrhea and constipation*, with bloating, *abdominal pain relieved by defecation*, and/or *mucus in the stool*. Look for psychosocial stressors in the history and normal physical findings and diagnostic tests. IBS is a diagnosis of exclusion; you must do at least basic lab tests, rectal and stool examination, and sigmoidoscopy or colonoscopy. Because it is extremely common, it is the most likely diagnosis if the question gives you no positive findings, especially in young adults (three times more common in women than in men). Common clinical criteria include >3 months of symptoms, abdominal pain relieved by a bowel movement, pain accompanied by a change in bowel pattern, and abnormality in bowel movement 25% of the time. Treat with increased fiber in the diet, avoidance of any triggering substances (e.g., lactose, caffeine), cognitive-behavioral therapy, and reassurance. Avoid medications or overtesting, and screen for depression.

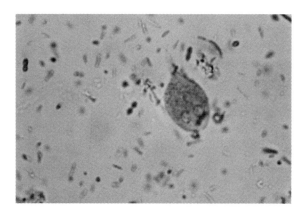

FIGURE 3-21 Giardiasis: typical appearance of *Giardia lamblia* trophozoites. *(From Auerbach P: Wilderness Medicine, 5th ed. Philadelphia, Mosby, 2007.)*

Liver disease

Acute liver disease: Elevated transaminases, jaundice, nausea and vomiting, right upper quadrant pain and tenderness, and/or hepatomegaly.

1. **Alcoholic hepatitis:** Elevated transaminases with aspartate aminotransferase (AST) more than twice as high as alanine aminotransferase (ALT).
2. **Viral hepatitis:** Acute symptoms are similar in all types; use serology to determine type.
   ○ **Hepatitis A** (Fig. 3-22): Look for outbreaks from food-borne source. No long-term sequelae. Serology: IgM anti-HAV-positive during jaundice or shortly thereafter. Usually self-limited, therefore requires only supportive care and reassurance. Report to health authorities.
   ○ **Hepatitis B** (Fig. 3-23): Prevention (vaccination) is the best treatment. The virus is acquired through needles, sex, or perinatal transmission. Transfused blood is now screened, but a history of transfusion years ago is still a risk factor. Use hepatitis B immunoglobulin for exposed neonates. Serology (Table 3-21): HBsAg-positive with any unresolved infection (acute or chronic). HBeAg is a marker for infectivity (i.e., a person with a positive HBeAb has a low likelihood of spreading disease). The first antibody to appear is IgM anti-HBc, which appears during the "window phase," when the patient presents with acute symptoms; both HBsAg and HBsAb are negative. Positive HBsAb means that the patient is immune (due either to recovery from infection or vaccination), and it never appears if the patient has chronic hepatitis. In most cases, no treatment is necessary as >90% spontaneously clear infection. Pegylated interferon-alfa and antiviral medications (lamivudine, adefovir, tenofovir, telbivudine, and entecavir) are the mainstay of therapy in chronic infection. Sequelae are cirrhosis and hepatocellular cancer (only with chronic infection). For prevention after exposure (needlestick, sexual exposure, birth), give HBV hyperimmune globulin (HBIG) and vaccination.

TABLE 3-21 General Interpretation of Serologic Markers in Hepatitis B

	HBsAg	ANTI-HBc IgM	ANTI-HBc IgG	ANTI-HBs
Acute hepatitis	+	+	+	–
Acute hepatitis, window period	–	+	–	–
Chronic hepatitis	+	–	+	–
Recovery from acute hepatitis, Immune	–	–	+	+
Vaccinated, Immune	–	–	–	+

HBsAg, Hepatitis B surface antigen; *anti-HBc IgM*, hepatitis B core antibody, IgM type; *anti-HBc IgG*, hepatitis B core antibody, IgG type; *anti-HBs*, hepatitis B surface antibody

   ○ **Hepatitis C** (Fig. 3-24): the most common cause of virus-induced chronic hepatitis and the most common reason for liver transplantation. Hepatitis C can also progress to chronic hepatitis, cirrhosis, and cancer. Serology: HCV Ab shows prior exposure but does not indicate recovery. The hepatitis C quantitative RNA test can detect virus in patients with chronic hepatitis C;

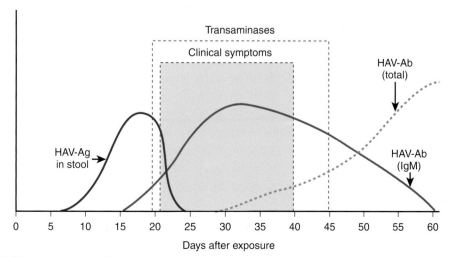

FIGURE 3-22 Hepatitis A: serologic tests. *(From Ferri FF: Ferri's Clinical Advisor 2012. Philadelphia, Mosby, 2012.)*

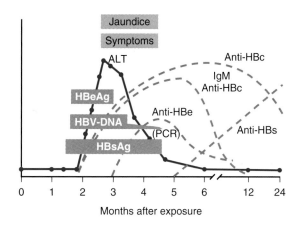

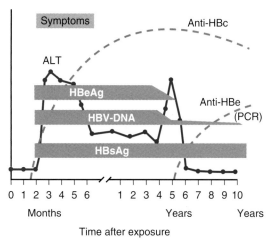

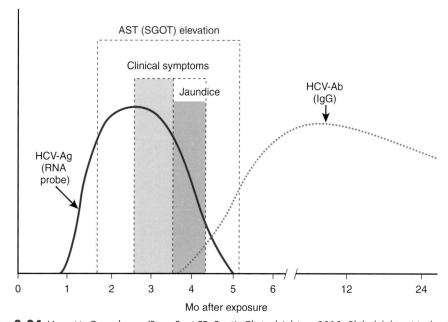

FIGURE 3-23 Hepatitis B serology in acute and chronic infection. *ALT,* Alanine aminotransferase; *anti-HBc,* total antibody to hepatitis B core antigen; *anti-HBe,* antibody to hepatitis B e antigen; *anti-HBs,* antibody to hepatitis B antigen; *HBeAg,* hepatitis B e antigen; *HBsAg,* hepatitis B surface antigen; *HBV,* hepatitis B virus; *IgM anti-HBc,* acute IgM antibody to hepatitis B core antigen; *PCR,* polymerase chain reaction. *(From Piccini JP, Nilsson KR: The Osler Medical Handbook, 2nd ed. Philadelphia, Saunders, 2006.)*

FIGURE 3-24 Hepatitis C serology. *(From Ferri FF: Ferri's Clinical Advisor 2012. Philadelphia, Mosby, 2012.)*

donated blood is now screened. Order an RNA test in any patient with hepatitis C antibody–positive serum and elevated liver enzymes. Recent studies demonstrate that early treatment with interferon alfa-2b during acute HCV infection prevents chronic infection. Patients with genotypes 1 and 4 have sustained virologic response, and cure rates are much lower than in patients with genotypes 2 and 3. The mainstay of therapy is pegylated interferon-alfa and ribavirin.

○ **Hepatitis D:** seen only in patients with hepatitis B. Infection can become chronic. The virus is acquired in the same ways as the hepatitis B virus. Superinfection in a patient already hepatitis B positive is worse than coinfection with hepatitis B and D. IgM antibody to hepatitis D antigen shows recent resolution of infection; presence of the hepatitis D antigen indicates chronicity.

○ **Hepatitis E:** similar to hepatitis A (food- or water-borne, no chronic state). Significantly increased risk of fatality in *pregnant women.*

3. **Drug-induced hepatitis:** Look for acetaminophen, isoniazid (and other TB drugs), or HMG-CoA reductase inhibitors (statins). Stop the drug!

4. **Reye syndrome:** Look for a child given *aspirin* for a fever.

5. **Acute fatty liver of pregnancy:** Occurs in third trimester. Treat with immediate delivery.

6. **Ischemia/shock:** Look for a history of shock.

7. **Idiopathic autoimmune hepatitis:** Look for a 20–40-year-old woman with *anti–smooth muscle, antinuclear antibodies, anti-LKM antibodies, anti-SLA/LP antibodies,* and no risk factors or lab markers of other causes for hepatitis. Treat with steroids.

8. **Biliary tract disease:** See below; look for markedly elevated *alkaline phosphatase* and *direct* (i.e., *conjugated) bilirubin.*

Chronic liver disease usually results from alcohol, viral hepatitis, or metabolic diseases (hemochromatosis, Wilson disease, α_1-antitrypsin deficiency). Classic signs of chronic liver disease include gynecomastia, testicular atrophy, palmar erythema, spider angiomas on the skin, ascites, and varices.

1. **Hemochromatosis:** the primary form is *autosomal recessive;* look for a family history. Excessive iron is absorbed through gut and deposited in the liver (cirrhosis, liver cancer); pancreas (diabetes); heart (dilated cardiomyopathy); skin (pigmentation; classically called "bronze diabetes"); and joints (arthritis). Impotence, amenorrhea, loss of libido, hair loss, and koilonychia ("spooning" of the fingernails) also occur. Men are symptomatic earlier and more often because women lose iron with menstruation. Suspect hemochromatosis on the basis of elevated transferrin saturation (best screening test), serum iron, and ferritin levels. Confirm with DNA testing of the *HFE* gene for the C282Y and H63D mutation. Treat with *phlebotomy* and genetic counseling with goal to bring ferritin <50 μg. Monitor cirrhotic patients by ultrasound imaging or CT for hepatocellular carcinoma. Screen first-degree relatives with *HFE* gene testing. Secondary iron overload can cause a hemochromatosis-like picture, usually seen with anemia from ineffective erythropoiesis (e.g., thalassemia) or excessive iron intake (thus do not prescribe iron for a microcytic anemia without confirming the diagnosis of iron-deficiency anemia).

2. **Wilson disease:** *autosomal recessive* disease of the *ATP7B* gene on chromosome 13 characterized by the presence of excessive copper. Serum *ceruloplasmin is low,* and urinary copper is elevated. Serum copper may be low, but liver biopsy reveals excessive copper and confirms the diagnosis. Patients also have *Kayser-Fleischer rings* found in the cornea, kidney disease, and central nervous system (CNS) or psychiatric manifestations due to copper deposits in the basal ganglia (thus another name for this disease is *hepatolenticular degeneration).* Treat with *penicillamine* (copper chelator); zinc and trientene are other agents used in treatment. If medications do not work, proceed to liver transplantation.

3. **α_1-Antitrypsin deficiency:** a younger adult develops *cirrhosis* and/or *emphysema* without risk factors for either. *Autosomal recessive* pattern of inheritance. Confirm the diagnosis with low blood levels of α_1-antitrypsin and DNA testing for the variant "Z" and "S" alleles of the *SERPINA1* gene. Homozygous ZZ and SS patients have severe deficiency, whereas heterozygous MS, MZ, and SZ patients have less severe disease. Replacement therapy is available to slow progression and delay complications.

Remember all of the metabolic derangements that accompany liver failure (classically seen in chronic liver disease, but most also can occur acutely).

1. **Coagulopathy:** prolonged prothrombin time (PT); with severe disease, partial thromboplastin time (PTT) also may be prolonged. Vitamin K is *ineffective* because it cannot be used by a damaged liver. Coagulopathy must be treated with *fresh frozen plasma* (FFP).

2. **Jaundice/hyperbilirubinemia:** elevated conjugated and unconjugated bilirubin with hepatic damage (vs. biliary tract disease with elevation primarily of direct bilirubin).

3. **Hypoalbuminemia:** A damaged liver cannot make albumin.

4. **Ascites:** due to portal hypertension and/or hypoalbuminemia. Ascites can be detected on physical exam by *shifting dullness* or a *positive fluid wave* (diagnosis can be confirmed with ultrasound or CT if in doubt). A possible complication is *spontaneous bacterial peritonitis;* infected ascitic fluid can

lead to sepsis. Look for fever and/or change in mental status in a patient with known ascites. Do a paracentesis and examine the ascitic fluid for WBCs (especially neutrophils). Other lab tests include Gram stain with culture and sensitivities, glucose level (low with infection), and protein level (high with infection). The usual cause is *E. coli, Streptococcus pneumoniae,* or miscellaneous enteric bugs. Treat with broad-spectrum antibiotics. Repeated therapeutic paracentesis may be necessary for some patients due to abdominal discomfort and/or respiratory difficulty.

5. **Portal hypertension:** causes ascites, hemorrhoids, esophageal varices, and caput medusae.
6. **Hyperammonemia:** The liver clears ammonia. Treat with decreased intake of protein (source of ammonia) and *lactulose,* which prevents absorption of ammonia. The last choice is neomycin, which kills bowel flora so that they cannot make ammonia.
7. **Hepatic encephalopathy:** at least in part due to hyperammonemia; often precipitated by protein ingestion, GI bleed, or infection.
8. **Hepatorenal syndrome:** Liver failure can cause kidney failure (for reasons that are still unclear). Essentially uniformly fatal without treatment. Due at least in part to altered cardiovascular hemodynamics with renal vasoconstriction and splanchnic vasodilatation. Treated with albumin, the α-adrenergic agent midodrine, octreotide, and/or vasopressin as well as consideration of transjugular intrahepatic portosystemic shunt creation (TIPS). Liver transplantation is a permanent/definitive "cure" when available.
9. **Hypoglycemia:** The liver stores glycogen.
10. **Disseminated intravascular coagulation:** because activated clotting factors are usually cleared by the liver.

Biliary tract disease

Jaundice can also be caused by bile duct obstruction. Look for marked elevation of *alkaline phosphatase* (or *gamma-glutamyl transpeptidase* [GGT] or *5'-nucleotidase*). Conjugated (i.e., direct) bilirubin is more elevated than unconjugated bilirubin. Other features include pruritus, *clay-colored stools,* and *dark urine,* which is strongly bilirubin positive. Unconjugated bilirubin is *not* excreted in the urine because it is tightly bound to albumin.

1. **Common bile duct obstruction with gallstone** (i.e., choledocholithiasis): Look for a history of gallstones or the four Fs (**f**emale, **f**orty, **f**ertile, **f**at) and abdominal pain in the right upper quadrant. Ultrasound may be able to image the stone; if not, use magnetic resonance cholangiopancreatography (MRCP) to diagnose and endoscopic retrograde cholangiopancreatography (ERCP) to treat (Fig. 3-25).
2. **Common bile duct obstruction from cancer:** usually pancreatic cancer (painless jaundice and palpable gallbladder = Courvoisier sign), occasionally cholangiocarcinoma or bowel cancer.
3. **Cholestasis:** often from medications (birth control pills, phenothiazines, androgens) or pregnancy.
4. **Primary biliary cirrhosis:** middle-aged woman with no risk factors for liver or biliary disease, marked *pruritus, jaundice,* and *positive antimitochondrial antibodies* (the rest of the workup is negative). Cholestyramine helps with symptoms, but no treatment is available other than liver transplantation.

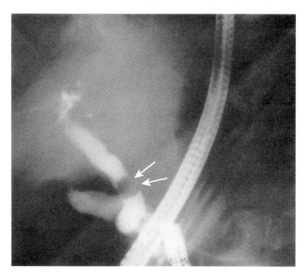

FIGURE 3-25 Endoscopic retrograde cholangiopancreatography reveals a single common bile duct stone *(arrows). (From Katz DS, Math KR, Groski SA [eds]: Radiology Secrets. Philadelphia, Hanley & Belfus, 1998.)*

5. **Primary sclerosing cholangitis:** seen in young adults with *ulcerative colitis;* manifests as with infectious cholangitis.
6. **Cholangitis:** infected bile, usually under pressure. Treat with antibiotics, and remove any stones/obstruction surgically, percutaneously, or endoscopically.

▢ **CASE SCENARIO:** A 39-year-old woman with a history of gallstones develops right upper quadrant pain, fever, shaking chills, and jaundice. What happened? An impacted gallstone in the common bile duct has led to cholangitis. *Charcot's triad* of cholangitis is jaundice, fever, and right upper quadrant pain.

Inflammatory bowel disease

Crohn disease and ulcerative colitis: main forms of inflammatory bowel disease (IBD); see Table 3-22 and Figure 3-26.

TABLE 3-22 Crohn Disease versus Ulcerative Colitis

	CROHN DISEASE	ULCERATIVE COLITIS
Site of origin	Any area of the gastrointestinal tract—distal ileum, proximal colon	Rectum and/or colon
Thickness of pathology	Transmural	Mucosa/submucosa only
Progression	Irregular (skip lesions)	Proximal, continuous from rectum; no skipped areas
Location	From mouth to anus	Involves only colon; rarely extends to ileum
Bowel habits change to	Obstruction, abdominal pain	Bloody diarrhea
Classic lesions	Fistulas/abscesses, cobblestoning, string sign on barium radiograph	Pseudopolys, lead-pipe colon on barium radiograph, toxic megacolon
Colon cancer risk	Slightly increased	Markedly increased
Serology	ASCA	p-ANCA
Surgery cures bowel disease?	No (may make worse)	Yes (proctocolectomy with ileoanal anastomosis)

ASCA, Anti–Saccharomyces cerevisiae antibodies; p-ANCA, perinuclear antineutrophil cytoplasmic antibody.

Patients with either form of IBD may develop *uveitis, arthritis, ankylosing spondylitis, erythema nodosum* or *multiforme, primary sclerosing cholangitis* (more common in ulcerative colitis), failure to thrive or grow (children), anemia of chronic disease, or fever. Both conditions are treated with some form of *5-ASA* (aspirin derivative) with or without a sulfa drug (e.g., sulfasalazine). Be sure to give folate supplementation with sulfasalazine. Corticosteroids and immunosuppresants

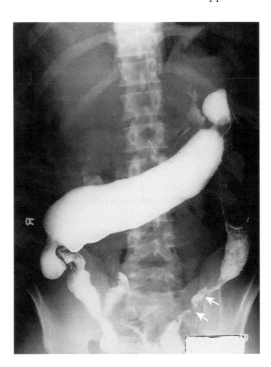

FIGURE 3-26 Foreshortened colon from long-standing ulcerative colitis. Note stricture of sigmoid colon from carcinoma *(arrows)*. *(From James EC, Corry RJ, Perry JF: Principles of Basic Surgical Practice. Philadelphia, Hanley & Belfus, 1987.)*

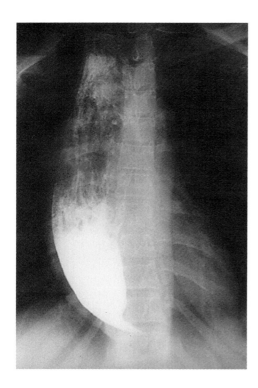

Figure 3-27 Anteroposterior radiograph from a barium esophogram, demonstrating the marked esophageal dilation with "beaked" narrowing distally that is characteristic of achalasia. Note lucency within the barium column, representing undigested food. *(From Katz DS, Math KR, Groski SA [eds]: Radiology Secrets. Philadelphia, Hanley & Belfus, 1998.)*

(e.g., infliximab, azathioprine) are used for severe disease flare-ups. Metronidazole may be useful for fistulas.

Although toxic megacolon is classically seen with ulcerative colitis, it also can occur in infectious colitis (especially with *Clostridium difficile*) or Crohn disease. It may be precipitated by the use of antidiarrheal medications. Patients have high fever, leukocytosis, abdominal pain, severe tenderness, and a very *dilated colon on radiograph with "thumbprinting"* (i.e., wall thickening with mucosal irregularity). Toxic megacolon is an emergency! Start treatment by discontinuing all antidiarrheal medications; then place the patient on NPO status, insert a nasogastric tube, administer intravenous fluids and antibiotics to cover bowel flora (e.g., ampicillin or cefazolin), and give steroids (if the cause is IBD). Proceed to surgery if perforation (as indicated by free air on radiograph and rebound tenderness) occurs.

Esophageal disorders

Patients usually present with dysphagia or atypical chest pain:

1. **Achalasia:** hypertensive LES, incomplete relaxation of LES, and loss or derangement of peristalsis. Achalasia is usually idiopathic but may be secondary to *Chagas disease* (South America). Patients have dysphagia for both solid foods and liquids. Barium swallow reveals a dilated esophagus with *distal "bird-beak" narrowing* (Fig. 3-27). The diagnosis can be made with esophageal manometry. Treat with local botulinum toxin injections, pneumatic balloon dilatation, calcium channel blockers, and, as a last resort, surgery (myotomy).

📁 **CASE SCENARIO:** A 32-year-old woman has dysphagia for solids and liquids, atypical chest pain, and severe heartburn. Can you rule out achalasia? Essentially, yes. Patients with achalasia do not have heartburn, because the LES will not open to allow reflux.

2. **Diffuse esophageal spasm/nutcracker esophagus:** Both have irregular, forceful, painful esophageal contractions that cause intermittent chest pain. Diagnose with esophageal manometry. Treat with nitroglycerin, calcium channel blockers, anticholinergics, and/or local botulinum toxin injections. Surgery (myotomy) used for cases that fail medical therapy.

3. **Scleroderma:** may cause aperistalsis due to fibrosis and atrophy of smooth muscle. Look for positive antinuclear antibody (ANA), masklike facies, and other autoimmune symptoms (calcinosis, Raynaud phenomenon, esophageal dysmotility, sclerodactyly, telangiectasias [CREST]).

📁 **CASE SCENARIO:** A 32-year-old woman has positive ANA and heartburn. Should you worry about scleroderma? Yes, because the LES usually becomes incompetent and patients develop severe reflux.

4. **Barrett esophagus:** columnar metaplasia due to acid reflux. Once detected, it should be followed with periodic endoscopy and biopsies to rule out progression to adenocarcinoma.
5. **Mallory-Weiss tears:** superficial esophageal erosions that may cause a GI bleed. They are usually seen with *vomiting and retching (alcoholism, bulimia)*. Diagnosis and treatment are done endoscopically; sclerose any bleeding vessels.
6. **Boorhave tears:** full-thickness esophageal ruptures. If not iatrogenic (from endoscopy), they are usually due to *vomiting and retching (alcoholism, bulimia)*. Diagnose with endoscopy or water-soluble contrast (i.e., Gastrografin) x-ray study, and treat with immediate surgical repair and drainage.

Pancreatitis

Causes: More than 80% of cases of acute pancreatitis are due to *alcohol* or *gallstones*. Other causes include hypertriglyceridemia; viral infections (mumps, coxsackievirus); trauma; and medications (e.g., steroids, thiazide diuretics, azathioprine).

Symptoms: Watch for abdominal pain radiating to the back; nausea; vomiting that fails to relieve the pain; leukocytosis; and *elevated amylase* and *lipase*. Perforated peptic ulcers also are associated with elevated amylase and can manifest similarly, but amylase elevation is mild, free air is classically seen on radiograph, patients often have a history of ulcer disease, and lipase is often normal with ulcer disease.

Grey Turner sign: Blue-black flanks; Cullen sign: blue-black umbilicus. Both result from hemorrhagic inflammatory exudate, and both indicate severe pancreatitis.

Diffuse calcifications within the pancreas may be seen on plain radiograph or CT scan in patients with chronic pancreatitis and are associated with alcoholism in >90% of cases. Gallbladder disease is not associated with chronic pancreatitis (because the gallbladder is removed after the first episode of gallstone pancreatitis).

Treatment of acute pancreatitis: NPO status, nasogastric tube, intravenous fluids, and narcotics (hydromorphone or meperidine). The contraindication to morphine is no longer accepted. Treat chronic pancreatitis with alcohol abstinence, oral pancreatic enzyme replacement, and fat-soluble vitamin supplements.

Complications: *Pseudocyst* (drain surgically if symptomatic), *abscess* or infection (antibiotics and CT-guided or open surgical abscess drainage), and diabetes and malabsorption (with chronic pancreatitis).

HEMATOLOGY

Anemia

Definition: hemoglobin <12 mg/dL in adult women or <14 mg/dL in adult men (or more pragmatically, hemoglobin below the limits of the normal range for the laboratory you are using).

Symptoms include fatigue, dyspnea on exertion, light-headedness, dizziness, syncope, palpitations, angina, and claudication. Signs include tachycardia, pallor (especially of the conjunctival and mucous membranes), systolic ejection murmurs (from high flow), and signs of the underlying cause (e.g., jaundice in hemolytic anemia, positive stool guaiac in GI bleed).

Important clues in the history:
1. **Blood loss:** trauma, surgery, GI bleed, menstrual blood loss.
2. **Chronic diseases:** anemia of chronic disease, seen especially in patients with long-term inflammatory and debilitating conditions such as autoimmune diseases, infections, and cancer (i.e., osteoarthritis does not cause anemia of chronic disease).
3. **Family history:** hemophilia, thalassemia, G6PD deficiency, etc.
4. **Alcoholism:** tendency to have iron, folate, and vitamin B_{12} deficiencies, as well as GI bleeds.
5. **Medications:** Many medications can cause anemia through various mechanisms. For example, *methyldopa* causes red blood cell (RBC) antibodies and hemolysis, chloroquine and *sulfa drugs* cause hemolysis in patients with glucose-6-phosphate dehydrogenase (G6PD) deficiency, *phenytoin* causes megaloblastic anemia, *chloramphenicol* causes aplastic anemia, and many chemotherapy agents can cause cell death and failure of cell growth/division in the bone marrow.

Steps in diagnosing the cause of anemia:
1. CBC with differential and RBC indices. First and foremost, the hemoglobin and hematocrit must be below normal. The mean corpuscular volume (MCV) tells you whether the anemia is microcytic (MCV <80), normocytic (MCV = 80–100), or macrocytic (MCV >100) (Table 3-23).

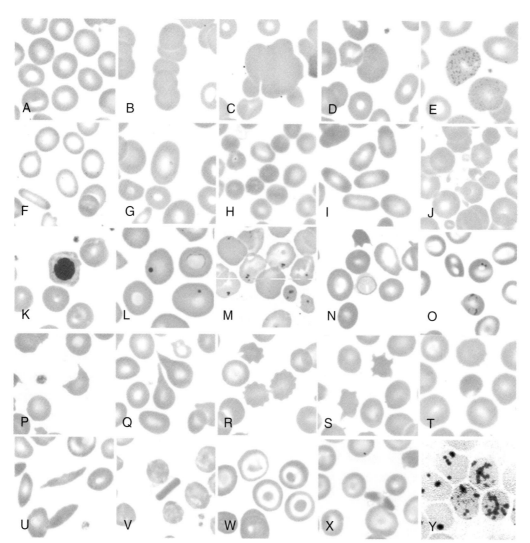

FIGURE 3-28 Classis red blood cell (RBC) morphology features and associated diseases. **A,** Normal RBCs. **B,** Rouleaux formation—mulitple myeloma. **C,** Agglutination—cold agglutinin disease. **D,** Polychromasia—equivalent to a reticulocyte. **E,** Basophilic stippling—lead poisoning, thalassemia. **F,** Hypochromic microcytic cells—iron deficiency anemia. Note the widened central pallor and the "pencil" cell in lower left. **G,** Macrocytes—megaloblastic anemia (vitamin B_{12}, folate deficiency) or myelodysplastic syndrome. **H,** Spherocytes—hereditary spherocytosis. **I,** Elliptocytes—hereditary elliptocytosis. **J,** RBC fragments in a burn patient. **K,** Nucleated RBC—marrow stress. **L,** Howell-Jolly bodies—splenic dysfunction or absence. **M,** Pappenheimer bodies—sideroblastic anemia. **N,** Cabot ring—megaloblastic anemia or MDS. **O,** Malarial parasites *(Plasmodium falciparum)*. **P,** Schistocyte—TTP, DIC. **Q,** Tear-drop cell—myelofibrosis. **R,** Echinocyte (Burr cell)—uremia. **S,** Acanthocyte (spur cell)—abetalipoproteinemia, liver disease, artifact. **T,** "Bite" cell—G6PD deficiency. **U,** Sickle cell—sickle cell anemia. **V,** Hemoglobin C crystal. **W,** Target cells—liver disease, thalassemia. **X,** Hemoglobin SC. Note red blood cell in center has condensed hemoglobin at each pole. **Y,** Heinz body preparation (supravital stain) from a patient with G6PD deficiency. *DIC,* Disseminated intravascular coagulation; *G6PD,* Glucose-6-phosphate dehydrogenase; *TTP,* thrombotic thrombocytopenic purpura. *(From Hoffman R, Furie B, Benz EJ, et al: Hematology, 5th ed. Philadelphia, Churchill Livingstone, 2009.)*

TABLE 3-23 Etiology of Anemia

MICROCYTIC	NORMOCYTIC	MACROCYTIC
Iron deficiency	Acute blood loss	Vitamin B_{12} deficiency
Thalassemia/hemoglobinopathy	Anemia of chronic disease —cancer, thyroid	Folate deficiency
Anemia of chronic disease	dysfunction, renal failure, liver disease	Medications (methotrexate,
Lead poisoning	Hemolytic	phenytoin)
Sideroblastic	Medications	Cirrhosis/liver disease
	Aplastic anemia	

2. Peripheral smear: Look for classic findings for an easy diagnosis (Fig. 3-28).
3. Reticulocyte index (RI) should be >2% with anemia; otherwise, the marrow is not responding properly. If the index is very high, consider hemolysis as the cause (the marrow is responding properly and is not the problem).

   Clues to presence of hemolytic anemia: Elevated lactate dehydrogenase (LDH); elevated bilirubin (unconjugated and conjugated if the liver functions properly); jaundice; *low or absent haptoglobin* (seen with *intravascular* hemolysis); and positive urobilinogen, bilirubin, or hemoglobin in urine. Only conjugated bilirubin appears in the urine, and hemoglobin appears in urine only when haptoglobin has been saturated, as in brisk intravascular hemolysis.

Microcytic anemias

1. **Iron deficiency anemia:** the most common cause of anemia in the United States. Best screening test is serum *ferritin.* Look also for *low iron* and *low total iron-binding capacity (TIBC) saturation.* Rarely patients have a craving for ice or dirt (pica) or *Plummer-Vinson syndrome* (iron deficiency anemia, glossitis, and an esophageal web producing dysphagia). Iron deficiency anemia is common in women of reproductive age because of menstrual irregularities. Considered a marker of colon/GI cancer "until proved otherwise" in all adults older than age 50. To treat iron deficiency anemia, correct the underlying cause, if possible, and treat with oral iron supplementation for at least 3–6 months.

🗀 **CASE SCENARIO:** A 22-year-old woman with menorrhagia presents with fatigue and has lab values consistent with iron deficiency anemia. How long should you treat her with iron? For roughly 3–6 months (then recheck lab values to see if it worked).

2. **Thalassemia must be differentiated from iron deficiency.** On CBC, look for increased RBC and normal RBC distribution width index (RDW). Serum ferritin is generally normal in thalassemia, and iron supplementation is contraindicated because it may cause iron overload. Look for *elevated hemoglobin A2* (β-thalassemia only) or *hemoglobin F* (β-thalassemia only); target cells, nucleated RBCs, or diffuse basophilia on peripheral smears; radiograph of the skull showing "crew-cut" or "hair-on-end" appearance (Fig. 3-29); splenomegaly; and/or family history. Thalassemia is more common in Blacks, Mediterraneans, and Asians. No treatment is required for minor thalassemia; patients are often asymptomatic because they are accustomed to living at a lower level of hemoglobin. Thalassemia major is more dramatic and severe (treated with transfusions as needed and iron chelation therapy to prevent hemochromatosis). Diagnosis is confirmed with hemoglobin electrophoresis.

🗀 **CASE SCENARIO:** If a child is asymptomatic at birth and develops symptoms of anemia around 6 months of age, could he or she have thalassemia? Yes. There are four gene loci for the α chain and only two for the β chain. Patients with severe α-thalassemia are symptomatic at birth or die in utero (due to fetal hydrops), but patients with β-thalassemia (see Fig. 3-29) have no symptoms until they run out of fetal hemoglobin (usually around 6 months).

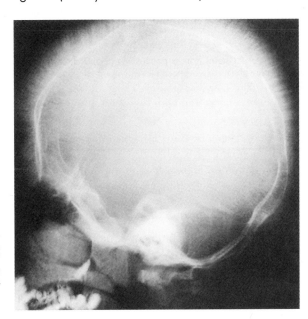

FIGURE 3-29 β-Thalassemia major. Lateral skull radiograph shows typical "hair-on-end" appearance, with thinning of cortical bone and expansion of the marrow cavity. *(From Hoffbrand AV, Pettit JE: Genetic disorders of haemoglobin. In Hoffbrand AV, Pettit JE [eds]: Color Atlas of Clinical Hematology, 3rd ed. St. Louis, Mosby, 2000, pp 85-106.)*

3. **Lead poisoning:** classically seen in children. With acute poisoning, look for vomiting; *ataxia; colicky abdominal pain;* irritability (aggression, behavioral regression); and *encephalopathy, cerebral edema,* or *seizures.* Usually poisoning is chronic. The history may include residence in an old or neglected building (paint chips and dust in old buildings may still contain lead) or residence near or family members who work at a lead-smelting or battery-recycling plant. Lab tests show microcytic anemia with *basophilic stippling.* Screen with venous blood level. If the level is >10 mg/dL, closer follow-up and intervention are necessary. The best first course of action is to *stop the exposure.* Lead chelation therapy may be necessary with *succimer (preferred in children)* or dimercaprol (for more severe cases) for lead levels >45 μg/dL. Levels >70 μg/dL require hospitalization with IV chelation.

4. **Sideroblastic anemia:** increased or normal iron, ferritin, and TIBC/ferritin saturation (which distinguish it from iron deficiency); polychromatophilic stippling on smear; and the classic *"ringed sideroblast"* in the bone marrow. Sideroblastic anemia may be related to myelodysplasia or future blood dyscrasia. Manage supportively. In rare cases, the anemia responds to *pyridoxine.* Do not give iron. Iron overload may require phlebotomy.

5. **Anemia of chronic disease** may be microcytic or normocytic. Look for diseases that cause chronic inflammation. Serum iron is low, but so is the TIBC (thus the % saturation may be near normal). Serum ferritin is usually elevated because ferritin is an acute-phase reactant. Elevated erythrocyte sedimentation rate and/or C-reactive protein often present (not usually true with iron deficiency anemia). Treat the underlying disorder (renal disease, liver disease, thyroid dysfunction, malignancy) to correct the anemia. Do not give iron.

Normocytic anemias

1. **Acute blood loss:** Immediately after blood loss, hemoglobin may be normal (takes a few hours to reequilibrate). Look for pale cold skin, tachycardia, and hypotension. Transfuse if indicated, even with a normal hemoglobin in the appropriate acute setting.

2. **Autoimmune hemolytic anemia has several possible causes:** Lupus (or medications that cause lupus-like syndrome such as *procainamide, hydralazine,* and *isoniazid*); drugs (classic is methyldopa, also penicillins/cephalosporins/sulfas and quinidine); and leukemia/lymphoma or infection (classic is mycoplasma, also Epstein-Barr virus [EBV] and syphilis). *Coombs test* is positive. May have spherocytes due to incomplete macrophage destruction. Cold agglutinin disease in which circulating antibodies bind at cooler body temperatures (e.g., fingers/toes in the winter); can result in acrocyanosis.

3. **Spherocytosis** (normochromic): Diagnosis is based on blood smear, family history (*autosomal dominant* inheritance), splenomegaly, *positive osmotic fragility test,* and an increased mean corpuscular hemoglobin concentration (MCHC). Treatment often involves splenectomy. Spherocytes also may be seen in extravascular hemolysis.

4. **End-stage renal disease:** The kidney makes erythropoietin; give erythropoietin to correct the anemia.

5. **Aplastic anemia** is usually idiopathic but may be caused by chemotherapy or radiation, malignancy (especially leukemias), benzene, and medications (e.g., chloramphenicol, carbamazepine, phenylbutazone, sulfa drugs, zidovudine). Look for decreased WBCs and platelets. Treat by stopping any possible causative medication. Patients may need antithymocyte globulin (ATG) or bone marrow transplant.

6. **Myelophthisic anemia** is usually due to myelodysplasia/myelofibrosis or malignant invasion and destruction of bone marrow (most common cause). Look for left-shifted granulocytes, *nucleated RBCs,* and *teardrop-shaped RBCs* on the peripheral smear. A bone marrow biopsy is usually done and may reveal no cells ("dry tap" due to fibrotic marrow in myelofibrosis) or malignant-looking cells.

7. **Glucose-6-phosphate dehydrogenase (G6PD) deficiency** is an *X-linked* recessive trait; clinically seen in males. It is most common in Blacks and Mediterraneans. Look for sudden hemolysis or anemia after exposure to *fava beans* or certain drugs (*antimalarials,* salicylates, *sulfa drugs*) or after infection. Diagnosis is based on the G6PD enzyme assay. Do not perform the assay immediately after hemolysis; you may get a false-negative result because all of the older RBCs have been destroyed and the younger RBCs are not affected in many patients. Treat by avoiding precipitating foods and medications. Discontinue the triggering medication first.

Macrocytic anemias

1. **Folate deficiency** is classically seen in alcoholics and pregnant women. Rare causes include poor diet (e.g., tea and toast), methotrexate, prolonged therapy with trimethoprim-sulfamethoxazole

(TMP-SMX), anticonvulsant therapy (especially phenytoin), and malabsorption. Check folate level (serum or RBC). Treat with oral folate.

2. **Vitamin B$_{12}$ deficiency** is most commonly due to *pernicious anemia* (antiparietal cell antibodies) but also may be due to gastrectomy, terminal ileum resection, diet (strict vegan), chronic pancreatitis, and *Diphyllobothrium latum* (fish tapeworm) infection. Look for *neurologic deficiencies* (loss of sensation or position sense, paresthesias, ataxia, spasticity, hyperreflexia, Babinski sign, dementia) and achlorhydria (no stomach acid secretion, elevated stomach pH). Check serum levels of vitamin B$_{12}$. A *Schilling test* usually determines the etiology.

▢ **CASE SCENARIO:** A 24-year-old woman with a history of hypothyroidism who eats a normal diet presents with tingling in her legs and macrocytic anemia with hypersegmented neutrophils. How should she be treated? With intramuscular vitamin B$_{12}$ injections (after confirming diagnosis with serum B$_{12}$ level), usually given monthly. Oral supplements cannot be used because the patient almost surely has pernicious anemia and cannot absorb oral supplements.

Other causes of anemia:
1. Mechanical heart valves (hemolyze red blood cells).
2. Hemolysis due to "microangiopathy" (e.g., disseminated intravascular coagulation, thrombotic thrombocytopenic purpura [see figure], hemolytic uremic syndrome). Look for schistocytes and RBC fragments.
3. Infections: *Clostridium perfringens*, malaria, babesiosis.
4. Hypersplenism: All patients have splenomegaly; other common findings include low platelets and low WBC count.

Miscellaneous hematologic abnormalities

Eosinophilia may be idiopathic or caused by allergy, eczema, atopy, angioedema, drug reactions, parasitic infections, blood dyscrasias (especially lymphoma), Löffler syndrome (pulmonary eosinophilia), autoimmune diseases, IgA deficiency, and adrenal insufficiency. Chronic eosinophilia may be due to a chronic myeloproliferative disorder.

Basophilia: Think of allergies, neoplasm, or blood dyscrasia. If neutrophilia with left shift is present, think of chronic myelogenous leukemia (CML).

Thrombocytopenia may be caused by idiopathic thrombocytopenic purpura, thrombotic thrombocytopenic purpura (TTP), hemolytic uremic syndrome, disseminated intravascular coagulation, HIV infection, splenic sequestration, heparin (treat by first stopping heparin), other medications (especially quinidine and sulfa drugs), autoimmune disorders, and alcohol. Bleeding from thrombocytopenia is in the form of *petechiae, nosebleeds,* and *easy bruising.* Do not give platelet transfusions to a patient with TTP or heparin-associated thrombocytopenia because this may cause thrombosis!

Transfusions
Different blood components have different indications:
1. **Whole blood**: rarely used today. Previously only for rapid, massive blood loss or exchange transfusions (poisoning, thrombotic thrombocytopenic purpura).
2. **Packed RBCs:** used instead of whole blood when the patient needs a transfusion.
3. **Washed RBCs:** free of traces of plasma, WBCs, and platelets. Good for IgA deficiency and allergic or previously sensitized patients.
4. **Platelets:** given for symptomatic thrombocytopenia (usually <10,000/μl).
5. **Granulocytes:** rarely used for neutropenia with sepsis caused by chemotherapy.
6. **Fresh frozen plasma** (FFP): contains all clotting factors; used for bleeding diathesis when the patient cannot wait for vitamin K to take effect (e.g., disseminated intravascular coagulation, severe warfarin poisoning) or when vitamin K is not effective (liver failure).
7. **Cryoprecipitate:** contains fibrinogen and factor 8; can be used in hemophilia, von Willebrand disease, disseminated intravascular coagulation, or blood loss with low fibrinogen.

▢ **CASE SCENARIO:** A 47-year-old man presents for a routine health visit. He is asymptomatic. A routine hemoglobin level is 6 mg/dL. How many units of blood should you transfuse? None. Transfusion should be based on clinical grounds. Treat the patient, not the lab value. There is no such thing as a "trigger value" for transfusion. An asymptomatic patient rarely needs a transfusion.

The most common cause of blood transfusion reaction is clerical error. Type O negative blood can be used to avoid reactions when you cannot wait for blood typing or the blood bank does not have the patient's type. Types of transfusion reactions are as follows:

1. **Febrile reaction** (chills, fever, and headache/back pain) from antibodies to WBCs.
2. **Hemolytic reaction** (anxiety/discomfort, dyspnea, chest pain, shock, jaundice) from antibodies to RBCs. Positive direct antiglobulin test (DAT).
3. **Allergic reaction** (urticaria, edema, dizziness, dyspnea/wheezing, anaphylaxis) from reaction to component in donor serum.
4. **Bacterial contamination**—Look for fever and chills immediately after beginning transfusion.
5. **Transfusion associated acute lung injury** (TRALI)—one of the leading causes of transfusion-related mortality. Look for shortness of breath, fever, hypotension, "white lung" on chest radiograph within 6 hours of transfusion. Treat with supportive care, oxygen, and intubation. If more transfusion products are necessary, use a different donor.

If the patient has associated oliguria, treat with IV fluids and diuresis (mannitol or furosemide). Massive transfusions may result in a bleeding diathesis from dilutional thrombocytopenia and citrate (a calcium chelator found in transfused blood; calcium is required for proper coagulation). Look for oozing from puncture or IV sites. The patient also may have hyperkalemia.

CASE SCENARIO: A 52-year-old man receives a transfusion for severe anemia due to a GI bleed. He develops chills, fever, and low back pain during the transfusion. What should you do? The first step is to stop the transfusion. Next, have the lab check to make sure that no clerical error or blood mix-up occurred while you monitor the patient and his urine output.

Coagulation

Disseminated intravascular coagulation (DIC) is most commonly due to *pregnancy* or obstetric complications (50%), *malignancy* (33%), *sepsis,* or *trauma* (especially head trauma, prostate surgery, and snake bites). DIC usually manifests with bleeding diathesis. Look for the classic *oozing or bleeding from puncture or IV sites.* However, it also may be associated with thrombotic tendencies. Look for prolonged prothrombin time (PT), partial thromboplastin time (PTT), and bleeding time (BT); positive D-dimer test; increased fibrin degradation products; thrombocytopenia; decreased fibrin; decreased clotting factors; and schistocytes. Treat the underlying cause (e.g., evacuate the uterus, give antibiotics). Patients may need transfusions/FFP or, rarely, heparin if thrombosis occurs.

Thrombophilia (tendency to form clots: see Table 3-24). Consider and test if thrombosis occurs in patients younger than age 50, is recurrent, is in an unusual location or with pregnancy/OCP. Treat the current episode with anticoagulant therapy to prevent further thrombosis and pulmonary embolism and prescribe long-term (life-long with significant inherited abnormalities) prophylaxis with anticoagulant therapy.

TABLE 3-24 Thrombophilias

	PREVALENCE	ARTERIAL OR VENOUS THROMBOSIS	RELATIVE RISK OF THROMBOSIS
Factor V Leiden (activated protein C resistance)	5% of whites; rare in nonwhites	Venous	Heterozygous: 5 Homozygous: 80
Prothrombin G20210A mutation	3% of whites; rare in nonwhites	Venous	3
Antiphospholipid antibody syndrome	1-2%	Venous + arterial (miscarriages)	8
Antithrombin III deficiency	0.02%	Venous	35
Protein C deficiency	0.3%	Venous	11
Protein S deficiency	0.05%	Venous	8
Hyperhomocysteinemia	6%	Venous + arterial	3

Antiphospholipid antibody syndrome requires the presence of a lupus anticoagulant or anticardiolipin antibodies to be present on two occasions at least 12 weeks apart.

Clotting tests: Use PT for extrinsic system (prolonged by warfarin), PTT for intrinsic system (prolonged by heparin), and bleeding time (BT) for platelet function (Table 3-25).

TABLE 3-25 Clotting Tests

DISEASE	PT	PTT	BT	PLATELET COUNT	RBC COUNT	OTHER
von Willebrand disease	Normal	High	High	Normal	Normal	Autosomal dominant (look for family history)
Hemophilia A/B	Normal	High	Normal	Normal	Normal	X-linked recessive; A = low factor 8; B = low factor 9
DIC	High	High	High	Low	Normal/low	Appropriate history, factor 8 level low
Liver failure	High	High	Normal	Normal/low	Normal/low	Jaundice, normal level of factor 8, do not give vitamin K (ineffective)
Heparin	Normal	High	Normal	Normal/low	Normal	Watch for thrombocytopenia/ thrombosis
Warfarin	High	Normal	Normal	Normal	Normal	Vitamin K antagonist (factors 2, 7, 9, and 10)
ITP	Normal	Normal	High	Low	Normal	Watch for preceding URI
TTP	Normal	Normal	High	Low	Low	Hemolysis, CNS symptoms; treat with plasmapheresis; do not give platelets
Scurvy	Normal	Normal	Normal	Normal	Normal	Fingernail and gum hemorrhages, bone hemorrhages

BT, bleeding time; *CNS,* central nervous system; *DIC,* disseminated intravascular coagulation; *ITP,* idiopathic thrombocytopenic purpura; *PT,* prothrombin time; *PTT,* partial thromboplastin time; *RBC,* red blood cell; *TTP,* thrombotic thrombocytopenic purpura; *URI,* upper respiratory infection.

📁 **CASE SCENARIO:** A 72-year-old man who eats "hot dogs and soda" for every meal complains of bleeding gums and muscle pain. On exam, you notice petechiae and splinter hemorrhages under his fingernails. Platelets and coagulation studies are normal. The patient takes no medications. What does the patient have? Vitamin C deficiency (scurvy). Treat with oral vitamin C (check level first to confirm diagnosis) and diet counseling.

IMMUNOLOGY AND INFECTIOUS DISEASE

Hypersensitivity reactions

1. **Type 1:** Immediate hypersensitivity reaction. Due to preformed IgE antibodies that cause release of vasoactive amines (e.g., histamine, leukotrienes) from mast cells and basophils. Examples are *anaphylaxis* (bee stings, food allergy [especially peanuts and shellfish], medications [especially penicillin and sulfa drugs], rubber glove allergy); *atopy; hay fever; urticarial;* allergic rhinitis; and some forms of asthma.

   ❍ With chronic type 1 hypersensitivity (atopy, some forms of asthma, allergic rhinitis), look for *eosinophilia,* elevated IgE levels, family history, and seasonal exacerbations. Patients also may have allergic "shiners" (bilateral infraorbital edema) and a transverse nasal crease (from frequent nose rubbing). Pale, bluish, edematous nasal turbinates with many eosinophils in clear, watery nasal secretions are also classic.

   ❍ Treat acute reactions immediately by securing the airway, if necessary. Laryngeal edema may prevent intubation, in which case a cricothyrotomy should be performed. Give *epinephrine and diphenhydramine.* Corticosteroids are not useful for acute episodes but are often given to prevent recurrence.

   ❍ Watch for *C1 esterase inhibitor (complement) deficiency* as a cause for hereditary angioedema. Patients have diffuse swelling of lips, eyelids, and possibly the airway, unrelated to any allergen exposure. The disorder is inherited in an autosomal dominant pattern; look for a family history.

C4 complement levels are low. Treat acutely as for anaphylaxis. Androgens are used for long-term treatment to increase liver production of C1 esterase inhibitor.

📁 **CASE SCENARIO:** What drug should be avoided in patients with asthma and nasal polyps? Aspirin, which may precipitate a severe asthmatic attack.

📁 **CASE SCENARIO:** What can be done if you suspect an allergy but are not sure of the trigger? Skin testing.

2. **Type 2:** cytotoxic. Due to preformed IgG and IgM, which react with antigen and cause secondary inflammation. Examples are *autoimmune hemolytic anemia* (classic causes are methyldopa or penicillin/sulfas) or other cytopenias caused by antibodies (e.g., ITP), *transfusion reactions,* erythroblastosis fetalis (Rh incompatibility), *Goodpasture syndrome* (watch for linear immunofluorescence on kidney biopsy), myasthenia gravis, Graves disease, pernicious anemia, pemphigus, and hyperacute transplant rejection (as soon as the anastomosis is made at transplant surgery, the transplanted organ deteriorates in front of your eyes).

📁 **CASE SCENARIO:** What test can be used to screen for suspected antibody-mediated hemolytic anemia? The Coombs test (direct antiglobulin test [DAT]).

3. **Type 3:** immune complex-mediated. Due to antigen-antibody complexes that are usually deposited in blood vessels and cause an inflammatory response. Examples are *serum sickness, lupus* and other autoimmune disorders, chronic hepatitis, cryoglobulinemia, and posttreptococcal glomerulonephritis.
4. **Type 4:** cell-mediated (delayed). Due to sensitized T lymphocytes that release inflammatory mediators. Examples are the *purified protein derivative (PPD) TB skin test; contact dermatitis* (especially poison ivy, nickel earrings, cosmetics, and topical medications); chronic transplant rejection; and *granulomatous diseases* (e.g., sarcoidosis).

HIV infection and AIDS

Initial seroconversion may manifest as a mononucleosis-type syndrome (fever, malaise, pharyngitis, rash, lymphadenopathy). Keep in the back of your mind as a consideration in the differential diagnosis for any sore throat or EBV-type presentation.

📁 **CASE SCENARIO:** How do you make the diagnosis of HIV infection? First order an enzyme-linked immunosorbent assay (ELISA); positive results should be confirmed with a Western blot test. If Western blot is positive, repeat with a new specimen to confirm. If Western blot is "indeterminate," repeat in 1 month. Do all tests before you tell the patient anything definitive!

📁 **CASE SCENARIO:** How long does it take for the HIV test to become positive once a person contracts the virus? Generally, it takes at least 1 month for antibodies to develop. If a patient presents because of specific recent risk-taking behavior and wants testing, you should retest the patient in 6 months if the initial test is negative.

📁 **CASE SCENARIO:** Once the diagnosis of HIV infection is made, how often should you check the CD4$^+$ count? Every 3–4 months.

📁 **CASE SCENARIO:** What HIV test should be ordered in a newborn? HIV proviral DNA polymerase chain reaction (PCR) testing. Conventional serologic testing is useless because maternal antibodies may persist for up to 9 months.

📁 **CASE SCENARIO:** When should you start antiretroviral therapy? All patients with AIDS-defining illness, pregnant patients, and when the CD4$^+$ count falls below 350/µL^3 (or sooner!).

AIDS-defining illnesses:
1. Candidiasis
2. Coccidioidomycosis
3. Cryptococcosis
4. Cryptosporidiosis

5. Cytomegalovirus (CMV) infection
6. Encephalopathy
7. Herpes simplex
8. Histoplasmosis
9. Isosporiasis
10. Kaposi sarcoma
11. Burkitt lymphoma and other types of lymphomas
12. *Mycobacterium* (*tuberculosis*, *avium* complex, *kansasii*) infections
13. *Pneumocystis jirovecii* pneumonia
14. Progressive multifocal leukoencephalopathy
15. *Salmonella* septicemia
16. Toxoplasmosis of the brain
17. Wasting syndrome due to HIV infection?
18. Cervical cancer
19. Pneumonia, recurrent
20. For children <13 years: recurrent bacterial infections and lymphoid interstitial pneumonia

▢ **CASE SCENARIO:** When should you start prophylaxis for *P. jirovecii* pneumonia (PCP)? When the CD4$^+$? count is <200/μL^3. What drug should you give for PCP prophylaxis? TMP-SMX. Use dapsone or pentamidine if the patient is allergic to TMP-SMX.

▢ **CASE SCENARIO:** When should you start prophylaxis for toxoplasmosis? When the CD4$^+$ count is <100/μL^3. Prophylaxis should begin when the CD4$^+$ count is <200/μL^3 if an opportunistic infection or malignancy develops. What drug should you give for prophylaxis? TMP-SMX if the patient is not already on it for PCP prophylaxis.

▢ **CASE SCENARIO:** When should you start prophylaxis for *Mycobactrium avium* infection (MAI)? When the CD4$^+$ count is <50 μL^3. What drug should you use for MAI prophylaxis? Azithromycin or clarithromycin. Also consider prophylaxis against *Candida* and *Cryptococcus* with fluconazole at this level. Consider prophylaxis against CMV with oral ganciclovir in patients with evidence of previous CMV infection to reduce invasive disease.

▢ **CASE SCENARIO:** Below what CD4$^+$ count is an HIV-seropositive person said to have AIDS even if he or she is asymptomatic? Below 200/μL^3.

▢ **CASE SCENARIO:** What is the only live vaccine given to HIV-positive patients? Measles, mumps, rubella (MMR).

▢ **CASE SCENARIO:** What are the two classic malignancies in patients with AIDS? Kaposi sarcoma and non-Hodgkin lymphoma (especially primary CNS B-cell lymphomas).

▢ **CASE SCENARIO:** AIDS plus a positive India ink preparation of the cerebrospinal fluid (CSF) indicates what infection? *Cryptococcus neoformans*.

▢ **CASE SCENARIO:** AIDS plus ring-enhancing lesions in the brain indicates which infection? *Toxoplasma* (or cysticercosis/*Taenia solium* in Latin American patients). Lymphoma is also usually in the differential for this finding in AIDS patients, however. Usually treated as presumptive toxoplasmosis and if the patient does not get better, think of other causes.

▢ **CASE SCENARIO:** What is the treatment of choice for CMV retinitis? Valganciclovir (foscarnet and cidofovir are second-line agents).

▢ **CASE SCENARIO:** What two protozoal causes of diarrhea are fairly unique to patients with AIDS? *Cryptosporidium* and *Isospora* spp.

▢ **CASE SCENARIO:** Should HIV-positive mothers be allowed to breast-feed? No. The virus can be transmitted through breast milk.

HIV sequelae include wasting syndrome (progressive weight loss), dementia, peripheral neuropathies, thrombocytopenia, and loss of delayed hypersensitivity (type 4) on skin testing (also known as *anergy*).

In any patient with AIDS and pneumonia, think of PCP first (although community-acquired pneumonia is more common). Look for severe hypoxia with normal-appearing x-ray or *diffuse, bilateral interstitial infiltrates.* Usually the patient has a dry, nonproductive cough.

You may be able to detect PCP with silver stains (Wright-Giemsa, Giemsa, or methenamine silver) after induced sputum; if not, bronchoscopy with bronchoalveolar lavage and brush biopsy can be used to make the diagnosis. In the correct clinical setting, patients are often treated empirically without securing a diagnosis.

Any adult patient with thrush should raise suspicion of HIV, leukemia, or diabetes, and any young adult who presents with herpes zoster should raise suspicion of HIV.

To prevent HIV transmission to infants, give a standard three-drug, highly active antiretroviral therapy (HAART) regimen to HIV-positive women in order to reduce the in utero transmission of HIV. Therapy is started either immediately or after completion of the first trimester. Efavirenz should be avoided in the first trimester. Give the infant AZT (or other antiretroviral) for 6 weeks after delivery. Cesarean section may also reduce transmission. The infant may have a positive HIV antibody test for 6–12 months because of maternal antibodies. Can check DNA or RNA PCR test (or culture) to detect HIV directly in such infants.

Standard treatment involves a three-drug regimen with two nucleoside/nucleotide reverse transcriptase inhibitors (nRTIs) and a nonnucleoside reverse transcriptase inhibitor (NNRTI) or a protease inhibitor (PI). One common regimen consists of zidovudine (AZT), lamivudine (3TC), and efavirenz. For postexposure prophylaxis after contact with an HIV-positive patient, the Centers for Disease Control and Prevention (CDC) recommends a two-drug nRTI regimen for less severe exposure and a standard three-drug regimen for more severe exposure.

Antibiotic therapy

Empiric therapy while awaiting culture and sensitivity results is summarized in Table 3-26.

TABLE 3-26 Summary of Empiric Therapy for Suspected HIV Infection Pending Definitive Diagnosis

CONDITION	MAIN ORGANISM(S)	EMPIRIC ANTIBIOTIC(S)
Bronchitis	Virus, *Haemophilus influenzae, Moraxella* spp.	Typically not recommended in acute bronchitis due to viral etiology in most cases. If COPD or severe exacerbation of chronic bronchitis, use a macrolide or doxycycline
Cellulitis	Streptococci, staphylococci	Cephalexin or dicloxacillin. Use trimethoprim-sulfamethoxazole, doxycycline, or clindamycin if MRSA is suspected
Endocarditis	Staphylococci, streptococci	Vancomycin + gentamicin
Meningitis (child or adult)	*Streptococcus pneumoniae, Neisseria meningitidis**	Ceftriaxone or cefotaxime + vancomycin
Meningitis (neonate)	group B streptococci, *Escherichia coli, Listeria* spp.	Ampicillin + aminoglycoside, third-generation cephalosporin that enters the CSF (cefotaxime)
Osteomyelitis	*Staphylococcus aureus, Salmonella* spp.	Oxacillin, cefazolin, vancomycin
Pneumonia (atypical)	*Mycoplasma, Chlamydia* spp.	Macrolid antibiotic, doxycycline
Pneumonia (classic)	*S. pneumoniae, H. influenzae*	Azithromycin ± third generation cephalosporin
Gonococci	Antistaphylococcal penicillin, vancomycin	Ceftriaxone or cefotaxime
Sepsis	Gram-negative organisms, streptococci, staphylococci	Third-generation cephalosporin or penicillin + gentamicin
Urinary tract infection	*E. coli*	Trimethoprim-sulfamethoxazole, amoxicillin, nitrofurantoin, quinolone

**H. influenzae* type b is no longer as common a cause of meningitis in children because of widespread vaccination. In a child with no history of immunization, *H. influenzae* is the most likely cause of meningitis.
†Examples: dicloxacillin, methicillin, nafcillin.
‡Think of staphylococci if the patient is monogamous or not sexually active. Think of gonorrhea for younger adults who are sexually active.
COPD, Chronic obstructive pulmonary disease; *CSF,* cerebrospinal fluid; *MRSA,* methicillin-resistant *Staphylococcus aureus.*

Empiric antibiotics of choice for different organisms are summarized in Table 3-27

TABLE 3-27 Summary of Empiric Antibiotics of Choice for Different Bugs*

BUG	ANTIBIOTIC	OTHER CHOICES
Bacteroides spp.	Metronidazole	Clindamycin
Borrelia spp.	Doxycycline (not recommended for children younger than 8 yr of age or pregnant or lactating women), amoxicillin, cefuroxime	Erythromycin
Chlamydia spp.	Azithromycin, doxycycline	Erythromycin, fluoroquinolone
Enterococci	Penicillin or ampicillin + aminoglycoside	Vancomycin + aminoglycoside
Escherichia coli	Third-generation cephalosporin, fluoroquinolone	Aminoglycoside
Gonococcus†	Ceftriaxone plus either doxycycline or azithromycin (to also cover asymptomatic chlamydial infection)	
Haemophilus spp.	Second- or third-generation cephalosporin	Ampicillin
Klebsiella spp.	Third-generation cephalosporin, fluoroquinolone	Third-generation penicillin + aminoglycoside
Meningococcus	Cefotaxime or ceftriaxone	Penicillin G if proven to be penicillin susceptible
Myobacterium tuberculosis	Isoniazide + rifampin + pyrazinamide + ethambutol	
Mycoplasma spp.	Macrolide	Doxycycline, levofloxacin, moxifloxacin
Pseudomonas spp.	Extended spectrum penicillin (ticarcillin or piperacillin) + aminoglycoside	Ceftazidime, cefipime, aztreonam, imipenem, ciprofloxacin
Streptococci A or B	Penicillin, cephazolin	Erythromycin
Treponema spp.	Penicillin	Doxycycline
Streptococcus pneumoniae	Third-generation cephalosporin	Fluoroquinolone
Staphylococci	Antistaphylococcal penicillin	Vancomycin (MRSA)

*Always use culture and sensitivity testing to guide therapy if available.
†With genital infections, treat for presumed *Chlamydia* coinfection with azithromycin or doxycycline.
MRSA, Methicillin-resistant *S. aureus.*

Tuberculosis

Important tuberculosis points:

1. The PPD (purified protein derivative) skin test is an intradermal injection given in the forearm, and the skin is assessed for diameter of induration at 48–72 hours after injection. Test is considered positive if:
   ○ >5 mm:
     ○ HIV infection or HIV risk factors
     ○ Close recent contact with active TB case
     ○ Those with chest radiograph suggesting prior TB
   ○ >10 mm:
     ○ Immigrants from high-prevalence areas—Asia, Africa, Latin America
     ○ Medically underserved low-income populations—Native Americans, Hispanics, Blacks
     ○ IV drug abusers
     ○ Health care workers, institutionalized persons
   ○ >15 mm:
     ○ All others
2. A two-step PPD is used to detect individuals with past TB infection and help improve detection of false negatives. If the initial PPD is negative, a second PPD is performed 1–3 weeks after the first one.
3. Perform sputum cultures and chest radiographs in patients with positive skin tests or suspected false-negative skin test.
4. If the patient is noncompliant, directly observed therapy (someone watches the patient take medications every day) is recommended.
5. Watch for liver dysfunction in patients on therapy.

6. Consider supplementation with vitamin B$_6$ (pyridoxine) for patients on isoniazid, and watch for signs of deficiency.
7. Multidrug-resistant TB is an increasing problem and requires the addition of a fourth (and sometimes fifth) drug, usually streptomycin or ethambutol, when treating active TB until sensitivities are known.

Tuberculosis therapy: see Table 3-28

TABLE 3-28 Summary of Tuberculosis Therapy

CLINICAL SETTING/FINDING	TREATMENT
Exposed adult with negative PPD test	None
Exposed child <5 yr old with negative PPD test	Isoniazid (INH) for 3 mo, then repeat the PPD test
Prophylaxis for PPD conversion (negative to positive) with no active disease or positive skin test of unknown duration	INH for 9 mo
Acute pulmonary disease/positive culture	4-drug regimen with INH/rifampin/pyrazinamide/ethambutol for 2 mo, then INH/rifampin for 4 mo in most patients

PPD, Purified protein derivative.

Streptococcal and staphylococcal infections

Skin infections often occur after a break in the skin due to trauma, scabies, or an insect bite. Watch for development of poststreptococcal glomerulonephritis.

1. **Impetigo:** maculopapules to vesicopustules or bullae to *honey-colored, crusted lesions.* Staphylococci are a more common cause than streptococci. Definitely think of staphylococci if a *furuncle* or *carbuncle* is present; if glomerulonephritis develops, think of streptococci. Impetigo is contagious: Look for sick contacts. Treat empirically with antistaphylococcal penicillin (e.g., dicloxacillin) to cover both organisms.
2. **Erysipelas:** a superficial cellulitis that is red, shiny, swollen, and tender. It may be associated with vesicles or bullae, fever, and lymphadenopathy. Treat with an antistaphylococcal penicillin (dicloxacillin) or cefazolin.
3. **Cellulitis:** involves subcutaneous tissues (deeper than erysipelas). Streptoccoci are the most common cause, but staphylococci also may be implicated. Treat empirically with antistaphylococcal penicillin or vancomycin to cover both. Other causes:
   ○ *Pseudomonas* spp. (diabetic patients with foot ulcers, burns, severe trauma): treat with broad-spectrum, "big-gun" antibiotics.
   ○ *Pasteurella multocida* (after dog/cat bites): treat with ampicillin.
   ○ *Vibrio vulnificus* (fishermen or other salt-water exposure): treat with tetracycline.
4. **Necrotizing fasciitis:** progression of cellulitis to necrosis and gangrene, crepitus, and systemic toxicity (tachycardia, fever, hypotension). Multiple organisms (aerobes and anaerobes) are often involved. Treat with intravenous fluids, debridement, hyperbaric oxygen, and broad-spectrum antibiotics.
5. **Endometritis** and puerperal fever usually result from streptococcal infection and cause postpartum fever and uterine tenderness. Treat with clindamycin + gentamicin.
6. *Streptococcus viridans:* causes subacute endocarditis and dental caries (*Streptococcus mutans*).
7. *Enterococcus faecalis:* normal bowel flora; causes endocarditis, urinary tract infection, and sepsis.
8. *S. pneumoniae:* common cause of pneumonia, otitis media, meningitis, sinusitis, and sepsis.
9. *Staphylococcus aureus* is a common cause of abscess (especially in the breast after breast-feeding or in the skin after a furuncle); *endocarditis* (especially in drug users); *osteomyelitis* (most common cause); *septic arthritis;* food poisoning (preformed toxin); *toxic shock syndrome* (preformed toxin; classically a woman who leaves a tampon in place too long and develops hypotension, fever, and rash that desquamates) (Fig. 3-30); scalded skin syndrome (preformed toxin, affects younger children who often start with impetigo, which then desquamates); impetigo; cellulitis; wound infections; pneumonia (often forms lung abscess/empyema); and furuncle/carbuncle. Health care workers who are chronic nasal carriers may cause nosocomial infections; treat carriers with

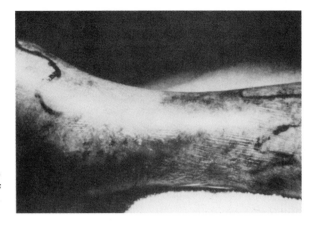

FIGURE 3-30 Skin desquamation secondary to toxic shock syndrome. *(From Cunha BA: Infectious Disease Pearls. Philadelphia, Hanley & Belfus, 1999.)*

antibiotics. Treat patients with an antistaphylococcal penicillin or vancomycin; abscesses require surgical drainage.

10. *Staphylococcus epidermidis:* causes IV catheter infections, infections of prosthetic implants (heart valves, vascular grafts), and sepsis. Treat empirically with antistaphylococcal penicillin or vancomycin.

11. *Staphylococcus saprophyticus:* causes urinary tract infections.

Miscellaneous infections

Endocarditis can either be *acute* (fulminant, most commonly caused by *S. aureus*) or *subacute* (insidious onset, most commonly caused by viridans streptococci). Look for general signs of infection (e.g., fever, tachycardia, malaise) plus *new-onset heart murmur;* embolic phenomena (stroke and other infarcts); *Osler nodes* (painful palpable nodules on tips of fingers); *Roth spots* (round retinal hemorrhages with white centers); *Janeway lesions* (*nontender,* erythematous lesions on palms and soles); *splinter hemorrhages* (small, asymptomatic linear hemorrhages under the nails); and septic shock (more dramatic with acute than with subacute disease). The diagnosis is made by blood cultures, and empiric treatment is begun until culture results are known.

○ Native heart valves or IV drug users: vancomycin (combination therapies are also sometimes used) is the agent of choice for empiric treatment until the exact etiology is identified. With methicillin-resistant *S. aureus* (MRSA): vancomycin.

○ Prosthetic heart valves or native heart valves allergic to penicillin: vancomycin + gentamicin + either cefepime or a carbapenem.

○ If HACEK organism: ceftriaxone, ampicillin-sulbactam, or ciprofloxacin.

○ If *S. viridans:* penicillin G or ceftriaxone (if penicillin-susceptible) with or without gentamicin

 People more likely to be affected include IV drug abusers (who classically develop right-sided valve lesions); patients with abnormal heart valves (prosthetic valves, rheumatic valvular disease, congenital heart defects); and postoperative patients (especially after genitourinary, gastrointestinal, or dental surgery–hence the recommendation for prophylaxis in susceptible people).

☐ **CASE SCENARIO:** If a patient has a secundum atrial septal defect (the more common type) or mitral valve prolapse, do you need to give endocarditis prophylaxis? No. The exception is patients with mitral valve prolapse who have an audible murmur (uncommon); consider prophylaxis in such patients.

Rabies is usually due to bites from bats, skunks, raccoons, or foxes in the United States (vaccination has eliminated dog rabies). The incubation period is usually around 1–2 months. The classic manifestations are hydrophobia and CNS signs (paralysis). After a bite, several steps should be taken:

1. **Local wound treatment.** Cleanse thoroughly with soap, and do not cauterize or suture the wound.

2. **Observe the animal.** If possible, capture and observe a dog or cat to see if it develops rabies. If a wild animal (bats, skunks, raccoons, foxes) is caught, it should be killed and the tissue should be examined for rabies.

3. **Prophylaxis and vaccination** with rabies immune globulin and rabies vaccine:
   ○ If a captured or killed animal has rabies, definitely give prophylaxis and vaccine.
   ○ If a wild animal (bats, skunks, raccoons, and foxes only) bites and escapes, give prophylaxis and vaccine.
   ○ If a dog or cat bites and escapes, do not give prophylaxis or vaccine unless the animal acted strangely and/or bit the patient without provocation and rabies is prevalent in the area (very rare).
   ○ Do not give prophylaxis or vaccine for bites by a rabbit or rodent (rats, mice, squirrels, chipmunks).

   Syphilis: Screen with Venereal Disease Research Laboratory (VDRL) or rapid plasmin reagin (RPR) test. If the result is positive, confirm with the fluorescent treponemal antibody, absorbed test (FTA-ABS) or the microhemagglutination-*Treponema pallidum* test (MHA-TP). *T. pallidum* can be seen with darkfield microscopy but not with Gram stain. Screen all pregnant women with VDRL/RPR. Treat with penicillin; use doxycycline or tetracycline in penicillin-allergic patients. Jarisch-Herxheimer reaction (fever, myalgia, tachycardia, hypotension) may occur within 24 hours of treatment. Notify partners and treat.

   Three stages are listed below:

1. **Primary:** Look for painless chancre (typically appears as a superficial ulcer with indurated, raised edges and a yellow base) that resolves on its own within 8 weeks.
2. **Secondary:** roughly 6 weeks to 18 months after infection. Look for condylomata lata, maculopapular rash (especially involving the palms of the hands and soles of the feet), and lymphadenopathy (Fig. 3-31). Between secondary and tertiary stages is the *latent phase*, in which the disease is quiet and asymptomatic.
3. **Tertiary:** occurs years after initial infection. Look for *gummas* (granulomas in many different organs); neurologic symptoms and signs (neurosyphilis, Argyll Robertson pupil, dementia, paresis, tabes dorsalis, Charcot joints); and/or thoracic aortic aneurysms.

🔲 **CASE SCENARIO:** What is the classic disease that can cause a false-positive result on the VDRL or RPR test? Lupus erythematosus.

Classic case scenarios and word associations
○ Elderly person with community-acquired, typical pneumonia: *S. pneumoniae*
○ Lung infection in a patient with cystic fibrosis: *Pseudomonas* spp., *S. aureus*

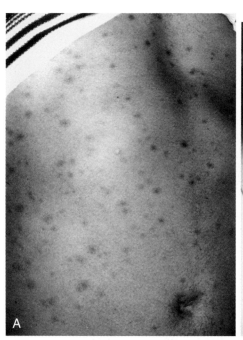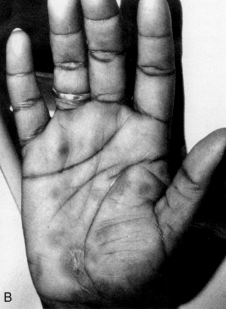

FIGURE 3-31 Syphiloderm of secondary syphilis. **A,** Hyperpigmented macules of secondary syphilis. The patient initially presented with a genital ulcer that was treated as chancroid. Note the strong similiarity of these lesions to pityriasis rosea. **B,** Characteristic papulosquamous lesions of secondary syphilis on the palm. *(From Fitzpatrick FE, Aeling JL: Dermatology Secrets. Philadelphia, Hanley & Belfus, 1996.)*

○ Atypical pneumonia in a college student: *Mycoplasma* spp. (positive cold-agglutinin titer), *Chlamydia* spp.

○ Lung infection in a child younger than 1 year: respiratory syncytial virus (RSV)

○ Lung infection in a person with AIDS: *Pneumocystis jirovecii*

○ Patient stuck with a thorn or gardening: *Sporothrix schenkii* (Fig. 3-32). Treat with itraconazole or fluconazole.

○ Aplastic crisis in sickle cell disease/other hemoglobinopathy: parvovirus B19

○ Sepsis after splenectomy (or autosplenectomy in sickle cell disease): *S. pneumoniae, Haemophilus influenzae, Neisseria meningitidis* (encapsulated organisms)

○ Pneumonia in the southwest (California, Arizona): *Coccidioides imitis.* Treat with itraconazole or fluconazole (use amphotericin B if severe).

○ Pneumonia after cave exploring (or exposure to bird droppings) in Ohio and Mississippi River valleys: *Histoplasma capsulatum*

○ Pneumonia after being around a parrot or exotic bird: *Chlamydia psittaci*

○ Fungus ball or hemoptysis after tuberculosis cavitary disease: *Aspergillus* spp.

○ Pneumonia in a patient with silicosis: tuberculosis

○ Diarrhea after hiking or drinking from a stream: *Giardia lamblia*

○ Pregnant women with cats: *Toxoplasma gondii*

○ Vitamin B_{12} deficiency and abdominal symptoms: *Diphyllobothrium latum*

○ Seizures with ring-enhancing brain lesion(s) on CT or MRI: *Taenia solium* (cysticercosis) or toxoplasmosis

○ Bladder cancer (squamous cell) in Middle East and Africa: *Schistosoma hematobium*

○ Worm infection in infants: *Enterobius* spp. (positive tape test, perianal itching)

○ Fever, muscle pain, eosinophilia, and periorbital edema after eating raw meat: *Trichinella spiralis* (trichinosis)

○ Gastroenteritis in infants/young children: rotavirus

○ Food poisoning after eating reheated rice: *Bacillus cereus*

○ Food poisoning after eating raw seafood: *Vibrio parahemolyticus*

○ Diarrhea after traveling to Mexico: *E. coli* (Montezuma's revenge)

○ Diarrhea after antibiotics: *Clostridium difficile* (treat with oral metronidazole or vancomycin)

○ Infant paralyzed after eating honey: *Clostridium botulinum* (toxin blocks acetylcholine release)

○ Genital lesions in children in the absence of sexual abuse or activity: molluscum contagiosum virus

○ Cellulitis from cat or dog bites: *Pasteurella multocida* (treat significant cat and dog bites with prophylactic ampicillin)

○ Slaughterhouse worker with fever: *Brucella* spp.

○ Pneumonia after being in a hotel or near air conditioner or water tower: *Legionella pneumophila* (treat with azithromycin or fluoroquinolone)

○ Burn wound infection with blue-green color: *Pseudomonas* spp. (*S. aureus* is also common but is not associated with a blue-green color)

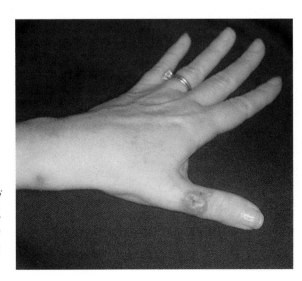

FIGURE 3-32 Sporotrichosis. *Sporothrix schenckii* is a dimorphic fungus that classically spreads via the lymphatics that can lead to lesion development in a linear manner along the lymphatic drainage pathway of the limb, as shown. *(From Bolognia JL, Jorizzo JL, Rapini RP, et al: Dermatology, 2nd ed. Philadelphia, Mosby, 2008.)*

Staining hints

- ❍ Gram-positive organisms: blue/purple; gram-negative organisms: red (as seen on a slide)
- ❍ Gram-positive cocci in chains = streptococci
- ❍ Gram-positive cocci in clusters = staphylococci
- ❍ Gram-positive cocci in pairs (diplococci) = *S. pneumoniae*
- ❍ Gram-negative coccobacilli (small rods) = *Haemophilus* spp.
- ❍ Gram-negative diplococci = *Neisseria* spp. (urethritis, septic arthritis, meningitis) or *Moraxella* spp. (lungs, sinusitis)
- ❍ Gram-negative rod that is plump and has thick capsule ("mucoid" appearance) = *Klebsiella* spp.
- ❍ Gram-positive rods that form spores = *Clostridium, Bacillus* spp. (food poisoning from reheated rice)
- ❍ Pseudohyphae = *Candida* spp.
- ❍ Acid-fast organisms = *Mycobacterium, Nocardia* spp.
- ❍ Gram-positive with sulfur granules = *Actinomyces* spp. (pelvic inflammatory disease in women who use intrauterine devices; rare cause of neck mass or cervical adenitis)
- ❍ Silver staining = *Pneumocystis jirovecii* and cat-scratch disease
- ❍ Positive India ink preparation (with thick capsule) = *Cryptococcus* spp. (Fig. 3-33)

 Spirochete = Treponema, Leptospira spp. (both seen only on darkfield microscopy), Borrelia spp. (seen with regular light microscope).

NEPHROLOGY

Acute renal failure (also known as acute kidney injury)

Look for a progressive rise in *serum creatinine* and *BUN*, metabolic acidosis, *hyperkalemia*, and often hypervolemia (pulmonary rales, elevated jugular venous pressure, dilutional hyponatremia, peripheral edema). Three categories to think about are as follows:

1. **Prerenal (most common):** hypovolemia (dehydration, hemorrhage), cardiac/"pump" failure, renovascular hypertension. Look for *BUN-to-creatinine ratio ≥15–20*. Patients usually have signs of hypovolemia (e.g., tachycardia, weak pulse) or congestive heart failure. Give IV fluids and/or blood (if needed) for hypovolemia and diuretics (e.g., furosemide) for heart failure. Other causes are sepsis (treat the sepsis and give IV fluids) and liver failure (hepatorenal syndrome; treat supportively).

   📁 **CASE SCENARIO:** A 45-year-old man has a massive heart attack and develops renal failure. How might the two conditions be related? If the massive heart attack caused heart failure (not uncommon), it would result in inadequate perfusion of the kidneys and cause prerenal kidney failure. Digitalis/dobutamine and diuretics may reverse the renal failure by optimizing cardiac function.

2. **Postrenal:** The classic cause is *BPH*. Watch for a man older than age 50 with symptoms of BPH (hesitancy, dribbling) and anuria; hydronephrosis is seen bilaterally on ultrasound. Treat with

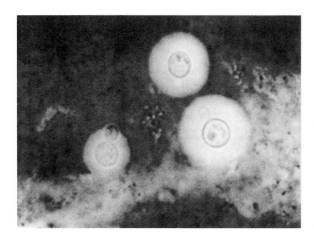

Figure 3-33 Positive India ink preparation of the cerebrospinal fluid in a patient with cryptococcal meningitis. Note the rounding of the yeast, which is classically budding. *(From Cunha BA: Infectious Disease Pearls. Philadelphia, Hanley & Belfus, 1999.)*

catheterization (suprapubic catheterization, if necessary) to relieve the obstruction and prevent further renal damage. Then consider surgery (transurethral resection of the prostate [TURP]).

📁 **CASE SCENARIO:** A patient has a left ureteral calculus and acute renal failure with no history of kidney disease. Did the stone cause renal failure? No—not unless the patient had bilateral ureteral stones or a bladder neck stone. A unilateral ureteral stone does not usually cause failure because the other kidney, if normal, picks up the slack (unless the patient has only a single kidney).

3. **Intrarenal:** *acute tubular necrosis* is the most common type. Examples of renal causes:
   ○ IV contrast: be careful in patients with diabetes and/or renal disease, as you may precipitate renal failure. Consider prehydrating the patient with IV fluids if contrast is necessary. Discontinue metformin before scanning in high-risk patients.
   ○ Lupus erythematosus: look for malar rash, arthritis, and other typical features. Renal failure is a major cause of morbidity and mortality in patients with lupus.
   ○ Toxins/medications: chronic NSAID use can cause *papillary necrosis* or acute tubular necrosis. Other implicated drugs include chemotherapy drugs (cyclosporine), HIV drugs (ritonavir), antibiotics *(aminoglycosides),* ACE inhibitors, cimetidine, and methicillin.
   ○ Mnemonic for causes of papillary necrosis: pyelonephritis, obstruction, sickle cell disease, tuberculosis, cirrhosis, analgesics, diabetes, systemic vasculitis (POSTCARDS).
   ○ Goodpasture syndrome: due to antiglomerular basement membrane antibodies *(linear IgG C3 immunofluorescence pattern* on renal biopsy with membranoproliferative glomerulonephritis), which also react with the lungs. Look for a young, white male smoker with hemoptysis, dyspnea, and renal failure. Eight percent are HLA-DR2–positive; look for a chest radiograph with diffuse alveolar disease. Treat acutely with plasma exchange, steroids (prednisone) and/or cyclophosphamide, and dialysis if renal failure is present.
   ○ Wegener granulomatosis also has lung and kidney involvement. Look for *sinonasal involvement* (bloody nose, nasal perforation, sinusitis) with necrotizing granulomatous lesions or hemoptysis and pleurisy as presenting symptoms. Patients have positive *antineutrophilic cytoplasmic antibody* (c-ANCA) titer. Kidney biopsy reveals crescentic glomerulonephritis with no immune deposits. Treat with cyclophosphamide. Other treatment aids include prednisone and TMP-SMX to prevent PCP, which can occur in 10% of patients.
   ○ Glomerulonephritis: The prototype is poststreptococcal disease; usually seen in children with a history of upper respiratory infection or streptococcal infection 1–3 weeks earlier. They present with edema, hypervolemia, hypertension, and hematuria/oliguria. *RBC casts* on urinalysis clinch the diagnosis. Kidney biopsy shows granular IgG C3 deposits. Treat supportively.

📁 **CASE SCENARIO:** A 22-year-old man comes into the emergency department with nausea and muscle pain after running a marathon in hot weather. His serum creatinine and BUN are high, but he has no history of renal failure. What is the cause of renal failure? What lab value goes with this condition? Rhabdomyolysis, which can result from strenuous exercise (e.g., marathon), alcohol, burns or muscle trauma, heat stroke, or neuroleptic malignant syndrome. Muscle breaks down and plugs up the renal filtration system. Look for very high levels of CK. Patients also may have myoglobinuria. Treat with hydration and diuretics.

In all cases of acute renal failure, dialysis may be required. Indications for dialysis include uremic encephalopathy, *pericarditis,* severe metabolic acidosis (roughly, pH <7.25), heart failure, and *hyperkalemia* severe enough to cause an arrhythmia.

📁 **CASE SCENARIO:** A 32-year-old thin woman with refractory hypertension is taking hydrochlorothiazide and metoprolol. A third drug, enalapril, is added and the patient develops a significant rise in creatinine shortly thereafter. What condition do you suspect as the cause of hypertension? Renal artery stenosis, probably due to fibromuscular dysplasia given the patient's age.

Chronic kidney disease

Basically, any of the disorders that cause acute renal failure can cause chronic kidney disease (CKD), also known as chronic renal failure (CRF) if the insult is severe or prolonged. Most cases of CKD are due to *diabetes* (number-one cause) or *hypertension* (many patients have both). Another fairly common cause is polycystic kidney disease. Look for multiple cysts in the kidney, family history (usually *autosomal dominant;* the autosomal recessive form presents in children), hypertension, hematuria, palpable renal masses, berry aneurysms in the circle of Willis, and cysts in the liver.

Metabolic derangements due to CKD:
1. Azotemia (high BUN/serum creatinine levels)
2. Metabolic acidosis
3. Hyperkalemia
4. Fluid retention (can cause hypertension, edema, heart failure, and pulmonary edema)
5. Hypocalcemia/hyperphosphatemia (impaired vitamin D production; bone loss leads to renal osteodystrophy)
6. Anemia due to lack of erythropoietin (synthetic erythropoietin may be given to correct the disorder)
7. Anorexia, nausea, and vomiting (from buildup of toxins)
8. CNS disturbances (mental status changes and even convulsions or coma from toxin buildup)
9. Bleeding (due to disordered platelet function)
10. Uremic pericarditis (*friction rub* may be heard on physical exam)
11. Skin pigmentation and pruritus (skin turns yellowish brown and itches due to metabolic byproducts)
12. Increased susceptibility to infection (due to impaired cellular immunity)

   Treatment: regular dialysis, water-soluble vitamins (removed during dialysis), phosphate restriction and phosphate binders (calcium carbonate), erythropoietin, and control of hypertension. The only cure is renal transplantation.

Urinary tract infection

Urinary tract infections (UTIs) in adults are much more common in women (by a 10–20:1 ratio). Most are caused by *E. coli;* other enteric organisms may also be implicated. Look for urinary *urgency, dysuria, suprapubic or low back pain,* and low-grade fever. The gold standard for diagnosis is urine culture. At the least, get a midstream urine sample; a catheterized sample or suprapubic tap is best (though rarely indicated in uncomplicated cases). Urinalysis shows white blood cells, bacteria, positive *leukocyte esterase,* and/or positive *nitrite.* Treatment can include TMP-SMX, amoxicillin, nitrofurantoin, or a first-generation cephalosporin for 3–10 days.

○ Some women get recurrent UTIs related to sexual activity and can be given antibiotics to take after intercourse.
○ Conditions that promote urinary stasis (enlarged prostate, pregnancy, stones, neurogenic bladder, vesicoureteral reflux) or bacterial colonization (indwelling catheter, fecal incontinence, surgical instrumentation) predispose to UTI. They also predispose to ascending UTI (pyelonephritis) and bacteremia/sepsis.
○ Pyelonephritis (Fig. 3-34) is also usually due to *E. coli.* The hallmark on physical exam is *costovertebral angle tenderness* with high fevers and shaking chills. Get blood and urine cultures. Most patients should be admitted to the hospital for inpatient treatment with intravenous antibiotics. If the patient does not improve within 48–72 hours, consider a CT scan to look for a renal abscess, which may need surgical drainage.

▭ **CASE SCENARIO:** An asymptomatic 40-year-old quadriplegic man with an indwelling urinary catheter has 3+ bacteriuria and 1+ WBCs in his urine on a routine urinalysis. Should you treat him? No. Asymptomatic bacteriuria is not treated, especially in chronically catheterized patients, who develop colonization and almost always have bacteria in the urine.

▭ **CASE SCENARIO:** On a routine urinalysis, a pregnant woman has 3+ bacteriuria on a midstream urine sample. She is asymptomatic and afebrile. Should you treat her? Yes. Asymptomatic bacteriuria has a high risk of progression to pyelonephritis in pregnancy. Use amoxicillin.

Other renal conditions

Nephrotic syndrome: Proteinuria (>3.5 g/day), hypoalbuminemia, edema (the classic example is morning periorbital edema), and hyperlipidemia/lipiduria. In children, nephrotic syndrome is usually due to *minimal change disease* (see loss of podocyte foot processes on electron microscopy), which is often postinfectious. Measure a 24-hour urine protein to clinch the diagnosis; treated with corticosteroids tapered over weeks with diuretics used if needed for fluid retention. Causes in adults include diabetes, hepatitis B, amyloidosis, lupus, and drugs (gold, penicillamine, captopril).

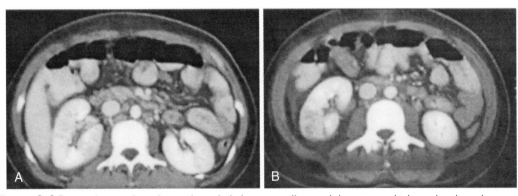

Figure 3-34 A and **B,** Pyelonephritis. The right kidney is swollen, and there are multiple wedge-shaped areas of decreased parenchymal enhancement. *(From Katz DS, Math KR, Groskin SA [eds]: Radiology Secrets. Philadelphia, Hanley & Belfus, 1998, p 187.)*

Nephritic syndrome: Oliguria, azotemia (rising BUN/creatinine), hypertension, and hematuria. Some proteinuria may be present, but not in the nephrotic range. Nephritic syndrome is classically due to poststreptococcal glomerulonephritis. Patients classically have *RBC casts* (a sign of glomerulonephritis).

NEUROLOGY

Delirium and dementia

Both may be associated with *hallucinations, illusions, delusions, orientation difficulties* (unawareness of time, place, or person), and "sundowning" (worsening symptoms at night) (Table 3-29). Memory impairment is usually global in delirium, whereas *remote memory is spared* in early dementia.

TABLE 3-29 Delirium versus Dementia		
FEATURE	**DELIRIUM**	**DEMENTIA**
Onset	Acute and dramatic	Chronic and insidious
Common causes	Illness, toxin, withdrawal	Alzheimer disease, multiinfarct dementia, HIV/AIDS
Reversible	Usually	Usually not
Attention	Poor	Usually unaffected
Arousal level	Fluctuates	Normal

AIDS, Acquired immunodeficiency syndrome; *HIV,* human immunodeficiency virus.

❍ Watch for *"pseudodementia"* in the elderly, a manifestation of depression that is reversible with treatment.
❍ Treatable causes of dementia include vitamin B$_{12}$ deficiency, endocrine disorders (especially thyroid and parathyroid disorders), uremia, syphilis, brain tumors, and normal pressure hydrocephalus. Treatment of Parkinson syndrome may also improve dementia.
❍ Watch for thiamine deficiency in alcoholics as the cause of delirium *(Wernicke encephalopathy).* The classic presentation includes *ataxia, ophthalmoplegia, nystagmus,* and *confusion.* If untreated, the delirium may progress to *Korsakoff syndrome,* which involves *anterograde amnesia* (inability to form new memories) and *confabulation* and is usually irreversible. Give thiamine before glucose in an alcoholic to prevent precipitating Wernicke encephalopathy.

Headaches

Tension headaches: Most common headache cause. Look for long history of headaches and *stress,* plus a feeling of tightness or stiffness, usually frontal or occipital and bilateral. Treat with stress reduction and acetaminophen or NSAID.

Cluster headaches: Male > female, unilateral, severe, associated with tearing/conjunctival injection, tender, and occur in clusters. Trying 100% *oxygen* inhalation for 15 minutes may abort an attack acutely.

Migraine headaches: Look for *aura, photophobia, nausea and vomiting,* and positive family history. Patients may occasionally have neurologic symptoms during an attack. Migraines usually begin between ages 10 and 30 years and are more common in females than in males (the gap lessens postmenopause). Treat or prevent acutely with antimigraine medication (e.g., *sumatriptan*). For prophylaxis, use β-blocker (propranolol), tricyclic antidepressant (nortriptyline), or antiepileptic (valproic acid).

Tumor/mass: Look for progressive neurologic symptoms; *papilledema;* intracranial hypertension (classically with nausea and vomiting, which may be projectile); mental status changes; and headaches every day that are classically *worse in the morning* (and increase in severity over time). MRI of the brain with contrast should be ordered; CT with contrast can be used if there is a contraindication to MRI.

Pseudotumor cerebri: May mimic tumor or mass because it also causes intracranial hypertension, papilledema, and daily headaches that are classically worse in the morning and also may be accompanied by nausea and vomiting. Pseudotumor cerebri is typically found in *young, obese women,* and a CT or MRI scan is negative. Lumbar puncture reveals markedly *elevated opening pressure* with no other abnormalities. Patients may have permanent vision loss without treatment. Initial conservative treatment includes acetazolamide, and *weight loss* usually helps. If this does not help, repeat lumbar punctures or a CSF shunt may be necessary to decrease pressure on the optic nerves (and reduce headache symptoms). Large doses of vitamin A, tetracyclines, and withdrawal from corticosteroids are possible causes.

Meningitis: Look for fever, leukocytosis, photophobia, Brudzinski and Kernig signs, and CSF findings (see table later in this section).

Subarachnoid hemorrhage: Often described as the "worst headache" of the patient's life; may be due to intracranial aneurysm rupture or trauma. The diagnosis is made with a noncontrast CT in the acute setting. Lumbar puncture is usually not indicated unless CT negative (because of the risk of uncal herniation) but reveals grossly bloody CSF. Treat injuries in the setting of trauma and order CT angiogram (or conventional catheter angiogram) to diagnose an aneurysm (or arteriovascular malformation) if no history of trauma. Tight blood pressure control with a drip if necessary is paramount.

Extracranial causes: Eye pain (optic neuritis, eyestrain from refractive errors, iritis, acute angle closure glaucoma); middle ear pain (otitis media, mastoiditis); sinus pain (sinusitis); oral cavity pain (toothache); herpes zoster infection with cranial nerve involvement; and malaise from any illness. Temporal arteritis can cause headache and vision loss.

Cranial nerves

Olfactory (CN 1): Rarely important clinically. *Kallman syndrome* is anosmia plus hypogonadism due to deficiency of gonadotropin-releasing hormone.

Optic (CN 2), oculomotor (CN 3), trochlear (CN 4), and abducens (CN 6): See Chapter 6, Ophthalmology section.

Trigeminal (CN 5): Innervates *muscles of mastication* and *facial sensation* (including the afferent limb of the corneal reflex). The classic disorder is *trigeminal neuralgia* (tic douloureux), an idiopathic disorder that causes *unilateral shooting facial pain in older adults* that is often triggered by minor activity (e.g., brushing teeth). It is best treated with *antiepilepsy medications* (carbamazepine). Other common disorders that can affect this nerve are tumors, stroke, and multiple sclerosis.

Facial (CN 7): Innervates *muscles of facial expression, taste in the anterior two-thirds of the tongue,* skin of the external ear, lacrimal and salivary glands (except parotid gland), and *stapedius muscle* (thus CN 7 lesions may cause hyperacusis). See Chapter 6, Ear, Nose, and Throat Surgery section.

☐ **CASE SCENARIO:** How can you tell the difference between an upper motor neuron (UMN) and lower motor neuron (LMN) facial nerve lesion using only physical examination? With a UMN (usually a stroke or tumor), the forehead is not involved on the affected side due to bilateral UMN innervation. With an LMN (usually Bell palsy), the forehead is involved on the affected side.

Vestibulocochlear (CN 8): Important for hearing and balance. Lesions cause *deafness, tinnitus,* and/or *vertigo.* See Chapter 6, Ear, Nose, and Throat Surgery section.

Glossopharyngeal (CN 9): Innervates pharyngeal muscles and mucous membranes (afferent limb of gag reflex), parotid gland, taste in posterior third of the tongue, skin of the external ear, and carotid body/sinus. Look for *loss of gag reflex* and loss of taste in posterior third of tongue.

Vagus (CN 10): Innervates muscles of palate, pharynx, larynx (efferent limb of gag reflex), taste buds in the base of the tongue, abdominal viscera, and skin of the external ear. Look for *hoarseness, dysphagia,* and *loss of gag or cough reflex.* Think of stroke or intracranial tumor, but thoracic aortic aneurysms or tumors (especially Pancoast lung tumors or esophageal cancers) can affect the recurrent laryngeal nerve in the upper thorax or neck.

Spinal accessory (CN 11): Innervates sternocleidomastoid and trapezius muscles. Patients with this lesion have difficulty in turning the head to the side opposite the lesion and ipsilateral shoulder droop.

Hypoglossal (CN 12): Innervates muscles of the tongue. Lesions produce deviation of a protruded tongue to the affected side.

Seizures

Six main types of seizures are likely to be tested on the boards:

1. **Simple partial (local, focal) seizures** may be motor (e.g., Jacksonian march), sensory (e.g., hallucinations), or "psychic" (cognitive or affective symptoms). The key point is that *consciousness is not impaired.* Treat with carbamazepine, lamotrigine, oxcarbazepine, or levetiracetam.

2. **Complex partial (psychomotor) seizures:** Any simple partial seizure followed by *impairment of consciousness.* Patients perform purposeless movements and may become aggressive if restraint is attempted. People who get in fights or kill other people, however, are not having a seizure! Common first-line agents are valproate, lamotrigine, and levetiracetam.

3. **Absence (petit mal) seizures:** Start *before the age of 20.* They are brief (duration of 10–30 seconds), generalized seizures of which the main manifestation is a *loss of consciousness,* often with *eye or muscle flutterings.* The classic description is that of a child in a classroom who stares off into space in the middle of a sentence and then 20 seconds later resumes the sentence where he or she left off. The child is having a seizure—*not* daydreaming. There is *no postictal state* (important differential point). Diagnosis can be aided by electroencephalogram (EEG) with hyperventilation and photic stimulation. First-line agents include ethosuximide and valproate.

4. **Tonic clonic (grand mal) seizures:** The classic seizures which may be associated with an *aura; tonic muscle contraction is followed by clonic contractions,* usually lasting 2–5 minutes. *Incontinence* (urine and/ or feces) is often an associated symptom, and the postictal state is characterized by *drowsiness, confusion, headache,* and muscle soreness. Common treatments for recurrent seizures include valproic acid (first-line), lamotrigine, and levetiracetam. Avoid valproic acid in women of child-bearing age due to the risk of teratogenicity.

5. **Febrile seizures:** Between the ages of 6 months and 5 years, children may have a seizure due to fever. The seizure is usually of the tonic-clonic, generalized type, and no specific seizure treatment is usually required. Treat the underlying cause of the fever, if possible, and give *acetaminophen.* Such children do not have epilepsy, and the chances of developing it are only slightly higher than in the general population. Make sure that the child does not have meningitis, tumor, or any other serious cause of seizure. The question should give clues in the case description if you are expected to pursue the workup of a serious condition. Lumbar puncture is often performed in children younger than 18 months to help exclude meningitis because such patients rarely demonstrate classic clinical findings of meningitis.

6. **Secondary seizure disorder:** Due to a *mass* (tumor, hemorrhage), *metabolic disorder* (hypoglycemia, hypoxia, phenylketonuria), *toxins* (lead, cocaine, carbon monoxide poisoning), *drug withdrawal* (alcohol, barbiturates, benzodiazepines, or too rapid a withdrawal from anticonvulsants), *cerebral edema* (severe hypertension, eclampsia), *CNS infections* (meningitis, encephalitis, toxoplasmosis [Fig. 3-35], cysticercosis), *trauma,* or *stroke.* Treat the underlying disorder. Use diazepam and/or phenytoin acutely to control seizures.

Important points:

1. For all seizures, secure the airway and, if possible, roll the patient onto his or her side to prevent aspiration.

2. A first unprovoked seizure with normal imaging, EEG, and lab workup requires no treatment. Recurrent seizures require treatment.

3. Cysticercosis is due to infection with the larval form of *Taenia solium,* the pork tapeworm. This infection is seen most commonly in patients with *AIDS* and in *immigrants* (most common cause of seizures in South America). CT often reveals calcified and/or "ring-enhancing" lesions. Treat with niclosamide or praziquantel.

4. Remember hypertension as a cause of *seizures* or convulsions, *headache, confusion,* and/or *mental status changes.*

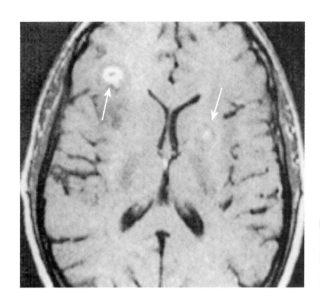

FIGURE 3-35 Toxoplasmosis in an immunosuppressed patient. Lesions on contrast-enhanced MRI may be either ring-enhancing *(left arrow)* or nodular *(right arrow)*. *(From Katz DS, Math KR, Groskin SA [eds]: Radiology Secrets. Philadelphia, Hanley & Belfus, 1998, p. 639.)*

5. Status epilepticus: when any type of seizure follows one after the other with *no intervening periods of consciousness.* Status epilepticus may occur spontaneously or result from too rapid a withdrawal of anticonvulsants. Treat with IV diazepam or lorazepam and phenytoin. Remember to protect the airway and intubate, if necessary.

Cerebrovascular disease

Cerebrovascular disease (stroke, cerebrovascular accident (CVA) is the most common cause of neurologic disability in the United States. Watch for classic causes: ischemia due to atherosclerosis (by far the most common), atrial fibrillation with resultant clot formation and emboli to the brain, and septic emboli from endocarditis.

Treatment for acute ischemic stroke in evolution is supportive (e.g., airway protection, oxygen, intravenous fluids). IV tPA may be used in the first 4.5 hours if criteria met. Treatment for acute hemorrhagic stroke involves blood pressure control, glucose control, seizure control, protamine sulfate if heparin-induced hemorrhage, vitamin K for warfarin-induced hemorrhage, or surgery for large bleeds.

📁 **CASE SCENARIO:** What is the first test usually performed for suspected acute stroke? Noncontrast CT scan to rule out hemorrhagic stroke, although MRI is a more comprehensive and sensitive test to detect CVA when available and can also detect hemorrhage.

📁 **CASE SCENARIO:** A patient has clinical symptoms of a stroke that started 2 hours ago, but the CT is negative. What does the patient probably have? A stroke or a transient ischemic attack (only time will tell which). Remember that the CT can be negative in the first 24–36 hours.

Transient ischemic attack (TIA): Focal neurologic deficit that lasts seconds to hours (classically lasts less than 2–3 minutes), then resolves spontaneously; often a precursor to a stroke. The classic symptoms are unilateral blindness *(amaurosis fugax)* and/or unilateral hemiplegia, hemiparesis, weakness, or clumsiness. Order a carotid duplex ultrasound scan or magnetic resonance angiography (MRA) to look for carotid stenosis. Heparin is somewhat controversial; avoid for board purposes unless the patient has atrial fibrillation. The best choice for therapy is aspirin and/or other antiplatelet medications. Recommend elective carotid endarterectomy for carotid stenosis with 70-99% blockage.

Localizing a stroke or other CNS lesion: see Table 3-30

TABLE 3-30 Localizing a Central Nervous System Lesion

SYMPTOMS/SIGNS	THINK OF THIS AREA
Decreased or no reflexes/fasciculations	Lower motor neuron lesion (or possibly a muscle problem)
Hyperreflexia	Upper motor neuron lesion (cord or brain)
Apathy/inattention/uninhibited/labile affect	Frontal lobes

TABLE 3-30 Localizing a Central Nervous System Lesion—cont'd

SYMPTOMS/SIGNS	THINK OF THIS AREA
Broca (motor) aphasia	Dominant frontal lobe*
Wernicke (sensory) aphasia	Dominant temporal lobe*
Memory impairment, aggression, hypersexuality	Temporal lobes
Inability to read, write, name, or do math	Dominant parietal lobe*
Ignoring one side of the body/difficulty in dressing	Nondominant parietal lobe*
Visual hallucinations or illusions	Occipital lobes
Cranial nerves 3 and 4	Midbrain
Cranial nerves 5, 6, 7, and 8	Pons
Cranial nerves 9, 10, 11, and 12	Medulla
Ataxia, dysarthria, nystagmus, intention tremor, dysmetria, scanning speech	Cerebellum
Resting tremor, chorea	Basal ganglia
Hemiballismus	Subthalamic nuclei
Locked-in syndrome (quadriplegic, cannot speak, fully conscious)	Basilar pontine stroke

*The left side is dominant in >95% of population (99% of right-handed people and 60-70% of left-handed people).

Movement disorders

Huntington disease: Autosomal dominant condition usually beginning between 35 and 50 years of age. Look for *choreiform movements* (irregular, spasmodic, involuntary movements of the limbs or facial muscles) and *progressive intellectual deterioration, dementia,* or *psychiatric disturbances.* Atrophy of the caudate nuclei may be seen on CT/MRI. Treatment is supportive; tetrabenazine may be used to treat chorea, and antipsychotics may help, but there is no cure.

Parkinson disease: Classic tetrad of *slowness or poverty of movement; muscular rigidity* ("lead pipe" or "cogwheel"); *resting tremor* ("pill-rolling" tremor that disappears with movement and sleep); and *postural instability* (shuffling gait and festination). Patients may also have dementia and depression. The mean age at onset is around 60. The cause is a loss of dopaminergic neurons, especially in the *substantia nigra,* which project to the basal ganglia; dopamine is thus decreased in the basal ganglia.

Drug therapy aims to increase dopamine. Options include dopamine precursors (levodopa with carbidopa), dopamine receptor agonists (ropinirole, pramipexole, bromocriptine, apomorphine, pergolide), monoamine oxidase–type B inhibitors (selegiline), COMT inhibitors (entacapone, tolcapone), anticholinergics (trihexyphenidyl, benztropine), and amantadine.

Besides Parkinson disease, a resting tremor may be due to hyperthyroidism, anxiety, drug withdrawal, or intoxication. A benign essential tremor is postural and accentuated by voluntary movement. Benign hereditary tremors are usually autosomal dominant. Look for a family history, and use β-blockers to reduce the tremor. Also watch for Wilson disease (hepatolenticular degeneration) as a cause of tremor. **Asterixis** *(outstretched hands flap slowly and involuntarily) occurs in patients with liver and kidney failure.*

Cerebellar disorders: Typically cause an *intention tremor* (tremor only during attempted voluntary movement; goes away at rest). In children, think of *brain tumor* (cerebellar astrocytoma, medulloblastoma), hydrocephalus (enlarging head in child younger than 6 months, may be related to Arnold-Chiari or Dandy-Walker malformations or prior meningitis), Friedreich ataxia (autosomal recessive disorder that starts between 5 and 15 years of age and also causes cardiomyopathy), or ataxia-telangiectasia (the diagnosis is in the name). In adults, think of *alcoholism,* tumor, ischemia/hemorrhage, or multiple sclerosis.

Amyotrophic lateral sclerosis (ALS), also known as Lou Gehrig disease: An idiopathic degeneration of both UMNs and LMNs. ALS is more common in men. The mean age at onset is 55 years. The key is to notice a *combination of UMN lesion signs* (spasticity, hyperreflexia, Babinski sign) and *LMN lesion signs* (fasciculations, atrophy, flaccidity). Treatment is supportive. Fifty percent of patients die within 3 years of onset.

Miscellaneous neurology topics

Know the classic CSF findings in different conditions (Table 3-31). Remember: Do not perform a lumbar puncture in patients with acute head trauma or signs of intracranial hypertension until you have a negative CT scan. You may cause the patient's death (from uncal herniation) if a space-occupying intracranial process is present. To check for the presence of CSF in fluid from the nose or ear, check β-2 transferrin.

TABLE 3-31 Classic Cerebrospinal Fluid Findings in Different Conditions

CONDITION	CELLS/mL*	GLUCOSE (mg/dL)	PROTEIN (mg/dL)	PRESSURE (mm Hg)
Normal cerebrospinal fluid	0-3 (L)	50-100	20-45	50-80
Bacterial meningitis	>1000 (PMN)	<50	Around 100	100-300
Viral or aseptic meningitis	>100 (L)	Normal	Normal or slightly increased	Normal or slightly increased
Pseudotumor cerebri	Normal	Normal	Normal	>200
Guillain-Barré syndrome	0-100 (L)	Normal	>100	Normal
Cerebral hemorrhage†	Bloody (RBC)	Normal	>45	>200
Multiple sclerosis‡	Normal or slightly increased (L)	Normal	Normal or slightly increased	Normal

*Main cell type is put in parenthesis after the number.
†Think of subarachnoid hemorrhage, but the same findings also can occur after an intracerebral hemorrhage.
‡On electrophoresis of cerebrospinal fluid, look for oligoclonal bands due to increased IgG production and an increased level of myelin basic protein (MBP) during active demyelination.
L, Lymphocytes; *PMN,* polymorphonuclear neutrophils; *RBC,* red blood cells.
Note: Bold type highlights the most important considerations for each disorder.

▢ **CASE SCENARIO:** A 32-year-old man with AIDS presents with gradual onset of lethargy, photophobia, low-grade fever, and headaches. Lumbar puncture reveals low glucose, high protein, and a high white blood cell count, which is due predominantly to high lymphocytes. What two types of meningitis should you consider? Tuberculous and fungal meningitis. Watch for a positive India ink preparation for cryptococcal meningitis or acid-fast stain for TB.

Multiple sclerosis: Look for insidious onset of neurologic symptoms in *women aged 20–40* years with *exacerbations and remissions.* Common presentations include paresthesias or numbness, weakness or clumsiness, *visual disturbances* (decreased vision and pain due to optic neuritis; diplopia due to cranial nerve involvement), gait disturbances, incontinence or urgency, and vertigo. Also look for emotional lability or other mental status changes. Internuclear ophthalmoplegia and scanning speech are classic symptoms, and patients may have a *Babinski sign. MRI* with and without contrast is the most sensitive diagnostic tool to show active demyelinating plaques (Fig. 3-36). Symptoms/lesions separated in space and time are necessary to make diagnosis. Also look for *increased IgG/oligoclonal bands* and *myelin basic protein* in the CSF. Evoked potential testing is also used to help confirm the diagnosis in many cases. The disease course is variable and unpredictable, although the long-term prognosis is generally poor. Treatment includes intravenous methylprednisolone for acute treatment, as well as azathioprine, cladribine, glucocorticoids, cyclophosphamide, interferons, and other agents for chronic treatment.

▢ **CASE SCENARIO:** In an African-American patient with clinical suspicion for multiple sclerosis, what should be considered? Neurosarcoidosis. Order chest radiograph and CSF ACE level.

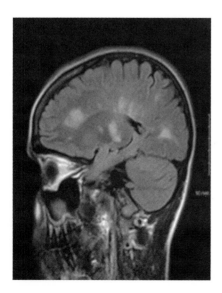

FIGURE 3-36 Multiple sclerosis. Sagittal fluid-attenuated inversion recovery image magnetic resonance scan shows multiple lesions in corpus callosum (periventricular and perpendicular to corpus callosum, known as "Dawson's fingers") along with lesions in right frontal, occipital lobes. *(From Ferri FF: Ferri's Clinical Advisor 2012. Philadelphia, Mosby, 2012.)*

Guillain-Barré syndrome: Look for a history of mild infection or immunization roughly *1 week before the onset of symmetric, distal lower extremity weakness or paralysis,* and *loss of deep tendon reflexes* in affected areas. Sensory disturbances (e.g., paresthesias) are mild or absent. As the ascending paralysis/weakness progresses in more severe cases, respiratory paralysis may occur; watch the patient carefully. Usually spirometry is used to follow inspiratory ability. Intubation may be required. Diagnosis is made by a combination of clinical symptoms, CSF analysis (usually normal except for markedly increased protein), and nerve conduction velocities (slowed). The disease usually stops spontaneously. Treatment with *plasmapheresis* and/or intravenous immunoglobulin (IVIG) can reduce the severity and duration of disease and is often used. Do not give corticosteroids; you may make the patient worse. Check IgA levels before IVIG to prevent anaphylaxis in IgA-deficient patients.

Electromyography (EMG): Measures the electrical (contractile) properties of muscle. LMN lesions are associated with fasciculations/fibrillations at rest. With disease in the muscle itself, there is little electrical activity at rest (which is normal), but amplitude is decreased with contraction of the muscle.

Syncope: The most common cause is *vasovagal* (e.g., after stress or fear). Other possibilities include cardiac events (especially arrhythmias; order an ECG and possibly an echocardiogram [e.g., aortic stenosis can cause syncope]) and neurologic disorders (especially seizures; consider EEG if appropriate setting and CT/MRI of head if other neurologic symptoms are present).

📖 **CASE SCENARIO:** A patient passes out. Should you worry about a stroke? Syncope is uncommon in the setting of stroke; if it occurs, it is usually due to a lesion in the posterior circulation (vertebrobasilar system) affecting the brainstem (classic is subclavian steal syndrome).

For delirious or unconscious patients in the emergency department with no history of trauma, first think of *hypoglycemia* (treat with glucose), *opioid overdose* (treat with naloxone), and *thiamine deficiency* (treat with thiamine before giving glucose in a suspected or known alcoholic). Other common causes are alcohol, illicit drugs, prescription medications, diabetic ketoacidosis, stroke, and epilepsy/postictal state.

Important causes of peripheral neuropathies:
1. **Metabolic disorders:** diabetes (autonomic and sensory neuropathy), uremia, hypothyroidism.
2. **Nutritional disorders:** deficiencies of vitamin B_{12}, B_6 (look for a history of isoniazid use), thiamine ("dry" beriberi), or vitamin E.
3. **Toxins/medications:** lead or other heavy metals, isoniazid, vincristine, ethambutol (optic neuritis). In patients with lead poisoning, the classic symptom is *wristdrop* or *footdrop;* look for coexisting CNS and abdominal symptoms.
4. **Postinfection, immunization, autoimmune disorders:** Guillain-Barré, systemic lupus erythematosus, polyarteritis nodosa, scleroderma, sarcoidosis, amyloidosis.
5. **Trauma:** carpal tunnel syndrome (median nerve entrapped at the wrist), pressure paralysis (radial nerve palsy in alcoholics), or fractures. Carpal tunnel syndrome is usually due to repetitive physical activity but may be a presentation of acromegaly or hypothyroidism; look for a *Tinel* or *Phalen sign.*
6. **Infection:** Lyme disease, diphtheria, HIV infection, tick bite, leprosy.

📖 **CASE SCENARIO:** What is the hallmark effect of peripheral neuropathies and demyelinating diseases on nerve conduction velocity? Nerve conduction velocity is slowed.

Myasthenia gravis (MG): Autoimmune disease that destroys acetylcholine receptors. MG usually presents in *women aged 20–40 years.* Look for *ptosis, diplopia,* and general muscle fatigability, especially *toward the end of the day* (eye involvement is classic). The diagnosis is suspected due to typical history and physical examination findings of increased muscle weakness with repetitive testing. The diagnosis is confirmed using a blood test to detect antiacetylcholine receptor antibodies (may be false negative with ocular forms of the disease) and nerve conduction velocity and electromyography can also be helpful. The Tensilon test is also a classic diagnostic method: muscle weakness improves after injection of *edrophonium* (Tensilon), a short-acting anticholinesterase. Watch for an associated *thymoma* (can be detected with a CT chest scan); most patients with MG improve after removal of the thymus (thymectomy considered part of treatment for those healthy enough and willing to undergo it). Treat medically with long-acting anticholinesterase (usually *pyridostigmine*); secondary agents include glucocorticoids, azathioprine, mycophenolate and cyclosporine; *plasmapheresis* is used in the setting of an acute crisis.

Eaton-Lambert syndrome (ELS): Paraneoplastic syndrome classically seen with *small cell lung cancer.* ELS is also associated with muscle weakness but *spares the extraocular muscles,* whereas in MG involvement of extraocular muscles is almost always a prominent feature. ELS also has a different mechanism of disease (impaired release of acetylcholine from nerves).

🗀 **CASE SCENARIO:** How can you tell the difference between MG and ELS by using repetitive muscle stimulation? In patients with MG, fatigue increases with stimulation, whereas in patients with ELS, fatigue decreases with stimulation.

Important points:
1. Do not forget organophosphate poisoning as a cause for myasthenic-like muscle weakness. It usually results from agricultural exposure. Look for parasympathomimetic effects (diarrhea, urination, miosis, bronchospasm, bradycardia, emesis, lacrimation, salivation DUMBBELLS). Treatment includes *atropine* and *pralidoxime*.
2. Aminoglycosides in high doses may cause myasthenic-like muscular weakness and prolong the effects of muscular blockade in anesthesia.

🗀 **CASE SCENARIO:** What conditions may occur in a patient with a port-wine stain over the right side of the face in the distribution of the first and second divisions of the trigeminal nerve? Seizures and glaucoma, as part of the *Sturge-Weber* syndrome.

ONCOLOGY

Cancer statistics: see Table 3-32. In children and younger adults, *leukemia* is the most common malignancy. *Age* has the most significant impact on the incidence and mortality of cancer (number-one risk factor, but not modifiable so rarely talked about). In the United States, the incidence of cancer roughly doubles every 5 years after age 25; therefore cancer most commonly affects older adults. Smoking is the most significant modifiable risk factor.

TABLE 3-32 Summary of Cancer Statistics

OVERALL HIGHEST INCIDENCE IN UNITED STATES		OVERALL HIGHEST MORTALITY RATE	
Male	**Female**	**Male**	**Female**
1. Prostate	1. Breast	1. Lung	1. Lung
2. Lung	2. Lung	2. Prostate	2. Breast
3. Colon	3. Colon	2. Colon	3. Colon

Tumor markers: see Table 3-33.

TABLE 3-33 Summary of Tumor Markers

MARKER	CANCER(S)
Alpha fetoprotein	Liver, testicular (yolk-sac)
β-HCG	Nonseminomatous germ cell tumors, gestational trophoblastic disease
Bladder tumor antigen, NMP 22	Bladder
CA 15-3, CA 27.29	Breast
CA 19-9	Pancreas, lung, breast
CA-125	Ovarian
Calcitonin	Thyroid medullary carcinoma
Carcinoembryonic antigen	Colon, pancreas, other GI tumors
Chromogranin A	Carcinoid tumors, neuroblastoma
Human chorionic gonadotropin	Hydatiform moles, choriocarcinoma
B_2-Microglobulin	Multiple myeloma, chronic lymphocytic leukemia
Prostate-specific antigen	Prostate
S-100	Melanoma, CNS tumors, nerve tumors
Thyroglobulin	Thyroid

CNS, Central nervous system; *GI*, gastrointestinal.

Genetic predisposition to cancer: See Table 3-34 and Figures 3-37 and 3-38. Other diseases associated with an increased incidence of cancer are immunodeficiency syndromes, Bloom syndrome, and Fanconi anemia. Breast, ovarian, and colon cancer are well known to have familial tendencies (as well as some other types of cancers) and sometimes a mendelian inheritance pattern can be shown (e.g., *BRCA1* gene for breast cancer).

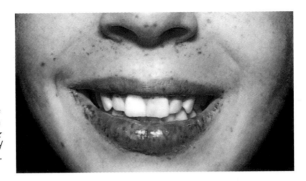

FIGURE 3-37 Peutz-Jeghers syndrome. Note the round, pigmented macules occur around the mouth and particularly on the lower lips. *(From Swartz MH: Textbook of physical diagnosis: history and examination, 4th ed. Philadelphia, 2002, WB Saunders, p 295.)*

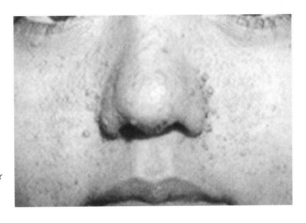

FIGURE 3-38 Adenoma sebaceum of face in a patient who has tuberous sclerosis. *(From Yanoff M, Duker JS: Ophthalmology, 3rd ed. Philadelphia, Mosby, 2009.)*

TABLE 3-34 Genetic Predisposition to Cancer

DISEASE/SYNDROME	INHERITANCE	TYPE OF CANCER (IN ORDER OF MOST LIKELY)/OTHER INFORMATION
Retinoblastoma	Autosomal dominant	Retinoblastoma, osteogenic sarcoma (later in life)
BRCA1, BRCA2	Autosomal dominant	Breast and ovarian cancer
MEN type 1	Autosomal dominant	Parathyroid, pituitary, pancreas (islet cell tumors)
MEN type 2a	Autosomal dominant	Thyroid (medullary cancer), parathyroid, pheochromocytoma
MEN type 2b	Autosomal dominant	Thyroid (medullary cancer), pheochromocytoma, mucosal neuromas
Hereditary nonpolyposis colon cancer (Lynch syndrome)	Autosomal dominant	Colon cancer, as well as endometrial, ovary, stomach, and other cancers.
Familial polyposis coli	Autosomal dominant	Hundreds of colon polyps that *always* result in colon cancer
Gardner syndrome	Autosomal dominant	Familial polyposis plus osteomas and soft tissue tumors
Turcot syndrome	Autosomal dominant	Familial polyposis plus central nervous system tumors
Peutz-Jeghers syndrome	Autosomal dominant	Look for perioral freckles and multiple noncancerous GI polyps; increased incidence of noncolon cancer (stomach, breast, ovaries); no increased risk of colon cancer
Neurofibromatosis type 1	Autosomal dominant	Multiple neurofibromas, café-au-lait spots; increased number of pheochromocytomas, bone cysts, meningiomas
Neurofibromatosis type 2	Autosomal dominant	Bilateral acoustic neuromas, meningiomas
Tuberous sclerosis	Autosomal dominant	Adenoma sebaceum, seizures, mental retardation, glial nodules in brain, increased renal angiomyolipomas, and cardiac rhabdomyomas
Von Hippel-Lindau	Autosomal dominant	Hemangioblastomas in cerebellum, renal cell cancer; cysts in liver and/or kidney
Xeroderma pigmentosum	Autosomal recessive	Skin cancers (basal cell carcinoma, melanoma, squamous cell carcinoma)
Ataxia-telangiectasia	Autosomal recessive	Lymphomas, leukemias, breast cancer
Bloom syndrome	Autosomal recessive	Lymphomas, leukemias, GI cancer
Fanconi anemia	Autosomal recessive	Acute myeloid leukemia, other carcinomas

GI, Gastrointestinal; *MEN,* multiple endocrine neoplasia.

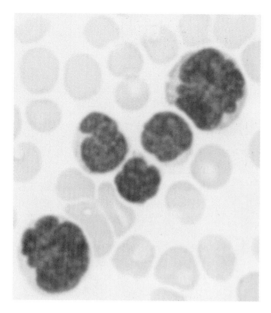

FIGURE 3-39 Mycosis fungoides/Sézary syndrome. Abnormal cells in the peripheral blood with characteristic cerebriform nuclei and scant cytoplasm (i.e., "butt" cells) are classic. *(From Hoffbrand AV, Pettit JE: Chronic lymphoid leukaemias. In Hoffbrand AV, Pettit JE [eds]: Color Atlas of Clinical Hematology, 3rd ed. St. Louis, Mosby, 2000, pp 177-190.)*

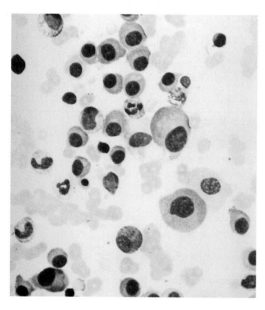

FIGURE 3-40 Multiple myeloma. A majority of cells seen in the bone marrow are atypical plasma cells. *(From Hoffbrand AV , Pettit JE: Myeloma and related conditions. In Hoffbrand AV, Pettit JE [eds]: Color Atlas of Clinical Hematology, 3rd ed. St. Louis, Mosby, 2000, pp 233-246.)*

Alterable risk factors for development of cancer: See Tables 3-35 to 3-37 and Figures 3-39 and 3-40.

TABLE 3-35 Avoidable Risk Factors for Cancer Development

CANCER TYPE	RISK FACTOR (GREATEST IMPACT LISTED FIRST)
All cancer overall	Smoking; second is alcohol
Bladder	Smoking, aniline dyes (rubber and dye industry), schistosomiasis (in immigrants)
Breast*	Combined estrogen/progesterone hormone replacement therapy, nulliparity, obesity, alcohol, high-fat diet (controversial), lack of exercise
Cervical	Smoking, sex (HPV infection), high parity
Clear cell cancer	Mothers should avoid diethylstilbestrol (DES) during pregnancy
Colorectal	High-fat and low-fiber diet
Endometrial	Unopposed estrogen stimulation, obesity
Esophagus	Smoking, alcohol, obesity, gastroesophageal reflux
Leukemia	Chemotherapy, radiotherapy, other immunosuppressive drugs, benzene
Liver	Alcohol, vinyl chloride (liver angiosarcomas), aflatoxins
Lung	Smoking, asbestos (also nickel, radon, coal, arsenic, chromium, uranium)
Mesothelioma	Asbestos
Oral cavity	Smoking, alcohol, oral sex (due to role of human papillomavirus)
Pancreas	Smoking
Pharynx, larynx	Smoking, alcohol
Skin	Ultraviolet light exposure (e.g., sun), coal tar, arsenic

TABLE 3-35 Avoidable Risk Factors for Cancer Development—cont'd

CANCER TYPE	RISK FACTOR (GREATEST IMPACT LISTED FIRST)
Renal cell	Smoking
Stomach	Alcohol nitrosamines, nitrites (from smoked meats and fish)
Thyroid	Childhood head, neck, or chest irradiation

*Order of importance for avoidable breast cancer risk factors is uncertain and remains controversial. This list is presented in a random order.

TABLE 3-36 Viral and Bacterial Causes of Cancer

AGENT	CANCERS ASSOCIATED
Epstein-Barr virus	Nasopharyngeal carcinoma, African Burkitt lymphoma, lymphoproliferative disorder, Hodgkin lymphoma
Helicobacter pylori	Stomach—MALT lymphoma
Hepatitis B and C	Hepatocellular carcinoma
Human herpesvirus 8	Kaposi sarcoma
Human papillomavirus	Anal, cervical, head and neck, penile, vaginal, and vulvar
Human T cell lymphotrophic virus type 1	Adult T cell leukemia and lymphoma

TABLE 3-37 Blood Dyscrasias

TYPE	AGE	WHAT TO LOOK FOR IN CASE DESCRIPTION/ BUZZ WORDS
Acute lymphoblastic leukemia (ALL)	Children (peak at 3-5 yr)	Pancytopenia (bleeding, fever, anemia), radiation therapy, blasts with TdT
Acute myelogenous leukemia (AML)	>30 yr	Pancytopenia (bleeding, fever, anemia), Auer rods, blasts with myeloperoxidase, disseminated intravascular coagulation
Chronic myelogenous leukemia (CML)	30-50 yr	WBC count >50,000 units, myelocyte bulge, basophilia, Philadelphia chromosome, blast crisis, splenomegaly
Chronic lymphocytic leukemia (CLL)	>50 yr	Male gender, lymphadenopathy, lymphocytosis with small round mature lymphocytes, infections, smudge cells, splenomegaly
Hairy cell leukemia	Adults	Blood smear with hairlike projections, TRAP stain, flow cytometry with CD11c, CD25, CD103, splenomegaly
Mycosis fungoides/ Sézary syndrome (see figure)	>50 yr	Plaquelike, itchy skin rash that does not improve with treatment, blood smear with cerebriform nuclei ("butt cells"), Pautrier abscesses in epidermis
Burkitt lymphoma	Children	Cytoplasmic vacuoles, associated with Epstein-Barr virus (in Africa)
Central nervous system B-cell lymphoma	Adults	HIV/AIDS
Hodgkin disease	15-34 yr	Reed-Sternberg cells, cervical lymphadenopathy, mediastinal mass, night sweats
Non-Hodgkin lymphoma	Any age	Low-grade lymphomas—CLL, follicular, marginal zone; High-grade lymphomas—diffuse large B-cell lymphoma, Burkitt
Myelofibrosis	>50 yr	Anemia, left shift granulocytes, teardrop cells, "dry tap" on bone marrow biopsy
Myelodysplasia	>60 yr	Anemia or cytopenias, hypercellular marrow, dysplasia
Multiple myeloma (see figure)	>40 yr	Bence Jones protein (IgG = 50%, IgA = 25%) osteolytic lesions, high calcium level, anemia, renal failure
Waldenstroms macroglobulinemia	>40 yr	Hyperviscosity, IgM spike, cold agglutins (Raynaud phenomenon with cold sensitivity)
Polycythemia vera	>40 yr	High hemoglobin, pruritus (after hot bath/shower). Use phlebotomy
Essential thrombocythemia	>50 yr	Platelet count usually >1,000,000/µL; patients may have bleeding or thrombosis

AIDS, Acquired immunodeficiency syndrome; *HIV,* human immunodeficiency virus; *MALT,* mucosa-associated lymphoid tissue.

Lung Cancer

Lung cancer is the number-one cause of overall cancer mortality in the United States. The incidence is rising in women because of a prior increase in smoking prevalence. Look for *change in a chronic cough in a smoker*—the more pack years of tobacco use, the more suspicious you should be. Patients also may present with hemoptysis, pneumonia, and/or weight loss. Chest x-ray (CXR) may show pleural effusion or mass; perform thoracentesis and examine for malignant cells when effusion present. After CXR, get a CT scan and tissue biopsy to confirm the diagnosis and define the histologic type.

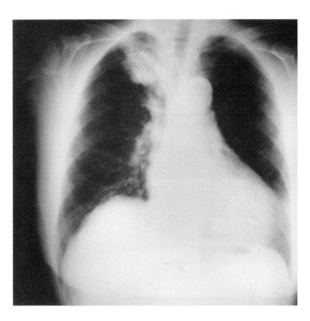

FIGURE 3-41 Right apical lung mass, also known as a *Pancoast tumor. (From Sahn SA, Heffner JE: Critical Care Pearls, 2nd ed. Philadelphia, Hanley & Belfus, 1998.)*

❍ Non–small cell lung cancer (NSCLC) may be treated with surgery if the cancer remains within one lung (ipsilateral hilar node involvement still allows resection, but not for contralateral mediastinal or hilar nodes and not when distant metastases are present). For unresectable NSCLC, treat with radiation and/or chemotherapy. Various chemotherapy regimens are available.

❍ Small cell cancer is treated with chemotherapy (cisplatin and etoposide) and/or radiotherapy only; early metastases make surgery inappropriate. Prophylactic cranial irradiation for patients in complete remission to decrease the risk of central nervous system metastasis.

Board-tested consequences of lung cancer:

1. **Horner syndrome:** due to invasion of cervical sympathetic chain by an apical (Pancoast) tumor (Fig. 3-41). Look for unilateral *ptosis, miosis,* and *anhidrosis* (no sweating).
2. **Diaphragm paralysis:** due to phrenic nerve involvement.
3. **Hoarseness:** due to recurrent laryngeal nerve involvement.
4. **Superior vena cava syndrome:** due to compression of superior vena cava with impaired venous drainage. Look for edema and plethora (redness) of the neck and face and CNS symptoms (headache, visual symptoms, altered mental status, nightmares).
5. **Cushing syndrome:** due to production of adrenocorticotropic hormone (ACTH) by a small cell carcinoma.
6. **SIADH:** due to ADH production by a small cell carcinoma.
7. **Hypercalcemia:** due to bone metastases or production of parathyroid-like hormone by a squamous cell carcinoma.
8. **Eaton-Lambert syndrome:** myasthenia gravis–like disease due to lung cancer that spares the ocular muscles. The muscles become stronger with repetitive stimulation (opposite of myasthenia gravis).

Solitary pulmonary nodule on CXR: The first step is to compare the current radiograph with previous chest radiographs. If the nodule has remained the same size for greater than 2 years, it is highly unlikely to be cancer. Use imaging surveillance only. If no old films are available and the patient is older than 35 or has a smoking history, order a CT scan. If the CT scan is not definitive, do a positron emission tomography (PET) scan of the nodule. If imaging studies suggest a benign lesion, short-interval follow-up CT scans are used to confirm stability. If imaging is indeterminate in a high-risk patient or suspicious in any patient, perform biopsy of the nodule (via bronchoscopy or transthoracic CT-guided biopsy, if possible) for a tissue diagnosis. If the patient is younger than 35 or has no smoking history, the cause is most likely infection (TB or fungal), hamartoma, or collagen vascular disease. Such patients can generally undergo observation and short interval follow-up with repeat CT or CXR. If following a nodule with imaging and it gets bigger, biopsy is usually recommended.

Breast cancer

Roughly 1 in 8–10 women will develop breast cancer in their lifetime. The most common histologic type of breast cancer is invasive ductal carcinoma. Each year there are 205,000 new patients. Annual mortality of 40,000.

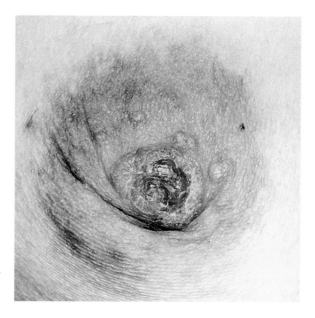

Figure 3-42 Paget disease of the nipple. *(From James EC, Corry RJ, Perry JF: Principles of Basic Surgical Practice. Philadelphia, Hanley & Belfus, 1987.)*

Risk factors for breast cancer:

1. Personal history of breast cancer, whether in situ or invasive
2. Family history of breast or ovarian cancer in first-degree relatives
3. Age (breast cancer is rare before age 30; the incidence increases with age)
4. Early menarche, late menopause, and late first pregnancy or nulliparity (more menstrual cycles = higher risk)
5. Personal history of abnormal breast biopsy: usual or atypical hyperplasia of the breast, sclerosing adenosis, papillomatosis
6. Radiation exposure to breasts before age 30
7. Genetic factors: *BRCA1* and *BRCA2* genes, p53 mutation (Li-Fraumeni syndrome). *BRCA-1* or *BRCA-2* genes carry lifetime risk as high as 85%.
8. Obesity
9. Alcohol
10. Prolonged use of combined estrogen and progesterone hormone replacement therapy

The debate about breast cancer and birth control pills for premenopausal women continues. A woman with a history of breast cancer should not receive estrogen.

Signs and symptoms that should make you think that a breast mass is cancer until proved otherwise: fixation of breast mass to the chest wall or overlying skin; satellite nodules or ulcers on the skin; lymphedema (also called *peau d'orange*); matted or fixed axillary lymph nodes; inflammatory skin changes (red, hot skin with enlargement of the breast due to inflammatory cancer of the breast); prolonged unilateral, scaling erosion of the nipple with or without discharge (may be Paget disease of the nipple) (Fig. 3-42); microcalcifications on mammography; and any new breast mass in a *postmenopausal woman*.

The conservative approach is best on the boards. In women older than 35, when in doubt, consider biopsy of a palpable breast mass, especially if the woman has any risk factors. If the question on the USMLE exam does not want you to biopsy the mass, it will give clues that the mass is not a cancer (such as bilateral, lumpy breasts that become symptomatic with every menses and have no dominant mass or age younger than 30 years old).

In women younger than 30, breast cancer is rare. With a discrete breast mass in this age group, think of a breast cyst. If it is a solid mass, think of *fibroadenoma*, which is usually round, rubbery-feeling, and freely movable.

In patients with a palpable breast mass, the decision to do a biopsy is a clinical one. A benign mammogram should not deter you from doing a biopsy. Furthermore, a lesion that is detected on mammography and looks suspicious should be biopsied, even if it is not palpable (needle localization biopsy).

Mammograms in women younger than 30 are rarely helpful (breast tissue is too dense to permit visualization of cancer), unless the mammogram is ordered to have a baseline before removal of a breast mass. Use ultrasound to image the breasts instead (and increasingly, MRI is being used).

Mammograms in women age 40–49 are controversial. The U.S. Preventive Services Task Force (USPSTF) recommends against "routine" screening of women 40–49. The task force recommends screening mammography every 2 years for women 50 to 74. The Task Force also discourages women from performing breast self-examination. The American Cancer Society, however, recommends annual mammograms beginning at age 40. Generally, these types of controversial questions are avoided on the boards.

Mastectomy versus breast-conserving surgery plus irradiation: Considered equal in efficacy. In either, do an axillary node dissection (or a sentinel node dissection) to determine spread to the nodes. If nodes are positive, give chemotherapy (hormonal and/or traditional chemotherapy depending on the specifics of the case). Whole body staging with a PET scan is normally done for node-positive disease or symptoms/signs suggestive of metastatic disease.

Aromatase inhibitors (e.g., letrozole, anastrozole) and tamoxifen generally improve breast cancer survival (and are routinely given) if a breast cancer is estrogen receptor–positive—they are even more beneficial if the tumor is also progesterone receptor positive. If the tumor is HER-2/neu receptor–positive, trastuzumab antibody therapy (against the receptor) is usually effective and recommended.

Prostate cancer

Risk factors:
1. Age (almost never seen in men younger than 40; the incidence increases with age; 60% of men older than 80 have prostate cancer)
2. Race: black > white > Asian
3. Family history

Patients present late if they are not in a screening program, because early prostate cancer is in the peripheral zone of the prostate, so it does not cause urinary symptoms until it is more advanced (BPH is more in the central zone, so it causes symptoms ealier). Look for BPH-like symptoms (hesitancy, dysuria, frequency) and hematuria. Look for prostate irregularities (nodule or nodules) on rectal exam. Patients may present with *back pain from vertebral metastases* (osteoblastic, not lytic lesions). Screening using prostate-specific antigen (PSA) is controversial. The American Cancer Society recommends offering the PSA test and DRE yearly to men aged 50 years old or older who have a life expectancy of at least 10 years. Earlier testing starts at age 45 years for African-American men and at age 40 for men with a first-degree relative with prostate cancer. Screening for prostate cancer in men aged 75 years or older is controversial and generally not recommended.

Treatment: Prostate cancer can be treated with surgery, radiation, or watchful waiting. Radical prostatectomy is generally performed in patients with localized prostate cancer and life expectancy >10 years. Radiation therapy (external-beam irradiation or brachytherapy) may be used in poor surgical candidates or patients with a high-grade malignancy. Watchful waiting is reasonable in patients who are too old or too ill to survive longer than 10 years. With metastases (usually detected using bone scan for bone mets and/or CT scan of the abdomen and pelvis for nodal mets), patients have several options for hormonal therapy: orchiectomy, gonadotropin-releasing hormone agonist (gosereline, *leuprolide*), androgen-receptor antagonist (flutamide), estrogen (diethylstilbesterol), and others (e.g., cyproterone). Standard chemotherapy rarely helps; radiation therapy is also used for local pelvic control and/or pain due to bone metastases.

Colorectal cancer

Risk factors: see Table 3-38.

TABLE 3-38 Colorectal Cancer (CRC) Screening and Surveillance Recommendations	
CLINICAL CATEGORY/FACTOR	**RECOMMENDATION**
All adults	Age 50 yr or older: Colonoscopy every 10 yr Flexible sigmoidoscopy every 5 yr Computed tomographic colonography every 5 yr FOBT FIT Stool blood testing annually or stool DNA testing acceptable but not preferred
History of colorectal adenoma	Colonoscopy every 3-5 yr after removal of polyps
History of inflammatory bowel disease	Colonoscopy every 1-2 yr beginning after 8 yr of pancolitis or after 15 yr if only left-sided disease

TABLE 3-38 Colorectal Cancer (CRC) Screening and Surveillance Recommendations—cont'd

CLINICAL CATEGORY/FACTOR	RECOMMENDATION
One or two first-degree relatives with CRC at any age or adenoma at age <60 yr	Colonoscopy every 5 yr beginning at age 40 yr, or 10 yr younger than earliest diagnosis, whichever comes first
Hereditary nonpolyposis colorectal cancer	Colonoscopy every 1-2 yr beginning at age 25 yr and then yearly after age 40 yr
Familial adenomatous polyposis and variants	Flexible sigmoidoscopy yearly beginning at puberty

From Andreoli TE, Ivor B, Griggs R, et al: Andreoli and Carpenter's Cecil Essentials of Medicine, 8th ed, Philadelphia, Elsevier, 2010.

1. Age (incidence begins to increase after age 40; peak incidence at 60–75 years)
2. Family history (especially with familial polyposis and Gardner, Turcot, or Lynch syndrome)
3. Inflammatory bowel disease (ulcerative colitis > Crohn disease, but both increase risk)
4. Low-fiber, high-fat diet (weak evidence)

Presentation: Patients may present with asymptomatic blood in the stool (visible streaks of blood or positive occult fecal blood test), *anemia* with right-sided colon cancer, and *change in stool caliber* ("pencil stool") or frequency (alternating constipation and frequency) with left-sided colon cancer. As with any cancer, look for weight loss. Colon cancer is a common cause of a large bowel obstruction in adults.

Occult blood in the stool of a person older than 40 years should be considered colon cancer until proven otherwise. To rule out colon cancer, do either a flexible sigmoidoscopy and barium enema or a colonoscopy. If you see any lesions with a flexible sigmoidoscope or barium enema, you need to do a total colonoscopy with removal and histologic examination of all polyps or lesions. For this reason, many physicians start with colonoscopy.

Carcinoembryonic antigen (CEA) is often elevated with colon cancer, and a preoperative level is usually measured. After surgery to remove the tumor, an elevated CEA due to colon cancer should return to normal levels. Periodic monitoring of CEA after surgery in such cases helps to detect recurrence before it is clinically apparent. CEA is not generally used as a screening tool for colon cancer because it can be increased in patients with many other conditions (smoking, IBD, alcoholic liver disease). A normal CEA result does not exclude the diagnosis of colorectal cancer.

Treatment depends on stage with CT and PET scans used to evaluate for metastatic disease. Treatment is primarily surgical for cases without distant metastatic disease, with resection of involved bowel and adjacent lymph nodes (palliative surgical resection may also be necessary in those with distant metastases). Adjuvant chemotherapy and/or radiation is used with locally advanced disease and with distant metastases.

Metastases frequently go to the liver; if the metastatic lesion is solitary, surgical resection is often attempted. With metastases elsewhere, chemotherapy or local ablative treatments (e.g., radiofrequency ablation, chemoembolization) have been used with moderate success.

Pancreatic cancer

The classic presentation for adenocarcinoma (the most common type of pancreatic cancer) (Fig. 3-43) is a smoker in the 40–80-year-old range who has *weight loss* and *jaundice*. Patients may have epigastric pain, migratory thrombophlebitis (*Trousseau syndrome,* which may also be seen with other visceral cancers), or a palpable, nontender gallbladder *(Courvoisier sign).* Pancreatic cancer is more common in men than women, in blacks than whites, and in diabetics than nondiabetics. CT scan makes the diagnosis and can assess for metastatic disease (most common to local lymph nodes and liver) and degree of local invasiveness. Surgery (Whipple procedure) is appropriate if the tumor is <5 cm, solitary, and without metastases. Overall prognosis remains dismal (<5% survival at 5 years).

Islet cell tumors:

1. **Insulinoma** (beta cell tumor): most common islet cell tumor (see Fig. 3-43). Look for fasting hypoglycemia (glucose <50 mg/dL), CNS symptoms due to hypoglycemia (confusion, stupor, loss of consciousness), and increased C-peptide and insulin levels. Abdominal CT or MRI detects most insulinomas. About 90% of insulinomas are benign; the cure is surgical resection (if possible).
2. **Gastrinoma:** *Zollinger-Ellison syndrome* is gastrinoma causing acid hypersecretion and peptic ulcers (gastrin causes acid secretion). Peptic ulcers are often *multiple and resistant to therapy;* they may be found in unusual locations (distal duodenum or jejunum). Surgery is curative in about 40%. More than half are malignant. Look for MEN-type 1 (hyperparathyroidism and pituitary tumors).

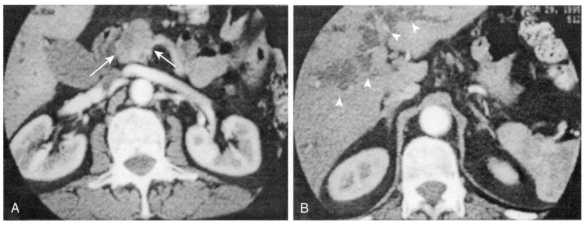

Figure 3-43 Small pancreatic head cancer (**A,** *arrows*) with resultant biliary dilatation (**B,** *arrowheads*). *(From Katz DS, Math KR, Groski SA [eds]: Radiology Secrets. Philadelphia, Hanley & Belfus, 1998.)*

3. **Glucagonoma** (alpha cell tumor): hyperglycemia with high glucagon level and *migratory necrotizing skin erythema.*

Ovarian cancer

Presentation: Ovarian cancer usually manifests as advanced disease with findings of weight loss, pelvic mass, *ascites,* and/or bowel obstruction in a postmenopausal woman. Any *ovarian enlargement in a postmenopausal woman is cancer until proved otherwise.* In women of reproductive age, most ovarian enlargements are benign. Risk factors include low parity, delayed childbearing, high-fat diet, hormone therapy, *BRCA1* mutation, and Lynch syndrome.

Ultrasound is a good first test to evaluate an ovarian/adnexal lesion and can distinguish between a benign cyst (most common) and complex cyst (indeterminate lesions; elevated CA-125 in 50% early-stage cancers; management depends on age and clinical situation, with younger reproductive women often followed on a short interval basis due to low cancer risk and surgical approach often favored in postmenopausal women) and solid mass (considered cancer until proven otherwise unless it has imaging features compatible with a dermoid).

Treatment consists of debulking surgery and cisplatin-based chemotherapy; the prognosis is usually poor. Most ovarian cancers arise from the ovarian epithelium. *Serous cystadenocarcinoma* is the most common type; *psammoma bodies* are often seen on histopathologic exam.

Germ cell and stromal tumors make good board questions:
1. **Teratoma/dermoid cyst:** Look for a description of the tumor to include skin, hair, sebum, fat, and/or teeth (which may show up on radiograph); can be diagnosed preoperatively using ultrasound imaging, CT, or MRI and are highly likely to be benign, though usually resected
2. **Sertoli-Leydig cell tumor:** can secrete androgen and thus cause virilization (hirsutism, receding hairline, deepening voice, clitoromegaly)
3. **Granulosa/theca cell tumor:** can secrete estrogens, leading to development of precocious puberty signs in pediatric age group
   Meigs syndrome: ovarian fibroma, ascites, and right hydrothorax
   Krukenberg tumor: stomach (or other gastrointestinal) cancer with metastases to the ovaries

Cervical cancer

Pap smears decrease the incidence and mortality of invasive cervical cancer. Give every female patient a Pap smear if she is due, even if she presents with an unrelated complaint.

Follow any dysplastic Pap smear with colposcopy-directed biopsies and endocervical curettage. If the Pap smear shows microinvasive cancer, proceed to conization. Invasive cervical cancer begins in the transformation zone and usually manifests with vaginal bleeding or discharge (postcoital bleeding, intermenstrual spotting, or abnormal menstrual bleeding). Women with invasive cancer require surgery (hysterectomy) and/or radiation.

The HPV vaccines Gardasil and Cervarix are approved for protection against HPV types 16 and 18, which cause 70% of cervical cancers. Gardasil is also approved for protection against HPV types 6 and 11, which cause 90% of genital warts.

Risk factors for cervical cancer:

1. Age younger than 20 years at first coitus, pregnancy, or marriage
2. Multiple sexual partners (role of *HPV* and possibly herpesvirus) or sexual relations with a promiscuous person
3. Smoking
4. Low socioeconomic status
5. High parity (which protects against endometrial and breast cancer)
6. Age (most commonly seen in women older than 40)

Uterine cancer

Presentation: *Postmenopausal vaginal or uterine bleeding is cancer until proved otherwise,* and endometrial cancer is the most common type to present in this fashion (fourth most common cancer in women). Any woman with unexplained gynecologic bleeding that persists needs a Pap smear, endocervical curettage, and endometrial biopsy.

Risk factors for endometrial cancer:

1. Obesity
2. Nulliparity
3. Early menarche and late menopause
4. Diabetes
5. Tamoxifen use
6. Endometrial atypical hyperplasia
7. Chronic, unopposed estrogen stimulation. Examples are *polycystic ovary* (i.e., Stein-Levinthal) *syndrome,* estrogen-secreting neoplasm (e.g., granulosa-theca cell tumor), and estrogen replacement therapy (only if taken without progesterone).

Most uterine cancers are endometrial *adenocarcinomas* and spread by direct extension (squamous cell carcinomas and leiomyosarcomas are rare). The usual treatment includes surgery with or without radiation or chemotherapy. Surgery generally consists of pelvic washings, total abdominal hysterectomy and bilateral salpingo-oophorectomy, omental biopsy, and selective pelvic and periaortic lymphadenectomy, depending on stage and grade. Hormonal therapy is an option for some young women who want to preserve fertility.

Miscellaneous neoplasms

Brain tumors: In adults, two-thirds of primary tumors are *supratentorial* (versus two-thirds infratentorial in pediatric patients); metastatic disease is as common as primary tumors (think metastases when more than one lesion or patient has known primary malignancy). Look for new-onset seizures, neurologic deficits, or signs of intracranial hypertension (headache, blurred vision, *papilledema,* nausea, and projectile vomiting). The most common primary type is a glioma (most are intraparenchymal astrocytomas, with little or no calcification) (Fig. 3-44). Treatment is surgical removal, which may be followed by radiation and chemotherapy, depending on the tumor. Meningiomas are the other common primary intracranial tumors, are benign, often contain calcium, are located external to the brain substance (i.e., a tumor of the meninges), and can be cured with surgical excision in most cases.

🔲 **CASE SCENARIO:** A 24-year-old obese woman has headaches, papilledema, and vomiting with negative CT/MRI scans. What is the likely diagnosis? Pseudotumor cerebri/idiopathic intracranial hypertension (not a neoplasm). Lumbar puncture reveals high pressure with no other abnormalities. Weight loss may help. Medical therapy includes acetazolamide and furosemide. Repeat lumbar punctures may be necessary to lower intracranial pressure and prevent optic nerve damage and visual field loss.

🔲 **CASE SCENARIO:** A 9-year-old boy presents with visual disturbances, headaches, and vomiting. A skull radiograph/CT scan shows calcified mass in the region of the sella turcica. What tumor does the child probably have? A craniopharyngioma (remnant of Rathke pouch), which is often heavily calcified.

Testicular cancer: Most common solid malignancy in adult men younger than 30 years old. The main risk factor is cryptorchidism. Other risk factors are family history, infertility, tobacco use, and white race. Transillumination and ultrasound help to distinguish *hydrocele* (which is fluid-filled and transilluminates) from cancer (which is solid). The most common type is *seminoma,* which is treated with surgery and radiation (tumor radiosensitive). Serum markers include hCG, AFP, and LDH.

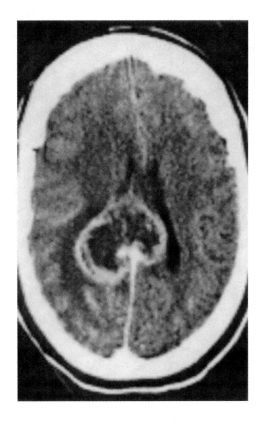

FIGURE 3-44 Contrast-enhanced computed tomography image of a butterfly glioma. This tumor has grown from the right side to the left, crossing through the splenium of the corpus callosum. *(From Katz DS, Math KR, Groski SA [eds]: Radiology Secrets. Philadelphia, Hanley & Belfus, 1998.)*

Pituitary tumors: Look for *bitemporal hemianopsia* due to mass effect on the optic chiasm; order an MRI to exclude a pituitary macroadenoma if it is present. Microadenomas cause no mass effect/local symptoms, and they are brought to clinical attention due to hormone secretion. The most common type is *prolactinoma* (high prolactin levels with galactorrhea and menstrual/sexual dysfunction). Other types may cause hyperthyroidism (high TSH) or Cushing disease (high ACTH).

📋 **CASE SCENARIO:** A 34-year-old schizophrenic man taking haloperidol presents with galactorrhea, decreased libido, and an elevated prolactin level. Why? Because of the haloperidol, a dopamine antagonist. Dopamine inhibits prolactin production.

Nasopharyngeal carcinoma: Most common in Asians; remember association with *EBV.*

Esophageal cancer (Fig. 3-45): Classically associated with dysphagia, weight loss, possible anemia, and complaints that "my food is sticking," which progresses to dysphagia for liquids. Adenocarcinoma and squamous cell carcinoma are the most common types with adenocarcinoma now accounting for more than 50% of new cancers. Adenocarcinoma is associated with obesity and gastroesophageal reflux and develops from Barrett metaplasia. It occurs in the distal one-third of the esophagus. Nonobese chronic smokers and drinkers older than age 40 usually develop squamous cell carcinoma in the middle one-third of the esophagus. Esophageal cancer typically manifests late, because early disease is asymptomatic and the extensive esophageal lymphatic system and lack of serosal layer facilitate early spread of malignancy. Staging evaluation includes CT of the chest and whole body PET scan, which help determine treatment. Surgery is the mainstay of treatment for cases without distant metastases, supplemented with chemotherapy and/or irradiation. Surgery is not indicated (unless for palliative measures) with distant metastases.

📋 **CASE SCENARIO:** In a 52-year-old man with severe heartburn, endoscopy reveals Barrett metaplasia in the distal esophagus. He begins taking omeprazole and feels better. What kind of follow-up does he need for the Barrett metaplasia? Periodic upper endoscopy with biopsies to make sure that he does not develop adenocarcinoma.

Thyroid cancer: Patients present with a nodule in the thyroid gland. Be suspicious for cancer in any of the following scenarios: *"cold nodule" on radionuclide scan,* male sex, history of *childhood irradiation,* nodule described as "stony hard," recent or rapid nodule enlargement, and increased *calcitonin* level (which indicates medullary thyroid cancer, classically in patients with MEN type 2). To evaluate a thyroid nodule, order thyroid function tests. Thyroid-stimulating hormone is the best screening test;

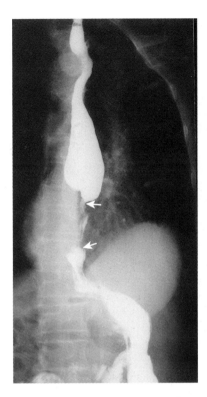

FIGURE 3-45. Obstructing carcinoma *(arrows)* of the lower esophagus. *(From James EC, Corry RJ, Perry JF: Principles of Basic Surgical Practice. Philadelphia, Hanley & Belfus, 1987.)*

"toxic" or functional nodules are unlikely to be cancer. Then order a thyroid ultrasound study and possibly a radionuclide scan ("cold" nodule or area of decreased uptake is more suspicious than a nodule with normal or increased uptake). The next step is ultrasound-guided fine-needle aspiration for any indeterminate or suspicious nodules.

Bladder cancer: Look for *persistent, painless hematuria.* The patient is often a *smoker* or worked in the rubber or dye industry (aniline dye exposure). CT scan with contrast or intravenous pyelogram may detect a lesion or nonmalignant cause of hematuria (e.g., urolithiasis). Cystoscopy is done to evaluate any suspicious lesions, to perform biopsy, or to investigate any persistent and/or unexplained hematuria.

Liver tumors: Hepatocellular carcinoma is caused by alcohol, chronic hepatitis (B or C), hemochromatosis, and essentially anything else that causes cirrhosis. *Alpha fetoprotein* is often elevated and can be measured postoperatively to detect recurrences. Patients have one of the previously mentioned histories and present with weight loss, right upper quadrant pain, and an enlarged liver. Surgery is usually the only hope for cure; prognosis is poor.

Other tumors of the liver:
- ◯ Hemangioma: most common primary tumor of the liver; benign, usually asymptomatic and generally left alone, but surgery may be done if the patient is symptomatic. CT or MRI can usually make the specific diagnosis and avoid the need for biopsy.
- ◯ Hepatic adenoma: uncommon benign tumor that appears most commonly in *women of reproductive age taking birth control pills.* Stop the pills! The tumor may then regress; if not, biopsy is necessary and surgical resection is often performed due to risk of rupture and low risk of malignant transformation. Also seen with higher frequency in patients with glycogen storage disease and pregnant women.
- ◯ Focal nodular hyperplasia: common benign usually asymptomatic tumor that is left alone. CT or MRI can often make the specific diagnosis.
- ◯ Cholangiocarcinoma: Up to 50% of patients have inflammatory bowel disease *(usually ulcerative colitis).* Liver flukes *(Clonorchis* spp.) increase the risk in immigrants.
- ◯ Angiosarcoma: Look for exposure to industrial vinyl chloride.
- ◯ Hepatoblastoma: the main primary liver malignancy in children.

Adrenal tumors may be functional in the cortex and cause primary hyperaldosteronism (Conn syndrome) or hyperadrenalism (Cushing syndrome). Another possibility is pheochromocytoma in the medulla (Fig. 3-46); look for intermittent, severe hypertension with mental status changes, headaches,

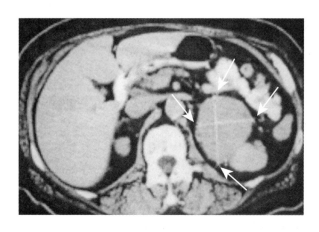

FIGURE 3-46 Magnetic resonance image showing a left adrenal pheochromocytoma (between the *arrows*) in a 71-year-old woman. *(From Katz DS, Math KR, Groski SA [eds]: Radiology Secrets. Philadelphia, Hanley & Belfus, 1998.)*

and diaphoresis. Check plasma-free metanephrines as the initial test. MRI is more sensitive than CT. Most adrenal tumors <3 cm are benign nonfunctional adenomas that are diagnosed using CT or MRI and can be left alone without the need for biopsy or removal. All patients with pheochromocytoma should be screened for MEN-type 2 (a or b) and von Hippel-Lindau disease.

Stomach cancer: Risk factors are Japanese ethnicity, increasing age, smoking, and ingestion of smoked meat. *Helicobacter pylori* infection has also been implicated in stomach mucosa-associated lymphoid tissue (MALT) lymphomas. A *Krukenberg tumor* is stomach cancer (or other GI malignancy) with ovarian metastases. A *Virchow node* is a left supraclavicular node enlargement due to visceral cancer spread via the thoracic duct (classically stomach cancer). If a gastric ulcer is seen on upper GI barium series or endoscopy, perform a biopsy to exclude malignancy. Treatment is surgical resection with or without chemotherapy and/or radiation unless distant metastases are detected with staging CT and PET scans, in which cases surgery is used only for palliation.

Carcinoid tumors: The most common locations are appendix, small bowel, rectum, and bronchi. Carcinoid syndrome consists of *episodic cutaneous flushing, abdominal cramps, diarrhea,* and *right-sided heart valve damage* from serotonin and other secreted substances. Urinary levels of *5-hydroxyindoleacetic acid (5-HIAA)*, a serotonin breakdown product, are increased. Treat with curative surgery only for local disease, with a combination of surgery, chemotherapy, octreotide, and adjunctive treatments (e.g., radiofrequency ablation of liver metastases) for cases with metastatic disease. Carcinoids can also occur outside the bowel, most commonly in the lung, where they are considered premalignant (i.e., are resected) and can cause carcinoid syndrome without liver metastases (because venous drainage reaches the systemic circulation before the liver).

Kaposi sarcoma: Most common in HIV-positive patients. Kaposi sarcoma is a vascular skin tumor that starts out as a papule or plaque, commonly on the upper body or in the oral cavity. The classic description is a *rash that does not respond to multiple treatments*. Associated with human herpesvirus 8 infection.

Skin cancer: Ultraviolet light increases the risk of basal cell, squamous cell, and melanoma skin cancer. The *ABCDs of melanoma* should make you suspicious of malignancy. Biopsy any lesion with any of these characteristics: asymmetry, borders (irregular), color (change in color or multiple colors), and diameter (the bigger the lesion, the more likely that it is malignant). Know the classic appearance of basal cell cancer: *pearly and umbilicated with telangiectasias*. Basal cell cancer is extremely common and can cause local bony erosion but almost never metastasizes. Metastasis is uncommon in squamous cell cancer but common in melanoma.

🗔 **CASE SCENARIO:** A 54-year-old woman reports that a mole on her back has changed in appearance and now itches. You note asymmetry, irregular borders, and multiple colors. What kind of biopsy should you perform—punch, excisional, needle, or shave? Excisional biopsy. You should cut out the entire lesion. New-onset itching in a mole that never itched before is a classic sign of melanoma.

Oropharyngeal cancer risk is increased by HPV infection (watch for history of oral sex with multiple partners), smoking or chewing tobacco, ethanol, and poor oral hygiene. Oral lesions often start as *leukoplakia* (white-colored plaquelike lesion), which must be differentiated from oral hairy leukoplakia, an EBV-associated disease that affects HIV-infected patients. Leukoplakia is rarely cancerous at presentation and often regresses if the person quits tobacco and alcohol use. *Erythroplakia* (red-colored plaque-like lesion) is more worrisome; if it is present, consider a biopsy. Almost all malignancies are of the squamous cell histologic type.

Histiocytosis: Symptoms can be variable, with bone lesions, skin lesions, and pulmonary involvement. Look for *Birbeck granules* (cytoplasmic inclusion bodies that look like tennis rackets) on electron microscopy. Perform curettage if isolated bone lesion. Smoking linked to pulmonary Langerhans cell histiocytosis.

Patients with cancer, like all other patients, have the *right to refuse any treatment.* However, watch for and treat depression, even in terminal patients.

📁 **CASE SCENARIO:** A 54-year-old man was diagnosed with pancreatic cancer and told of his odds for survival. He refuses all treatment, "even for a sore throat." The patient mentions insomnia, lack of appetite, and loss of interest in his hobbies. He mentions that the world would "probably be better off without me" and starts crying. He hands you an advance directive that states he refuses any type of medical treatment whatsoever under any circumstances. What should you do with his advance directive? Refuse to honor it until his depression has been treated and offer the patient antidepressants and counseling.

📁 **CASE SCENARIO:** What is the most common malignancy seen in the liver? Metastatic disease! Do not be fooled into saying that hepatocellular carcinoma is the most common malignancy of the liver if metastatic cancer is a choice. Do not assume that the question refers to a primary tumor unless it specifically says so.

📁 **CASE SCENARIO:** A 73-year-old man with known stage IV prostate cancer presents with local spinal pain and acute onset of hyperreflexia and muscle weakness in the lower extremities. What should you do first? What factor is most closely linked to final outcome? Metastases to the spine can cause cord compression (local spinal pain, reflex changes, weakness, sensory loss, paralysis). This scenario is an emergency. The first step is to start high-dose corticosteroids, and then order an MRI. If there is metastatic disease in the spine, the next step is treatment with radiation. Surgical decompression is used if radiation fails or the tumor is known not to be radiosensitive. The final outcome is most closely linked to pretreatment function. Do not wait to give corticosteroids.

PULMONOLOGY

Asthma
High-yield pearls:
○ Usually manifests during childhood.
○ The "atopic triad" is classic: *wheezing, eczema,* and *seasonal rhinitis.* If one parent has asthma, the child has a 25% risk; if both parents have asthma, the child's risk is 50%.
○ Do not forget other causes of wheezing such as bronchiolitis, foreign body, and cystic fibrosis.
○ The best way to make the diagnosis is with spirometry and pulmonary function tests. A decreased ratio of forced expiratory volume in 1 second (FEV_1) to forced vital capacity (FVC) that should reverse (at least partially) with bronchodilators.

📁 **CASE SCENARIO:** What class of medications should be avoided in patients with asthma or chronic obstructive pulmonary disease? β-blockers, which block the $β_2$ receptors that are necessary to open the airways.

📁 **CASE SCENARIO:** What infection should you suspect when wheezing occurs in children younger than 2 years old? Respiratory syncytial virus causing bronchiolitis. Look for coexisting fever.

📁 **CASE SCENARIO:** What should you suspect in a young child with unilateral wheezing of acute onset and no prior history of symptoms? Foreign body inhalation.

📁 **CASE SCENARIO:** A child has symptoms of wheezing only during gym class and soccer practice. What test should you use to confirm a suspicion of asthma? Have the child exercise immediately before performing spirometry (exercise challenge or provocation). Alternatively, have the child use albuterol one-half hour before exercise and see if the symptoms improve. The child's trigger is probably exercise.

Management issues:
- Avoid any known triggers, and ask the patient's parents to stop smoking (at least in the home and around the child).
- In one-half of children with asthma, the symptoms resolve by early adulthood. No symptoms = no treatment.
- Treatment is based on age and severity of symptoms. The 2007 Expert Panel Report 3 (EPR-3) guideline for the management of asthma lists specific step-wise approaches to therapy. In general, treat patients with intermittent asthma with a short acting β-2 agonist. If the asthma is persistent, start a low-dose inhaled corticosteroid. Then proceed to a medium- or high-dose inhaled corticosteroid or a long-acting β-agonist.
- Children who need hospitalization because asthma does not respond to emergency treatment commonly receive IV steroids.
- Cromolyn, nedocromil, and leukotriene inhibitors (zafirlukast, zileuton) are alternatives or additional agents for prophylaxis, not acute attacks.
- Follow children who have frequent exacerbations with peak flow measurements. The child should have a peak flow meter at home, and the parents should call the physician when values start to drop so that early treatment can be initiated.

■ **CASE SCENARIO:** A child in the emergency department with a severe asthma attack is no longer hyperventilating. The patient seems calm and sleepy. What should you do? Check arterial blood gas immediately for hypoxemia. The patient may be crashing and require intubation. Fatigue alone is sufficient reason to intubate an asthmatic patient.

Emphysema/chronic obstructive pulmonary disease
High-yield pearls:
- The cause is almost always smoking.
- In COPD, the FEV_1/FEV ratio is less than normal (<0.70), whereas in restrictive lung disease, the FEV_1/FEV is often normal. *FEV_1 may be equal in both conditions, but the ratio of FEV_1 to FEV is different.*
- Treat with bronchodilators, usually $β_2$ agonists or anticholinergics (e.g., albuterol, ipratropium, salmeterol, tiotropium). Consider steroids for acute exacerbations and antibiotics for signs of infection (change in sputum color or amount).
- Remember pneumococcal and annual influenza vaccines.
- Long-term oxygen therapy reduces mortality and should be used when oxygen saturation is <90% (or partial arterial oxygen tension [Pao_2] is <60) while the patient is breathing room air. Oxygen saturation needs to desaturate to 88% in order to qualify for home oxygen therapy.
- Consider pulmonary rehabilitation (supervised exercise), if given the option, for its long-term benefit.

■ **CASE SCENARIO:** What is the best way to reduce mortality in a patient with emphysema? Stop smoking.

■ **CASE SCENARIO:** A 72-year-old man with severe emphysema comes to the emergency department because of a stubbed toe. Oxygen level = 50 mm Hg, carbon dioxide level = 50 mm Hg. He denies respiratory complaints and says that his toe hurts. Should you admit the patient and intubate him? No. Treat the patient, not the lab value. Remember that a patient with chronic COPD may normally live at higher carbon dioxide and lower oxygen levels. If the patient is asymptomatic and talking to you calmly, the lab value should not make you panic (also: could we have accidentally gotten venous blood on this one?).

■ **CASE SCENARIO:** What should you suspect in a smoker with chronic bronchitis who has a "change" in his chronic cough but no other symptoms of infection? Lung cancer.

As a rough rule of thumb, you should prepare to intubate any patient whose carbon dioxide is >50 mm Hg or whose oxygen is <50 mm Hg, especially if the pH in either situation is <7.30 while the patient is breathing room air (this is a guideline—treat the patient, not the lab). Usually, unless the patient is crashing rapidly, a trial of supplemental oxygen by nasal cannula and/or nonrebreather mask is given first. If this approach fails or the patient becomes too tired (using accessory muscles is a good clue to the work of breathing), consider intubation.

Miscellaneous conditions

Solitary pulmonary nodule: Certain clues point to the underlying cause:

○ Immigrant: Think of tuberculosis, and do a skin test.

○ Southwest United States: think of *Coccidioides immitis.*

○ Cave explorer, exposure to bird droppings, or Ohio/Mississippi River valleys (Midwest): Think of histoplasmosis.

○ Smoker older than the age of 40: Think of lung cancer; do CT scan, PET scan, and/or bronchoscopy and biopsy.

○ Person younger than 40 with none of the above: Think of hamartoma.

🗀 **CASE SCENARIO:** What is the first step you should take if a patient has a single pulmonary nodule on a CXR? Check for old CXRs. If the lesion has not changed in 2 years, it is likely to be benign. If no old films are available or there is a change, get a CT scan. If CT scan is indeterminate or suspicious, get a PET scan. If the PET scan is positive, get tissue diagnosis with biopsy. If the PET scan is negative, do short interval follow-up imaging of nodule with CT scan and think biopsy if nodule enlarges.

Aggressive pulmonary toileting, incentive spirometry, minimal narcotics, and early ambulation help to minimize or prevent postoperative pulmonary complications.

🗀 **CASE SCENARIO:** What is the best way to reduce postoperative pulmonary complications in a smoker? Preoperative smoking cessation.

 The most common cause of a postoperative fever in the first 24 hours is **atelectasis.**

Acute respiratory distress syndrome (ARDS): Results in *noncardiogenic pulmonary edema,* respiratory distress, and *hypoxemia.* Common causes are sepsis, major trauma, pancreatitis, shock, near drowning, and drug overdose. Look for ARDS to develop within 24–48 hours of the initial insult. Classic patients have mottled or cyanotic skin, intercostal retractions, rales or rhonchi, and *no improvement in hypoxia with oxygen administration.* Radiographs show bilateral patchy pulmonary opacities with normal cardiac silhouette and no vascular congestion (i.e., not a congestive heart failure pattern). Treat with intubation, mechanical ventilation with high percentage of oxygen, and positive end-expiratory pressure (PEEP), while addressing the underlying cause if possible.

Pneumonia is usually diagnosed on the basis of clinical findings plus elevated WBC count and CXR abnormalities. With x-ray findings, history, and physical exam, try to differentiate between typical (*S. pneumoniae*) and atypical (other organisms) community-acquired pneumonia, although the distinction is not always clear (Tables 3-39 and 3-40).

TABLE 3-39 Typical versus Atypical Pneumonia

	TYPICAL PNEUMONIA	ATYPICAL PNEUMONIA
Prodrome	Short (<2 days)	Long (>3 days); headache, malaise, aches
Fever	High (>102°F)	Low (<102°F)
Age	>40 yr	<40 yr
Chest radiograph	One distinct lobe involved	Diffuse or multilobe involvement
Organism	*Streptococcus pneunoniae*	Many (*Haemophilus influenzae, Mycoplasma* or *Chlamydia* spp.)
Medications*	Third-generation cephalosporin or broad-spectrum fluoroquinolone	Azithromycin

*Avoid the temptation to pull out the "big-gun" antibiotics (with a wide spectrum) unless the patient is crashing or unstable.

TABLE 3-40 Clinical Clues Suggestive of Certain Organisms

CLINICAL CATEGORY/FACTOR	THINK OF THESE BUGS
College student	*Mycoplasma* spp. (cold agglutinins) or *Chlamydia* spp.
Alcoholic	*Klebsiella* spp. ("currant jelly" sputum), *Staphylococcus aureus,* other enteric organisms (aspiration)
Cystic fibrosis	*Pseudomonas* spp. or *S. aureus*
Immigrant or silicosis	Tuberculosis
Chronic obstructive pulmonary disease	*Haemophilus influenzae, Moraxella* spp.

Continued

TABLE 3-40 Clinical Clues Suggestive of Certain Organisms—cont'd

CLINICAL CATEGORY/FACTOR	THINK OF THESE BUGS
Patient with TB and pulmonary cavitation	*Aspergillus* spp.
Exposure to air conditioner	*Legionella* spp.
HIV/AIDS	*Pneumocystis jirovecii* or cytomegalovirus (with koilocytosis)
Exposure to bird droppings	*Chlamydia psittaci* or *Histoplasma capsulatum*
Child <1 yr old	Respiratory syncytial virus
Child 2-5 yr old	Parainfluenza (croup) or epiglottitis (less common)

AIDS, Acquired immunodeficiency syndrome; *HIV,* human immunodeficiency virus.

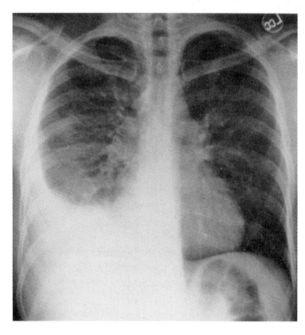

FIGURE 3-47 Pleural effusion. *(From Sahn SA, Heffner JE: Pulmonary Pearls II. Philadelphia, Hanley & Belfus, 1995.)*

🗀 **CASE SCENARIO:** A young child has recurrent pneumonia in the right middle lobe, with no other signs of immune deficiency. What should you suspect? Foreign body aspiration or congenital malformation in the affected lung segment. Remember that an aspirated foreign body is most likely to go down the right bronchus.

Pleural effusion: If you do not know the cause, always consider thoracentesis and examine the fluid by doing a Gram stain, culture (including tuberculosis), cell count with differential, cytology, glucose level (low in infection), and protein level (high in infection). A pleural effusion can occur in the setting of pneumonia and often resolves with the pneumonia, but watch for possible progression to an empyema (infected, loculated pleural fluid), which requires chest tube drainage (Fig. 3-47).

RHEUMATOLOGY

Arthritis

The large majority of cases of arthritis in adults (especially the elderly) are due to osteoarthritis (OA). Obtain radiographs of the affected joint to confirm. When in doubt, or if you suspect something other than OA, consider aspirating fluid from the affected joint for examination if an effusion is present. Examine the fluid for cell count and differential, glucose, bacteria (Gram stain and culture), and crystals.

🗀 **CASE SCENARIO:** A 50-year-old man presents with an acutely painful, hot, swollen, stiff right knee with no history of trauma or musculoskeletal problems. What should you do next? Arthrocentesis and joint fluid examination.

Arthritis key differences/points:

1. **Osteoarthritis (OA):** little evidence of inflammation on exam (no hot, red, tender joints as in most other rheumatologic/arthritic disorders). Classic signs and symptoms include *Heberden nodes* at the distal interphalangeal (DIP) joint and *Bouchard nodes* at the proximal interphalangeal (PIP) joint

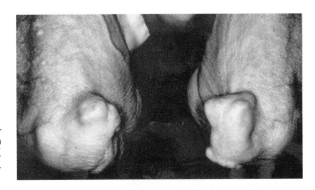

Figure 3-48 Unusually large dermal and subcutaneous rheumatoid nodules in a patient with severe rheumatoid arthritis. *(From Fitzpatrick JE, Aeling JL: Dermatology Secrets. Philadelphia, Hanely & Belfus, 1999.)*

(both relate to palpable bone hypertrophy/osteophyte formation), as well as worsening symptoms in the evening or after use. Radiographs reveal joint space narrowing and osteophyte formation. The incidence increases with age. Treat with weight reduction when appropriate and as-needed NSAIDs or acetaminophen.

2. **Rheumatoid arthritis (RA):** Diagnosis involves number and size of affected joints, positive rheumatoid factor (RF) and anticyclic citrullinated protein (CCP) antibody testing, elevated ESR or C-reactive protein, and symptom duration >6 weeks (Fig. 3-48). Children with RA are often RF-negative. Look for systemic symptoms (fever, malaise, subcutaneous nodules, pericarditis/pleural effusion, uveitis), prolonged morning stiffness, and *swan neck* and *boutonniére* deformities. The buzz word is *pannus* (articular cartilage looks like granulation tissue due to chronic inflammation). Radiographs reveal joint space narrowing with no osteophytes and periarticular erosions. There are five general classes of medications used for the treatment of rheumatoid arthritis, with disease-modifying antirheumatic drugs (DMARDs) forming the backbone of treatment. Treatment options include the following: analgesics (from acetaminophen to narcotics); NSAIDs; glucocorticoids; nonbiologic DMARDs (methotrexate, sulfasalazine, leflunomide, hydroxychloroquine, and minocycline); and biologic DMARDs. Biologic DMARDs include tumor necrosis factor (TNF) inhibitors (etanercept invliximab, and adalimumab), an interleukin-1 receptor antagonist (anakinra), a monoclonal antibody (rituximab), and biologic response modifiers (abataept).

3. **Gout:** classically starts with *podagra* (gout in the big toe). Look for *tophi* (subcutaneous uric acid deposits on exam or radiograph, cause "punched-out" erosions on bone radiograph) and *needle-shaped urate crystals* (often inside leukocytes) with *negative birefringence*. Gout is more common in men than in women. Patients should avoid alcohol, which may precipitate an attack. Colchicine or NSAIDs (not aspirin, which causes decreased excretion of uric acid by the kidney) or intraarticular corticosteroid injection are used for acute attacks. For maintenance therapy, high fluid intake, alkalinization of the urine, and colchicine or *allopurinol*.

🗀 **CASE SCENARIO:** A 58-year-old obese man presents with acute onset of pain, redness, and swelling in the big toe. Joint aspiration reveals needle-shaped crystals with negative birefringence. Should you use low-dose or high-dose allopurinol? Neither. Allopurinol should not be given for acute attacks because it makes matters worse.

4. **Pseudogout:** *rhomboid-shaped* calcium pyrophosphate dihydrate crystals with *weakly positive birefringence*. Mnemonic: pseudogout = pyrophosphate and positive birefringence. Treat with NSAIDs or colchicine.

5. **Septic arthritis:** Synovial fluid shows bacteria on Gram stain. *S. aureus* is the most common organism, except in sexually active young adults (in whom the most common organism is *Neisseria gonorrhoeae*). Do blood cultures in addition to joint cultures because the organism usually reaches the joint via the hematogenous route. Do urethral swabs and cultures in appropriate patients.

Other causes of arthritis:

1. **Psoriasis:** In the presence of classic skin lesions, always consider psoriatic arthritis. The disease usually affects hands and feet. The arthritis resembles rheumatoid arthritis, but rheumatoid factor is negative. Treat with NSAIDs (first-line therapy), methotrexate, PUVA, retinoic acid derivatives, cyclosporine, sulfasalazine, azathioprine, antimalarials, etanercept, or infliximab.

2. **Lupus erythematosus or inflammatory bowel disease:** Look for other symptoms of the primary disease to make the diagnosis. Both can cause an inflammatory arthritis that can be treated similar to RA.

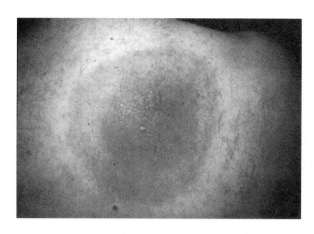

Figure 3-49 Erythematous, annular rash known as erythema (chronicum) migrans, which is characteristic of Lyme disease. *(From Cunha BA: Infectious Disease Pearls. Philadelphia, Hanley & Belfus. 1999.)*

3. **Ankylosing spondylitis:** Remember the association with *HLA-B27*. Most often a 20–40-year-old man with a positive family history presents with back pain and morning stiffness. The patient may assume a bent-over posture. Sacroiliac joints are primarily affected, and radiographs may show a *"bamboo spine."* Watch for other autoimmune symptoms such as fever, elevated sedimentation rate, anemia, and *uveitis.* Treatment is exercise and NSAIDs, methotrexate, sulfasalazine, or TNF antagonists (etanercept, infliximab, adalimumab).

4. **Reactive arthritis** is also associated with *HLA-B27*. The classic triad of symptoms is urethritis (due to chlamydial infection), conjunctivitis/uveitis, and arthritis (the patient *"can't pee, can't see, and can't climb a tree"*). Reactive arthritis, previously known as Reiter syndrome, also may follow enteric bacterial infections. Superficial oral and penile ulcers may occur. Diagnose and treat the sexually transmitted disease (particularly HIV), if present; also treat the patient's sexual partners. Use NSAIDs for mild arthritis and methotrexate and/or sulfasalazine for more severe symptoms.

5. **Hemophilia:** Recurrent hemarthroses can cause a debilitating arthritis. Treat with acetaminophen; avoid antiplatelet agents.

6. **Lyme disease:** Look for tick bite, *erythema chronicum migrans* (Fig. 3-49), and migratory arthritis later. Treat with doxycycline (amoxicillin in pregnant women and children younger than the age of 8 years); use parenteral ceftriaxone for carditis or other serious complications.

7. **Rheumatic fever:** Look for previous streptococcal pharyngitis. *Migratory polyarthritis* is one of the major Jones criteria.

8. **Sickle cell disease:** Patients frequently have arthralgias and may develop *avascular necrosis* of the humeral or femoral head, which can lead to severe arthritic changes and deformities, as well as a propensity to develop bone infarcts in long bones.

9. **Trauma:** generally causes osteoarthritis due to altered biomechanics.

10. **Childhood orthopedic problem:** slipped capital femoral epiphysis, congenital hip dysplasia, and Legg-Calvé-Perthes disease may cause arthritis as an adult. Use history (age of onset) and radiograph to figure out which disease the patient had (see Chapter 2, Pediatric Orthopedics section).

11. **Charcot joint:** most commonly seen in *diabetics;* also seen in other neuropathies. Lack of sensation causes the patient to overuse or misuse joints, which become deformed and painful. The best treatment is prevention. After even seemingly mild trauma, patients with neuropathy need radiographs to rule out fractures.

12. **Hemochromatosis/Wilson disease:** Both may cause arthritis due to deposition of iron or copper, respectively.

Autoimmune diseases

Autoimmune diseases affect women of reproductive age unless otherwise specified. For board purposes, classic disease findings differentiate one condition from the other. Almost all have systemic signs of inflammation (elevated sedimentation rate/C-reactive protein, fever, anemia of chronic disease, fatigue, weight loss).

1. **Systemic lupus erythematosus:** Diagnosis requires 4 or more of the following 11 criteria: malar rash; discoid rash; photosensitivity; kidney damage; arthritis; pericarditis or pleuritis; positive *antinuclear antibody* (ANA); positive *anti-Smith antibody* or false-positive syphilis test (VDRL, RPR); hematologic disorder (thrombocytopenia, leukopenia, anemia, hemolysis); neurologic disturbances

(depression, psychosis, seizures); or oral ulcers. Use ANA titer as a screening test; confirm with the anti-Smith antibody test. Treat with NSAIDs, hydroxychloroquine, corticosteroids, and/or other immunosuppresants (e.g., methotrexate, cyclophosphamide, azathioprine, or mycophenolate). Use cyclophosphamide for lupus nephritis.

2. **Scleroderma/progressive systemic sclerosis:** Look for CREST symptoms (calcinosis, Raynaud phenomenon, esophageal dysmotility, sclerodactyly, telangiectasias); *heartburn*/GERD; and mask-like, leathery facies. The screening test is the ANA assay; confirmatory tests are *anticentromere antibody* (for CREST) and *antitopoisomerase* (for scleroderma). Treat with corticosteroids and/or methotrexate.

3. **Sjögren syndrome:** autoimmune disorder characterized by lymphocytic and plasma cell infiltration and destruction of salivary and lacrimal glands with subsequent diminished lacrimal and salivary gland secretions. Symptoms include dry eyes (*keratoconjunctivitis sicca*) and dry mouth (xerostomia); often associated with other autoimmune disease. Positive ANA with autoantibodies anti-SS A and anti-SS B may be present. Treat with eye drops and good oral hygiene. The most serious complication is the development of non-Hodgkin's lymphoma and other lymphoproliferative disorders.

4. **Dermatomyositis:** polymyositis (see Table 3-41) plus skin involvement (*heliotrope rash around the eyes with associated periorbital edema* is classic). Patients classically have difficulty in rising out of a chair or climbing steps because the disease affects proximal muscles. Muscle enzymes (i.e., CK) are elevated, and electromyography is irregular. Muscle biopsy establishes the diagnosis. Corticosteroids are the mainstay of therapy. Patients have an increased incidence of *malignancy* (ovary, lung, GI, breast) and this disorder can be seen as a paraneoplastic syndrome.

5. **Polyarteritis nodosa:** a vasculitic syndrome involving medium-sized to small arteries associated with *hepatitis B* infection and cryoglobulinemia. Patients present with fever, abdominal pain, weight loss, livedo reticularis, testicular pain, renal disturbances, and/or peripheral neuropathies. Lab abnormalities include high sedimentation rate, leukocytosis, anemia, and hematuria/proteinuria. Vasculitis involves medium-sized vessels and may cause aneurysms. Biopsy is the gold standard for diagnosis. Treat with steroids and cyclophosphamide.

6. **Wegener granulomatosis:** resembles Goodpasture syndrome, but instead of antiglomerular antibodies, look for positive *ANCA* titer. Also look for *sinonasal involvement* (nose bleeds, nasal perforation), which is not seen in Goodpasture syndrome, as well as involvement of lungs (hemoptysis, dyspnea) and kidneys (hematuria, acute renal failure). Treat with cyclophosphamide.

7. **Kawasaki syndrome:** typically affects *children younger than 5 years old* and is more common in Japanese children and boys (5:1 M:F). Patients present with truncal rash, high fever (lasting >5 days), conjunctival infection, cervical lymphadenopathy, *"strawberry" tongue*, late *skin desquamation* of palms and soles, and/or arthritis. Patients can develop coronary vessel vasculitis and subsequent aneurysms, which may thrombose and cause an MI. You should consider Kawasaki disease in any child who experiences an MI. Treat during the acute stage with aspirin (one of the few times to use aspirin in children) and IV immunoglobulins to reduce the risk of coronary aneurysm.

8. **Takayasu arteritis:** tends to affect Asian women between 15 and 30 years of age. It is also called *"pulseless disease"* because you may not be able to feel the patient's pulse or get a blood pressure measurement on one side. Vasculitis affects the aortic arch and the branches that arise from it; carotid involvement may cause neurologic signs or stroke. Heart failure is not uncommon. A CT or MR angiogram shows characteristic lesions. Treat with corticosteroids and/or cyclophosphamide.

9. **Behçet syndrome:** idiopathic multisystem vascular-inflammatory disease. The classic patient is a man in his 20s with *painful oral and genital ulcers*. May also have uveitis, arthritis, and other skin lesions (especially erythema nodosum). Corticosteroids may help.

10. **Henoch-Schönlein purpura** (HSP) is a small-vessel vasculitis characterized by purpura (rash on the legs), arthritis, abdominal pain, and hematuria. The typical patient is a child or young adult with a recent history of an upper respiratory infection. It is characterized by IgA, C3 and immune complex deposition in arterioles, capillaries, and venules. Treatment is supportive.

Fibromyalgia versus polymyositis versus polymyalgia rheumatica

See Table 3-41 and Figure 3-50.

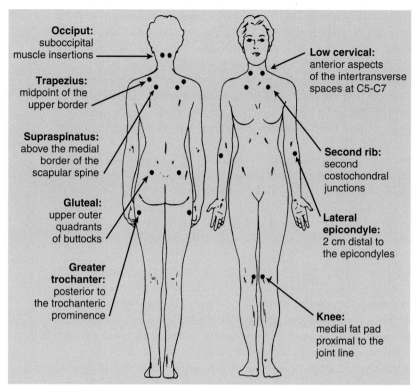

Occiput: suboccipital muscle insertions

Trapezius: midpoint of the upper border

Supraspinatus: above the medial border of the scapular spine

Gluteal: upper outer quadrants of buttocks

Greater trochanter: posterior to the trochanteric prominence

Low cervical: anterior aspects of the intertransverse spaces at C5-C7

Second rib: second costochondral junctions

Lateral epicondyle: 2 cm distal to the epicondyles

Knee: medial fat pad proximal to the joint line

FIGURE 3-50 Location of the 18 (9 pairs) specific tender points in patients with fibromyalgia. *(From Freundlich B, Leventhal L: The fibromyalgia syndrome. In Schumacher HR Jr, Kippel JH, Koopman WJ [eds]: Primer on the Rheumatic Diseases, 10th ed. Atlanta, Arthritis Foundation, 1993, pp 247-249.)*

TABLE 3-41 Fibromyalgia versus Polymyositis versus Polymyalgia Rheumatica

FEATURE	FIBROMYALGIA	POLYMYOSITIS	POLYMYALGIA RHEUMATICA
Classic age/sex	Young adult woman	40-60-yr-old woman	Woman >50 yr old
Location	Various (see figure)	Proximal muscles	Pectoral and pelvic girdles, neck
ESR	Normal	Elevated	Markedly elevated (often >100)
Muscle biopsy/EMG	Normal	Abnormal	Normal
Classic findings	Anxiety, stress, insomnia; point tenderness over affected muscles; negative work-up	Elevated CK; abnormal EMG and biopsy; greater risk of cancer	Temporal arteritis; great response to steroids, very high ESR; elderly patient
Treatment	SSRIs, NSAIDs, exercise	Steroids	Steroids

CK, Creatine kinase; *EMG,* electromyography; *ESR,* erythrocyte sedimentation rate; *NSAIDs,* nonsteroidal antiinflammatory drugs; *SSRIs,* selective serotonin reuptake inhibitors.

📁 **CASE SCENARIO:** A 65-year-old woman presents with unilateral scalp tenderness, fatigue, and muscular weakness. Her sedimentation rate is markedly elevated. She mentions that she is having trouble seeing out of her right eye. What should you do next? Start corticosteroids immediately. Do not wait to confirm the diagnosis of temporal arteritis with a biopsy because the patient may go blind while you are waiting for the biopsy results.

Paget disease: a disease of bone in which bone is broken down and regenerated, often simultaneously. The disease is seen in patients older than *40 years of age,* more commonly in men, and often discovered in an asymptomatic patient on radiograph. Classic signs include pelvic and skull involvement; watch for a patient who has had to buy larger-sized hats. Patient may have bone pain, arthritis, or nerve deafness (with skull base involvement). *Alkaline phosphatase* is classically markedly elevated in the presence of *normal calcium and phosphorus levels.* Bone scintigraphy is the most sensitive test for determining the extent of disease. Patients have an increased risk of osteosarcoma in affected bones. Treat with NSAIDs for pain relief and bisphosphonates. If the GFR is <35, use calcitonin instead of bisphosphonates.

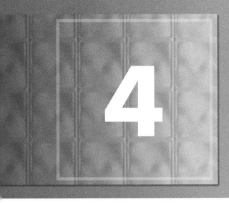

4 GYNECOLOGY AND OBSTETRICS

GYNECOLOGY

Infections

Pelvic inflammatory disease (PID): Look for a female patient aged 13–35 years with *abdominal pain, adnexal tenderness,* and *cervical motion tenderness* (all three should be present). Patients also have at least one of the following: elevated sedimentation rate, leukocytosis, fever, or *purulent cervical discharge.* Treat with more than one antibiotic (e.g., cefoxitin/ceftriaxone and doxycycline on an outpatient basis; clindamycin and gentamicin on an inpatient basis) to cover multiple organisms (e.g., *Neisseria gonorrhoeae, Chlamydia* spp., *Escherichia coli*). In patients with a history of intrauterine device use, think of *Actinomyces israelii* (Table 4-1).

Table 4-1 Vaginal Infections

ORGANISM/DISEASE	FINDINGS	TREATMENT
Candida albicans	"Cottage cheese" discharge, pseudohyphae on KOH preparation, history of diabetes mellitus, antibiotic treatment	Azole cream vaginal. With recurrent infection or in HIV+ patient, use oral azole
Gardnerella vaginalis	Malodorous discharge; fishy smell on KOH preparation, clue cells	Metronidazole
Trichomonas vaginalis	Pale green, frothy, watery discharge; motile protozoa on wet mount; "strawberry cervix"; sexually transmitted	Metronidazole Treat partners
Chlamydia trachomatis	Most common sexually transmitted disease; dysuria, positive PCR-DNA test, culture, or antibody test	Doxycycline or azithromycin
Neisseria gonorrhoeae	Mucopurulent cervicitis; gram-negative bugs on Gram stain, positive PCR-DNA test	Ceftriaxone or cefixime
Herpes simplex virus	Multiple shallow, painful ulcers; recurrence and resolution	Acyclovir, valacyclovir
Human papillomavirus	Genital warts, koilocytosis on Pap smear; high risk include types 16, 18. Low risk include types 6, 11	Many—observation, acid, cryotherapy, laser, podophyllin)
Molluscum contagiosum	Characteristic appearance of lesions (pearly papule with central umbilication), intracellular inclusions	Many—observation, curettage, cryotherapy
Pediculosis	"Crabs"; itching, lice on pubic hairs	Permethrin cream
Primary syphilis	Painless chancre, spirochete on dark field microscopy	Penicillin
Secondary syphilis	Condylomata lata, maculopapular rash on palms, serology	Penicillin

DNA, Deoxyribonucleic acid; KOH, potassium hydroxide; PCR, polymerase chain reaction.

❍ PID is the most common cause of preventable infertility (causes scarring of the fallopian tubes) and the most likely cause of infertility in a woman younger than 30 years of age with normal menstrual cycles.

❍ Watch for progression to tubo-ovarian abscess (palpable on exam and/or visible on ultrasonography [US]) and abscess rupture. Rupture is treated with emergent laparotomy and excision of the affected tube (with unilateral disease) or hysterectomy and bilateral salpingo-oophorectomy (with severe bilateral disease). An unruptured abscess may respond to antibiotics (unlike many abscesses) alone, with percutaneous drainage sometimes used.

📁 **CASE SCENARIO:** A 19-year-old woman presents with a purulent cervical discharge. Culture reveals gonorrhea. What should the treatment be? Ceftriaxone plus doxycycline or azithromycin (the doxycycline or azithromycin is given to treat presumed chlamydial coinfection). The reverse is not true, however; do not treat patients with chlamydial infection for gonorrhea unless you know they have both.

📁 **CASE SCENARIO:** A 24-year-old woman with purulent vaginal discharge tests positive for *Chlamydia* by polymerase chain reaction (PCR testing). A urine human chorionic gonadotropin (HCG) test is positive for pregnancy. What is the preferred treatment? Erythromycin is preferred over doxycycline in pregnant or breast-feeding patients because doxycycline has the potential for fetal harm including tooth discoloration and bone malformation.

📁 **CASE SCENARIO:** A woman presents with a malodorous vaginal discharge, and a fishy odor is evident when you perform a potassium hydroxide preparation of a swab sample. How should you handle treatment of the woman's sexual partner? The patient is infected with *Gardnerella* spp. You do not need to treat the patient's sexual partners. The same is true for candidal infection. Remember to treat partners and give counseling (e.g., condoms) for the other infections in the chart provided earlier.

Amenorrhea

Primary amenorrhea: Any female who has not menstruated by age 16 has primary amenorrhea. In the absence of secondary sexual characteristics by age 14 or absence of menstruation within 2 years of developing secondary sex characteristics, patients should be evaluated. *First get a pregnancy test* (pregnancy can cause primary amenorrhea!). If it is negative and no abnormalities are seen on physical exam (e.g., absent uterus, Turner syndrome phenotype), *administer progesterone.* If bleeding occurs, estrogen and a normal uterus are present. If bleeding does not occur, the patient probably has either an absence of estrogen or an anatomic abnormality. See the following list for specifics.

○ If the patient is older than 14 and has no secondary sexual characteristics, there is most likely a genetic problem.

○ In a phenotypically normal female (normal breast development) with an absence of both axillary and pubic hair who is tall for her age, think of *androgen insensitivity syndrome.* The uterus is absent, and the patient is XY or a genotypic male but should be treated as a female. Check for undescended testes, and consider removal of the testes due to a high risk of malignancy. Treat with estrogens to advance secondary sexual characteristics.

○ *Transverse vaginal septum/imperforate hymen* manifests in a menarche-aged patient with blood in the vagina that cannot escape. On exam, the hymen bulges outward. Treatment is surgical opening of the hymen.

📁 **CASE SCENARIO:** A mother brings in her 14-year-old daughter who has cyclical abdominal pain but has never had menses. A bulging membrane is seen on pelvic exam. What is the diagnosis? Primary amenorrhea secondary to a transverse vaginal septum or imperforate hymen.

Secondary amenorrhea This diagnosis requires absence of menses for 6 months in a woman with prior normal menstruation. In a sexually active woman of reproductive age, the cause should be considered *pregnancy until proven otherwise* with a negative HCG assay. If the pregnancy test is negative and no obvious abnormality is apparent on the history or physical exam, administer progesterone, which will tell you the patient's estrogen status:

○ If the patient has vaginal bleeding within 2 weeks, she has sufficient estrogen. Next, check the luteinizing hormone (LH) level. If it is high, think of *polycystic ovary syndrome.* If it is low or normal, think of three possibilities: (1) pituitary adenoma (check *prolactin*); (2) *hypothyroidism* (check thyroid-stimulating hormone [TSH]); or (3) low gonadotropin hormone levels due to drugs, stress, *exercise,* or *anorexia nervosa* (normal prolactin and TSH). With any of these disorders, the patient can try *clomiphene* to become pregnant.

○ If the patient has no bleeding, estrogen is insufficient. Check follicle-stimulating hormone (FSH) next. If it is elevated, the patient has *premature ovarian failure/menopause;* check for an autoimmune disorder, karyotype abnormalities, and history of chemotherapy. If FSH is low or normal, the patient may have a neoplasm affecting the hypothalamus; consider magnetic resonance imaging (MRI) of the brain.

📁 **CASE SCENARIO:** What is the first test to order in any woman of reproductive age who has amenorrhea, whether primary or secondary? A pregnancy test.

Other menstrual disorders

Endometriosis: Ectopic endometrial glands that are outside the uterus. Patients are classically *nulliparous* and *older than age 30*, with the following symptoms: *dysmenorrhea, dyspareunia* (painful intercourse), *dyschezia* (painful defecation), and/or perimenstrual spotting. The most common site of occurrence is the *ovaries;* look for tender adnexae in a patient without other evidence of PID. Other exam findings include nodularities of the broad/uterosacral ligaments and retroverted uterus. The gold standard of diagnosis is laparoscopy with visualization of the lesions of endometriosis (described as raised blue-colored *"mulberry spots";* flat, brown-colored *"powder burns";* or blood-filled *"chocolate cysts"*).
○ Endometriosis is the most likely cause of infertility in a menstruating woman older than 30 years of age.
○ Treat first with *birth control pills* (danazol and gonadotropin-releasing hormone ([GnRH] agonists are second-line agents).
○ Surgery/cautery can be used to destroy endometriomas, which often improves fertility. In an older patient, consider hysterectomy with bilateral salpingo-oophorectomy for severe symptoms.

Adenomyosis: ectopic endometrial glands that are within the uterine musculature. Patients are usually *older than age 40*, with *dysmenorrhea* and menorrhagia. Physical exam reveals a *large, boggy uterus.* Do D&C (D&C) to rule out endometrial cancer, and consider hysterectomy to relieve severe symptoms. GnRH agonists may also relieve symptoms.

Dysfunctional uterine bleeding (DUB): Defined as abnormal uterine bleeding not associated with tumor, inflammation, or pregnancy. DUB is the most common cause of abnormal uterine bleeding and is a diagnosis of exclusion. More than 70% of cases are associated with anovulatory cycles (unopposed estrogen). The age of the patient is important. After menarche and just before menopause, DUB is common and, in fact, physiologic. Most other women have *polycystic ovary syndrome.* Perform D&C to rule out endometrial cancer in women older than 35. Also get a complete blood count to make sure that the patient is not anemic from excessive blood loss. Uncommon causes of DUB are infections, endocrine disorders (thyroid, adrenal, pituitary/prolactin), coagulation defects, and estrogen-producing neoplasms.
○ In the absence of pathology, treat first with nonsteroidal anti-inflammatory drugs (NSAIDs), which are first-line agents for DUB and dysmenorrhea.
○ Birth control pills are also a first-line agent for menorrhagia/DUB if the patient does not desire pregnancy and her menstrual cycles are irregular.
○ For severe bleeding, progesterone is sometimes given. If the patient does not desire pregnancy, consider endometrial ablation or hysterectomy.

Polycystic ovary syndrome (PCOS): Look for an *overweight* woman who has *hirsutism, amenorrhea,* and/or *infertility* (i.e., "heavy, hirsute, and [h]amenorrheic"). PCOS is the most likely cause for infertility in a woman younger than 30 with abnormal menstruation. Impaired glucose tolerance and diabetes are common. Multiple ovarian cysts are often seen on US. The primary event is thought to be *androgen excess;* the *LH-to-FSH ratio is greater than 2 : 1.* Unopposed estrogen increases risk for *endometrial hyperplasia* and *carcinoma.* Treatment can include surgery (laparoscopic wedge resection), birth control pills, weight loss, or cyclic progesterone. Metformin improves ovulation and insulin sensitivity. Spironolactone may help the hirsutism. If the woman desires pregnancy, clomiphene may be used, alone or in combination with other treatments.

Premenstrual dysphoric disorder (aka PMS): Occurs every month just before menstruation. The patient is symptom free at other times. Classic signs and symptoms include bloating, breast swelling/tenderness, headaches, irritability, and depression. Treat with NSAIDs; consider antidepressants (selective serotonin reuptake inhibitors [SSRIs]) for depression symptoms.

Menopause: The average age at menopause is around 50. Patients have irregular cycles or *amenorrhea, hot flashes, mood swings,* and an *elevated FSH level.* See "Obstetric Pharmacology and Teratogenesis" later for information about hormone replacement therapy (HRT). A bone density test may show osteoporosis. Patients may also complain of *dysuria, dyspareunia, incontinence,* and/or *vaginal itching, burning, or soreness*—symptoms often due to atrophic vaginitis in this age group. Look for vaginal mucosa to be thin, dry, and atrophic, with increased parabasal cells on cytology. Estrogen, either topical or systemic, improves these symptoms.

Leiomyoma (fibroid): Can also cause painful or excessive menstrual bleeding. Uterine enlargement is common on exam. Diagnosis can be confirmed with pelvic US. Rarely these may be malignant leiomyosarcoma (watch for rapid growth, hemorrhage, necrosis, invasion, and metastasis).

Breast disorders

Breast discharge: Watch for history of birth control pills, hormone therapies, antipsychotic medications, or hypothyroidism symptoms, all of which can cause discharge. When the discharge is *bilateral and nonbloody*, the cause is not breast cancer. The patient may have a prolactinoma (check prolactin level) or endocrine disorder. When the discharge is unilateral, whether bloody or not, and/or associated with a mass, it should raise concern for breast cancer or intraductal papilloma (benign, but associated with increased risk for subsequent development of breast cancer). Biopsy any mass in this setting (Table 4-2).

TABLE 4-2 Breast Masses		
LESION	**CHARACTERISTICS**	**TREATMENT**
Fibrocystic disease	Most common breast disorder. *Bilateral,* multiple, nodular, tender areas on the breast that may vary with the menstrual cycle	Generally, no further work-up necessary—just routine follow-up and reassurance. Danazol may help relieve pain
Fibroadenoma	Most common benign tumor of the female breast. Painless, discrete, *sharply circumscribed, rubbery, mobile mass. Pregnancy and estrogen-containing medicines* (e.g., oral contraceptives) *may stimulate growth* (tumors are estrogen dependent). Watch out for phylloides tumor, a potentially malignant tumor that can masquerade as a rapidly growing fibroadenoma	Observation is the generally preferred treatment. Excision is curative but not often required unless the patient desires or there is clinical concern for cancer
Mastitis/abscess	Lactating woman with reddish, painful, fluctuant mass, typically within first 3 mo post partum. Cracked, fissured, or sore nipples. The most common organism is *Staphylococcus aureus.* Less common are group A beta-hemolytic streptococci, *Streptococcus pneumoniae,* and *Escherichia coli*	Mainstay of therapy is effective milk removal through continued breast-feeding. Antibiotics (cephalexin, dicloxacillin, or amoxicillin-clavulanate) are often used, as well as pain relief with NSAIDs. If abscess is present, surgical drainage is indicated
Breast cancer	Classic presentation of *nipple retraction* and/or *peau d'orange* may or may not be seen in a *nulliparous* woman with a *strong family history.* Always consider biopsy in a woman older than 35. In addition, get a baseline mammogram	See Chapter 3, Oncology section, for more information on management of breast cancer

 Mammography in women younger than 30 is rarely useful, because the breast tissue is too dense to allow characterization of masses. If cancer (rare in this age group) is suspected, use US of the breast for further evaluation.

☐ **CASE SCENARIO:** What is a new breast mass in a postmenopausal female? Cancer until proven otherwise. Perform a biopsy.

In patients with a clinically evident breast mass, mammography and US are secondary tools. The decision to perform a biopsy is a *clinical decision* based on risk factors, physical exam, history, and imaging characteristics. Mammography is best used to detect nonpalpable breast masses (as a screening tool) and is only one of many tools used to evaluate a palpable mass. On the other hand, if a suspicious lesion is found on mammogram, it should be biopsied even if physical exam findings are benign.

Miscellaneous

Uterine leiomyomata (fibroids): Benign tumors are the most common indication for hysterectomy (when they grow too large or cause symptoms). Malignant transformation is rare (<1%), and some believe it is nonexistent. Look for *rapid growth during pregnancy or use of estrogen* (e.g., birth control pills) or regression after menopause (estrogen-dependent). Fibroids may cause infertility (which may be restored by myomectomy), pain, or menorrhagia/metrorrhagia; anemia due to fibroids is an indication for hysterectomy. Perform D&C to rule out endometrial cancer and malignant transformation in women older than 40. Patients may present with a polyp protruding through the cervix. US can confirm the diagnosis and help exclude an adnexal mass when the exam is difficult due to uterine size.

Pelvic relaxation/vaginal prolapse: Due to weakening of pelvic ligaments. Look for a history of several vaginal deliveries, a feeling of heaviness or fullness in the pelvis, backache, worsening of symptoms with standing, and resolution with lying down.

○ Cystocele: Bladder bulges into the *upper anterior vaginal wall.* Symptoms include urinary urgency, frequency, and incontinence.

○ Rectocele: Rectum bulges into *lower posterior vaginal wall.* The major symptom is difficulty in defecating.
○ Enterocele: Loops of bowel bulge into the *upper posterior vaginal wall.*
○ Urethrocele: Urethra bulges into the *lower anterior vaginal wall.* Symptoms include urinary urgency, frequency, and incontinence.

 Conservative treatment involves pelvic strengthening exercises and/or use of a **pessary** *(artificial, removable device that provides support). Surgery is used for refractory or severe cases.*

Infertility: Inability to achieve pregnancy after 1 year of trying. One in eight couples experience infertility. Forty percent of cases are due to a female problem, 40% are due to a male problem, and the remainder are due to a combined or unexplained cause. Age, history of sexually transmitted diseases (STDs), being overweight, and smoking are factors that can impair fertility. If nothing is apparent after the history and physical exam, the first step is a *semen analysis* (cheap, noninvasive test that may lead to an easy diagnosis).
○ Consider ovulation disorders in women with irregular menstrual cycles. Check TSH, FSH, LH, prolactin, and US (PCOS) as initial tests.
○ Consider a tubal problem in patients with a history of PID or previous ectopic pregnancy.
○ Consider a uterine problem in patients with a history of D&C (which may cause intrauterine synechiae), fibroids, or signs or symptoms of endometriosis or adenomyosis.
○ Consider cervical factors in patients with a history of cervicitis, birth trauma, or previous cone biopsy of the cervix.
○ Laparoscopy is a last result or is done in patients with a history suggestive of endometriosis. Lysis of adhesions and destruction of endometriosis lesions may restore fertility.

🗀 **CASE SCENARIO:** What test can be used to look for structural abnormalities of the uterus and tubes? A hysterosalpingogram. MRI and three-dimensional US are viable alternatives.

🗀 **CASE SCENARIO:** In which women can clomiphene be used to induce ovulation? Women who produce adequate estrogen. If the woman is hypoestrogenic, use human menopausal gonadotropin (hMG), which is a combination of FSH and LH. If these approaches fail, consider in vitro fertilization.

If a patient does not desire sterilization, the most effective form of birth control is an intrauterine device or hormonal implant (etonogestrel implant) followed by injectable hormone depot preparations, then birth control pills/patch, and a hormonal vaginal ring. Only condoms (male or female) protect from STDs. Intrauterine devices (IUDs) were previously used only in older women, but use among nulliparous young women has gained popularity. IUDs are preferably placed in patients who are monogamous, to prevent complications such as PID. IUDs do not increase the risk of ectopic pregnancy but rather are more effective at preventing intrauterine implantation than ectopic implantation. Postcoital contraception is essentially a high dose of birth control pills taken within 72 hours after intercourse.

OBSTETRICS

Preventive care/normal pregnancy

Consider pregnancy in all women of reproductive age before treating any condition: Do not give a teratogenic drug or order a radiograph/computed tomography (CT) scan without knowing whether the woman is pregnant. A patient who says that she is on birth control may still be pregnant; no contraception is 100% effective, especially when compliance is taken into account. The standard HCG pregnancy test becomes positive roughly 2 weeks after conception.

Give folate to all women of reproductive age to prevent neural tube defects. This prevention is most effective in the first trimester, when many women do not even know that they are pregnant.

Signs of pregnancy: amenorrhea, morning sickness with nausea or vomiting, *Hegar sign* (softening and compressibility of the lower uterine segment), *Chadwick sign* (dark discoloration of the vulva and vaginal walls), linea nigra (Fig. 4-1), *melasma* (Fig. 4-2), and weight gain.

Changes and complaints associated with normal pregnancy: nausea and vomiting (morning sickness), heavy (possibly even painful) feeling of the breasts, increased pigmentation of the nipples and areolae,

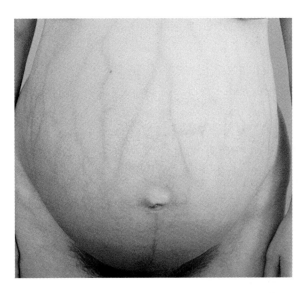

Figure 4-1 Linea nigra. The typical vertically oriented line of increased pigmentation in the midline of the lower abdomen is shown. *(From Seidel HM, Ball JW, Dains JE, Benedict W: Mosby's Physical Examination Handbook, 6th ed. Philadelphia, Mosby, 2006.)*

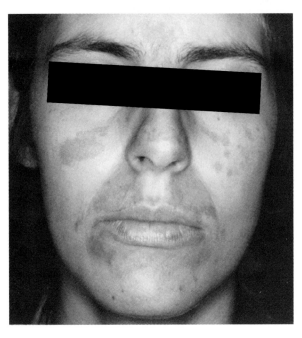

Figure 4-2 Melasma. This photodistributed macular hyperpigmentation of the face has also been termed *chloasma* or the *mask of pregnancy.*

backache, striae gravidarum, and mild ankle edema. Heartburn and increased frequency of urination are also frequent symptoms associated with pregnancy. *Quickening* (the mother's first perception of fetal movements) usually occurs at 18–20 weeks in a primigravida and at 16–18 weeks in a multigravida.

Routine prenatal tests in pregnancy: see Table 4-3.

Table 4-3 Routine Prenatal Tests in Pregnancy

VISIT	TEST	NOTES
Initial visit	CBC	To see whether the patient is anemic (pregnancy aggravates anemia). Give iron supplements (in prenatal vitamin formulations) to prevent anemia
	Blood type and screen	To identify possible isoimmunization/Rh incompatibility
	Urinalysis	Should be done at every visit to screen for preeclampsia, bacteriuria, and diabetes. *Treat asymptomatic bacteriuria in pregnancy;* 20% of pregnant women develop cystitis or pyelonephritis if untreated, at least in part because progesterone decreases the tone of the ureters and the uterus compresses the ureters
	Pap smear	If the patient is due. Also do routine chlamydial and gonorrhea cultures for any sexually active woman younger than 25, especially if she has multiple partners or is indigent, even if she is asymptomatic

TABLE 4-3 Routine Prenatal Tests in Pregnancy—cont'd

VISIT	TEST	NOTES
	Syphilis test (RPR or VDRL)	Mandated in most states for the first visit and should be performed at subsequent visits in high-risk patients
	Rubella antibody screen	If negative, patients should avoid exposure. Do not offer rubella vaccine during pregnancy because it may cause congenital rubella syndrome. Recommend rubella vaccination after delivery
	HIV test	The American College of Obstetrics and Gynecology (ACOG) advocates an "opt-out" approach to screening rather than an "opt-in" approach in order to increase screening. Identification and treatment of affected mothers improves outcomes and reduces risk of transmission to the child. Treat the mother with standard three-drug HAART. Avoid nevirapine, efavirenz, didanosine, and stavudine due to fetal toxicity. The infant should be treated with zidovudine for 6 wk after birth. Recommend cesarean section to reduce vertical transmission. Advise against breast-feeding
	Hepatitis serology	If positive for hepatitis B (HBsAg) or hepatitis C, recommend cesarean section to reduce vertical transmission and advise against breast-feeding
10-24 wk	Screening for Down syndrome, neural tube defects and aneuploidy	For patients who present in the **first trimester**, options include: • **Sequential screen**: PAPP-A, total β-HCG and ultrasound NT in 1st trimester. If high risk, offer CVS. If low risk, quad test in 2nd trimester. • False positive rate - 2% (1/50 women) • **Full integrated screen:** PAPP-A, total β-HCG and ultrasound NT in first trimester combined with quad test in 2nd trimester • Lowest false positive rate - 1% (1/100 women) • Results not available until second trimester, so early CVS not an option. • **Serum integrated screen**: PAPP-A and total β-HCG in 1st trimester, followed by Quad test in 2nd trimester. • False positive rate - 3.6% (1/28 women). • Used in places where ultrasound is not available. Results are not available until second trimester, so early CVS not an option. For patients who present in the **second trimester**: Use quad screen plus ultrasound

Quad Test

Condition	AFP	β-HCG	Estriol	Inhibin A
Neural tube defect	High	Normal	Normal	Normal
Down syndrome (trisomy 21)	Low	High	Low	High
Edwards syndrome (trisomy 18)	Low	Low	Low	Low/normal

VISIT	TEST	NOTES
		If the sequential screen, integrated screen, or second trimester screen is positive, order level II ultrasound to check the dates first and then offer genetic counseling and diagnostic testing (amniocentesis or CVS)
24-28 wk	Diabetes screening 50 g/1 hr GTT	Gestational diabetes results from increased placental hormones, primarily human placental lactogen. Positive 1-hr test result >185 mg/dL. If 1-hr GTT is indeterminate (140-185 mg/dL), perform a fasting glucose and then 3-hr 100 g GTT. Recommend dietary therapy first line. If fasting glucose or 1-hr GTT remains abnormal after 2 wk of diet therapy, use NPH insulin or lispro insulin. Avoid long-acting insulin (glargine) and oral hypoglycemics (metformin, glyburide). Perform glucose testing 1 mo after delivery to watch for development of diabetes mellitus
35-37 wk	Group B streptococcal cultures	If the culture is positive, treat during labor with IV penicillin or ampicillin to prevent neonatal meningitis

AFP, Alpha-fetoprotein; *CBC,* complete blood count; *CVS,* chorionic villus sampling; *GTT,* glucose tolerance test; *HAART,* highly active antiretroviral therapy; *β-hCG,* β-human chorionic gonadotropin; *HIV,* human immunodeficiency virus; *IV,* intravenous; *NT,* nuchal translucency; *PAPP-A,* pregnancy-associated plasma protein A; *RPR,* rapid plasma reagin; *VDRL,* Venereal Disease Research Laboratory.

☐ **CASE SCENARIO:** What is the most likely cause of macrosomia in a term infant? Maternal diabetes.

☐ **CASE SCENARIO:** What is the most common cause of an abnormal triple or quadruple screen? Error in gestation age dating.

At every prenatal visit, listen for fetal heart tones and evaluate uterine size for any size-dates discrepancy. Fetal heart tones can be heard with Doppler at 10–12 weeks and with a stethoscope at 16–20 weeks. Uterine size is evaluated by measuring the distance from the symphysis pubis to the top of the fundus in centimeters. At 12 weeks' gestation, the uterus enters the abdomen, and at 20 weeks, it reaches the umbilicus. Between roughly 20 and 35 weeks, the measurement in centimeters should equal the number of weeks' gestation. A discrepancy greater than 2–3 cm is called a size-dates discrepancy, and US should be done. A size-dates discrepancy may indicate problems such as intrauterine growth retardation, multiple gestation, or inaccurate dates.

HCG levels roughly double every 2 days in the first trimester of pregnancy, and an HCG that stays the same or increases only slowly with serial testing indicates a fetus in trouble, ectopic pregnancy, or fetal demise. A rapidly increasing HCG or one that does not decrease after delivery may indicate a hydatidiform mole or choriocarcinoma.

The average weight gain in pregnancy is 28 lb (12.5 kg). With larger gains, think of diabetes. With smaller gains, think of hyperemesis gravidarum, psychiatric disorder, or major systemic disease.

Normal physiologic changes in pregnancy:

○ Lab tests
1. Sedimentation rate is markedly elevated (not a useful test in pregnancy).
2. Overall levels of thyroxine (T_4) and thyroid-binding globulin increase, but the level of free T_4 remains normal.
3. Hemoglobin increases, but plasma volume increases more; the net result is a decrease in hematocrit and hemoglobin.
4. Blood urea nitrogen (BUN) and serum creatinine decrease as the glomerular filtration rate increases. Levels of BUN and serum creatinine at the high end of normal indicate renal disease in pregnancy.
5. Alkaline phosphatase increases markedly.
6. Mild proteinuria and glycosuria are normal in pregnancy.
7. Electrolytes and liver function tests remain normal.

○ Cardiovascular changes
1. Blood pressure decreases slightly.
2. Heart rate increases by 10–20 beats/minute.
3. Stroke volume and cardiac output increase (up to 50%).

○ Pulmonary changes
1. Minute ventilation increases because of increased tidal volume with same or only slightly increased respiratory rate.
2. Residual volume decreases.
3. Carbon dioxide decreases *(physiologic hyperventilation/respiratory alkalosis)*.

Abortion and ectopic pregnancy

Abortion is defined as termination of a pregnancy at less than 20 weeks (fetal size <500 g). Most abortions occur in the first trimester and are spontaneous (i.e., a miscarriage). Treat all patients with intravenous (IV) fluids and/or blood, if needed, and give Rh immune globulin (RhoGAM) in the setting of Rh incompatibility.

○ Threatened abortion: uterine bleeding without cervical dilation and no expulsion of tissue. Treat with pelvic rest (no sex/tampons/douching). Half of affected women go on to have a normal pregnancy.
○ Inevitable abortion: uterine bleeding with cervical dilation, crampy abdominal pain, and no tissue expulsion. Treat with observation, often followed by D&C of the uterine cavity.
○ Incomplete abortion: passage of some products of conception through the cervix. Treat with observation, often followed by D&C.
○ Complete abortion: expulsion of all products of conception from the uterus. Treat with serial HCG testing to make sure it goes down to zero. Consider D&C with pain or open cervical os.
○ Missed abortion: fetal death without expulsion of fetus. Most women will go on to have spontaneous miscarriage, but D&C commonly performed.
○ Induced abortion: intentional termination of pregnancy, 20 weeks (may be elective, which is requested by patient, or therapeutic if done to maintain the health of the mother).
○ Recurrent abortion: two or three successive, unplanned abortions. Causes include inherited or acquired prothrombotic states (e.g., factor V Leiden, protein C or S deficiency)
○ Infectious (syphilis, *Listeria*, *Mycoplasma*, *Toxoplasma* spp.)
1. Environmental (alcohol, tobacco, drugs)
2. Metabolic (diabetes, hypothyroidism)
3. Autoimmune (lupus and/or antiphospholipid antibodies/lupus anticoagulant)

4. Anatomic abnormalities (cervical incompetence, congenital female tract abnormalities, fibroids)
5. Chromosomal abnormalities (e.g., maternal/paternal translocations)

CASE SCENARIO: What condition classically causes painless, recurrent abortions in the second trimester? *Cervical incompetence.* Future pregnancies can be treated with cervical cerclage (suture to keep cervical os closed) at 14–16 weeks. Other anatomic abnormalities such as septate uterus should also be considered.

Classic symptoms of ectopic pregnancy (which usually manifests between 4 and 10 weeks and ends in spontaneous or therapeutic abortion, sometimes with catastrophic tubal rupture) are *amenorrhea, vaginal bleeding*, and *abdominal pain* with *a positive HCG* test. Palpation of an adnexal mass may indicate an ectopic pregnancy or a corpus luteum cyst. Transvaginal US in combination with β-HCG ≥1500 mIU/mL is generally used for diagnosis. When you are in doubt and the patient is crashing (e.g., hypovolemia, shock, severe abdominal pain/rebound tenderness), consider laparotomy. If the patient is stable, laparoscopy with salpingostomy can be performed. Medical abortion (e.g., with methotrexate treatment) can be performed if there are no contraindications to methotrexate (hepatic disease, renal disease, low blood counts); ectopic pregnancy less than 3.5 cm is present; HCG is <15,000 mIU/mL; the fetus has no cardiac activity; and the patient is compliant.

Transvaginal US can detect intrauterine pregnancy at roughly *5 weeks* or when the HCG level is greater than 2000 mIU. Use this information when trying to determine the possibility of an ectopic pregnancy. If the patient's last menstrual period was 3 weeks ago and the pregnancy test is positive, you cannot rule out an ectopic pregnancy. If, however, the patient's last menstrual period was 8 weeks ago and an US of the uterus does not show a gestational sac, be highly suspicious of ectopic pregnancy.

CASE SCENARIO: What is the major risk factor for ectopic pregnancy? A previous history of *pelvic inflammatory disease* (10-fold increased risk). Other risk factors include previous ectopic pregnancy, history of tubal sterilization or tuboplasty, and pregnancy that occurs with an intrauterine device in place.

Prenatal evaluation

Consider US for all women with a size/dates discrepancy greater than 2–3 cm and all women who have risk factors for a complicated pregnancy (e.g., hypertension; diabetes; renal disease; lupus erythematosus; cigarette, alcohol, or drug use; history of previous problems). There are fewer and fewer women who do not have an indication (or desire) for an US exam.

Intrauterine growth retardation (IUGR) is defined as size below the tenth percentile for age. The causes are many and are best understood in broad terms as due to one of three types of factors: *maternal* (e.g., smoking, alcohol or drugs, lupus); *fetal* (e.g., TORCH infections, congenital anomalies); or *placental* (e.g., hypertension, preeclampsia). The US parameters measured for determination of IUGR determination are biparietal diameter, head circumference, abdominal circumference, and femur length.

The biophysical profile (BPP) is used to evaluate fetal well-being. It consists of a heart tracing and US to measure four parameters:
○ Nonstress test: fetal heart rate tracing is obtained for 20 minutes to look for normal variability.
○ Amniotic fluid index: measures the amount of amniotic fluid to screen for oligohydramnios or polyhydramnios
○ Fetal breathing movements
○ Fetal body movements
Use the BPP if there is any concern about fetal well-being and in high-risk pregnancies near term. If the fetus scores low on the BPP, the next test is the contraction stress test for uteroplacental dysfunction. The mother is given oxytocin, and the fetal heart strip is monitored. If late decelerations are seen on the fetal heart strip with each contraction, the test is positive; usually a cesarean section is done.

Oligohydramnios: Decreased amniotic fluid (<500 mL at 32–36 weeks' gestation or amniotic fluid index [AFI] below the 5th percentile). Causes include *IUGR, premature rupture of membranes* (PROM), postmaturity, and renal agenesis (Potter disease). Oligohydramnios may cause fetal problems such as *pulmonary hypoplasia*, cutaneous or skeletal abnormalities due to compression, or hypoxia due to cord compression.

Polyhydramnios: Too much amniotic fluid (1700–2000 mL, or amniotic fluid index above the 95th percentile). Causes include *maternal diabetes, multiple gestation, neural tube defects* (anencephaly, spina bifida), *GI anomalies* (omphalocele, esophageal atresia), and *hydrops fetalis* (e.g., Rh incompatibility, fetal heart failure). Polyhydramnios can cause postpartum *uterine atony* (with resultant postpartum hemorrhage) and maternal dyspnea (the overdistended uterus compromises pulmonary function).

Monitoring of fetal heart and uterine contraction patterns during labor is routinely done, but the benefit is controversial. At term, the normal fetal heart rate is 110–160 beats/minute. Any value outside this range is worrisome. The following abnormalities are fair game, and you may be shown a fetal heart strip:

❍ Early deceleration, in which the nadir (low point) of fetal heart deceleration and the peak of uterine contraction coincide, signifies *head compression* (probable vagal response) and is *normal.*

❍ Variable deceleration (variable with relation to uterine contractions) is the most commonly encountered abnormality and signifies *cord compression.* Place the mother in the lateral decubitus position, administer oxygen by face mask, and stop any oxytocin infusion. If bradycardia is severe (<80–90 beats/min) or the variable pattern fails to resolve, measure fetal oxygen saturation and/or fetal scalp pH.

❍ Late deceleration, in which fetal heart deceleration occurs after uterine contraction, signifies *uteroplacental insufficiency* and is the most worrisome pattern (Fig. 4-3). First, place the mother in lateral decubitus position, give oxygen by face mask, and stop oxytocin. Next, give a tocolytic agent (β_2 agonist such as ritodrine or magnesium sulfate) and IV fluids if the mother is hypotensive (especially with epidural anesthesia!). If late decelerations persist, measure fetal oxygen saturation and/or scalp pH.

❍ Loss of variability in heart rate: if the fetal heart rate stays constant, consider checking fetal scalp pH. Any loss of variability associated with significant late or variable decelerations is a worrisome pattern and typically indicates the need for delivery.

❍ Fetal tachycardia or bradycardia is worrisome if it is prolonged or if the heart rate is well outside the normal range.

❍ Any recurrent or prolonged (>2 minutes) decelerations are worrisome.

 Any fetal scalp pH less than 7.2 or abnormally decreased fetal oxygen saturation is an indication for delivery. If the pH is greater than 7.2 or fetal oxygen saturation is normal, you may consider continuing to observe or deliver.

Labor and delivery

In true labor, normal contractions occur at least every 3 minutes, are fairly regular, and are associated with cervical changes (effacement and dilation) (Table 4-4). In false labor (Braxton-Hicks contractions), contractions are irregular and associated with no cervical changes.

TABLE 4-4 Stages of Labor			
STAGE	**CHARACTERISTICS**	**NULLIGRAVIDA**	**MULTIGRAVIDA**
First	Onset of true labor to full cervical dilation	<20 hr	<14 hr
Latent phase	From 0 to 3-4 cm dilation (slow, irregular)	Highly variable	Highly variable
Active phase	From 3-4 cm to full dilation (rapid, regular)	>1 cm/hr dilation	>1.2 cm/hr dilation
Second	From full dilation to birth of baby	30 min to 3 hr	5-30 min
Third	Delivery of baby to delivery of placenta	0-30 min	0-30 min
Fourth	Placental delivery to maternal stabilization	Up to 48 hr	Up to 48 hr

Term labor

Protraction disorder occurs once true labor has begun if the mother takes longer than Figure 4-4 indicates . Arrest disorder occurs once true labor has begun if no change in dilation occurs over 2 hours (as opposed to slow change in protraction disorder) or no change occurs in descent over 1 hour. First, rule out *abnormal lie* and *cephalopelvic disproportion.* If neither is present, treat with labor augmentation (oxytocin, prostaglandin gel, amniotomy). If this approach fails, observe and do a cesarean section at the first sign of trouble.

The most common cause of "failure to progress" (protraction or arrest disorder), also known as dystocia ("difficult birth"), is cephalopelvic disproportion (CPD), defined as disparity between the size of the baby's head and the mother's pelvis. Labor augmentation is contraindicated in this setting.

When oxytocin is given to augment ineffective uterine contractions, watch out for uterine hyperstimulation (painful, overly frequent, and poorly coordinated uterine contractions); *uterine rupture;* fetal heart rate decelerations; and *water intoxication (hyponatremia* from the antidiuretic hormone–like effect of oxytocin). Treat all of these problems by first discontinuing oxytocin infusion (half-life <10 minutes).

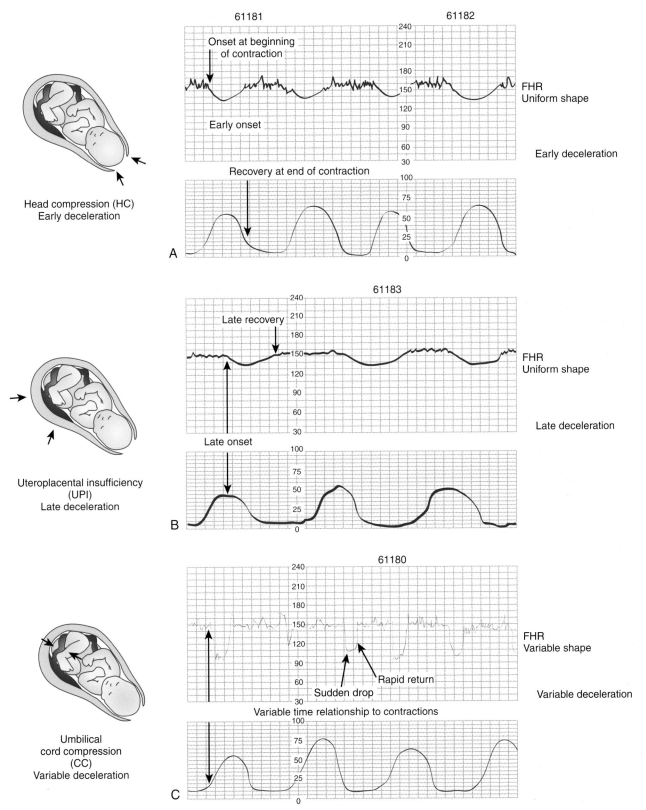

FIGURE 4-3 Deceleration patterns of the fetal heart rate (FHR). **A,** Early deceleration caused by head compression. **B,** Late deceleration caused by uteroplacental insufficiency. **C,** Variable deceleration caused by cord compression. *(From Marx J, Hockberger R, Walls R: Rosen's Emergency Medicine: Concepts and Clinical Practice, 7th ed. Philadelphia, Mosby, 2009.)*

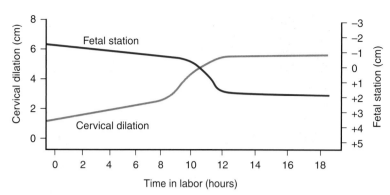

FIGURE 4-4 Arrested labor. A normal course of cervical dilatation and fetal station is present until 12–13 hours, when complete arrest is evident because of a "flattening out" of parameter lines. *(From Brochert A: Platinum Vignettes: Obstetrics and Gynecology. Philadelphia, Hanley & Belfus, 2002, p 75.)*

Prostaglandin E$_2$ (PGE$_2$), or dinoprostone, may also be used locally to induce the cervix ("ripening") and is highly effective in combination with oxytocin. PGE$_2$ may also cause uterine hyperstimulation. *Amniotomy* hastens labor but exposes the fetus and uterus to possible infection if labor does not occur.

Contraindications to labor induction/augmentation are placenta previa, vasa previa, umbilical cord prolapse or presentation, prior classic (vertical) uterine cesarean section incision, transverse fetal lie, active genital herpes, known cervical cancer, and known CPD (similar to contraindications for vaginal delivery).

When the mother has genital herpes simplex virus (HSV) infection, delay the decision about whether to do a cesarean section until the mother goes into labor. If, at the time of true labor, the mother has lesions of HSV, do a cesarean section. Otherwise, allow vaginal delivery.

After a cesarean section with a classic (vertical) uterine incision, the mother must have cesarean sections for all future deliveries because of increased rate of uterine rupture. After a cesarean section with a lower (horizontal) uterine incision, a woman may attempt to deliver future pregnancies vaginally.

Epidural anesthesia is preferred in obstetric patients. General anesthesia involves a higher risk of aspiration and resulting pneumonia because the gastroesophageal sphincter is relaxed in pregnancy and most patients have not been put on NPO (nothing-by-mouth) status for long. There are also concerns that general anesthetic agents may cross the placenta and affect the fetus. Spinal anesthesia can interfere with the mother's ability to push and is associated with a higher incidence of hypotension than epidural anesthesia.

Signs of placental separation: Fresh blood appears from the vagina, the umbilical cord lengthens, and the fundus rises and becomes firm and globular.

🔲 **CASE SCENARIO:** What is the first maneuver to try if shoulder dystocia occurs during delivery? *The McRobert maneuver.* Have the mother sharply flex her thighs against her abdomen, which may free the impacted shoulder. If this maneuver does not work, your options are limited. An extended episiotomy or other more complex maneuvers are generally necessary.

🔲 **CASE SCENARIO:** What is the correct order of labor positions? Descent, flexion, internal rotation, extension, external rotation, and expulsion.

Fetal malpresentations: Although under specific guidelines some frank and complete breeches may be delivered vaginally, it is acceptable to do a cesarean section for any breech presentation. With shoulder presentation or incomplete/footling breech, cesarean section is mandatory. For face and brow presentations, watchful waiting is best because most convert to vertex presentations. If they do not convert, do a cesarean section.

Preterm and postterm labor

Preterm labor: Labor occurring between 20 and 37 weeks with cervical dilatation and more than three contractions over 30 minutes. Treat with lateral decubitus position, bed/pelvic rest, oral or IV fluids, and oxygen administration (all may stop the contractions). Then give a tocolytic agent: IV magnesium sulfate (avoid in renal disease or myasthenia gravis), the calcium channel blocker nifedipine (avoid in CHF), or the β$_2$ agonist terbutaline (avoid in diabetes, cardiac disease, hyperthyroidism). The patient can be discharged on oral tocolytics. The many contraindications to tocolysis include heart

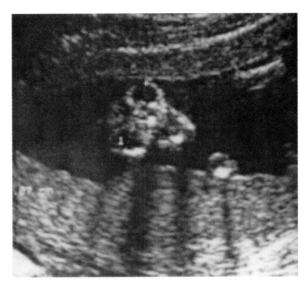

Figure 4-5 Anencephalic fetus with froglike appearance. *(From Katz DS, Math KR, Groskni SA: Radiology Secrets. Philadelphia, Hanley & Belfus, 1998, p 229.)*

disease, hypertension, diabetes, hemorrhage, preeclampsia, chorioamnionitis, IUGR, ruptured membranes, cervical dilation greater than 4 cm, fetal demise, and fetal anomalies incompatible with survival. Tocolysis allows for time for fetal lung maturity with intramuscular betamethasone.

Fetal fibronectin may be detected in vaginal secretions of women presenting with signs and symptoms of preterm labor. Secretions negative for fibronectin between 22 and 34 weeks indicate a low likelihood of delivery in the next 2 weeks. Thus a more conservative, observational approach can be used. If fetal fibronectin is positive, the woman remains at a higher risk for delivery in the next 2 weeks and a more aggressive approach to tocolysis and fetal lung maturity hastening is employed.

If fetal lungs are immature (can use *lecithin-to-sphingomyelin [L-to-S] ratio <2 : 1* or lamellar body count) and the fetus is between 26 and 34 weeks of age, corticosteroid administration may hasten lung maturity and thus reduce the risk of respiratory distress syndrome.

Premature rupture of the membranes (PROM) is rupture of the amniotic sac before the onset of labor. Diagnosis of rupture of membranes (whether premature or not) is based on history and sterile speculum exam, which shows (1) *pooling of amniotic fluid*, (2) *ferning pattern* when the fluid is placed on a microscopic slide and allowed to dry, and/or (3) *positive nitrazine test* (nitrazine paper turns blue in the presence of amniotic fluid). US should be done to assess amniotic fluid volume (as well as gestational age and any anomalies that may be present). Spontaneous labor often follows membrane rupture. If labor does not occur within 6–8 hours and the mother is at term, consider inducing labor.

Chorioamnionitis is a prenatal/natal infection that presents with fever and a *tender, irritable uterus*. The classic cause is PROM or preterm PROM. Do a culture and Gram stain of the amniotic fluid, and treat with ampicillin while awaiting culture results. Chorioamnionitis may result in neonatal sepsis and/or maternal sepsis or endomyometritis.

Preterm PROM is premature rupture of the membranes before 36–37 weeks. Risk of infection increases with the duration of ruptured membranes. Do a culture and Gram stain of the amniotic fluid. If the results are negative, treat with pelvic/bed rest and frequent follow-up. If the results are positive for group B streptococci, treat the mother with amoxicillin/ampicillin even if she is asymptomatic.

Postterm pregnancy is defined as one lasting beyond than *42 weeks'* gestation. Generally, if the gestational age is known to be accurate, such patients are induced into labor (e.g., with oxytocin). If dates are uncertain, do twice-weekly BPP. At 43 weeks, most physicians induce labor or do a cesarean section. Remember that both prematurity and postmaturity increase perinatal morbidity and mortality.

📁 **CASE SCENARIO:** Prolonged gestation is classically associated with what congenital anomaly? Anencephaly (Fig. 4-5).

Third-trimester bleeding

Always do an ultrasound scan before a pelvic exam. The differential diagnosis includes:

○ **Placenta previa:** Predisposing factors include multiparity, increasing age, multiple gestation, and prior previa. This condition is why you do a US before a pelvic exam. *Bleeding is painless and may be profuse.* US is 95–100% accurate in diagnosis. If patient is hemodynamically unstable, cesarean section is mandatory for delivery. If patient is stable, consider bed/pelvic rest and tocolysis if the patient is preterm and the bleeding stops.

○ **Abruptio placentae:** Predisposing factors include hypertension (with or without preeclampsia), trauma, polyhydramnios with rapid decompression after membrane rupture, *cocaine* or tobacco use, and preterm PROM.

> *The patient can have this condition without visible bleeding, because the blood may be contained behind the placenta. Watch for* **uterine pain and tenderness** *and increased uterine tone with* **hyperactive contraction pattern.** *Fetal distress is apparent. Abruptio placentae also may cause disseminated intravascular coagulation if fetal products enter the maternal circulation. Ultrasound appearance may be falsely normal. Treat with rapid delivery (vaginal preferred).*

○ **Uterine rupture:** Predisposing factors include previous uterine surgery, trauma, *oxytocin*, grand multiparity (several previous deliveries), excessive uterine distention (e.g., multiple gestation, polyhydramnios), abnormal fetal lie, cephalopelvic disproportion, and shoulder dystocia. Look for sudden onset of severe pain, often accompanied by maternal hypotension or shock. Fetal parts may be palpated in the abdomen, or the *abdominal contour may change.* Treat with immediate laparotomy and usually hysterectomy after delivery.

○ **Fetal bleeding:** usually results from *vasa previa* or velamentous insertion of the cord. The major risk factor is *multiple gestation* (the higher the number of fetuses, the higher the risk). *Bleeding is painless,* and the mother is completely stable, whereas the fetus shows worsening distress (tachycardia initially, then bradycardia as the fetus decompensates). The *Apt test* is positive on uterine blood (differentiates fetal from maternal blood cells). Treat with immediate cesarean section.

○ **Cervical or vaginal lesions:** herpes, gonorrhea, *Chlamydia, Candida* spp.

○ **Cervical or vaginal trauma:** usually from intercourse.

○ **Bleeding disorder:** Antepartum presentation is rare (more common postpartum).

○ **Cervical cancer:** can occur in pregnant patients, too!

○ **"Bloody show":** With cervical effacement, a blood-tinged mucous plug may be released from the cervical canal and heralds the onset of labor (this is a normal occurrence and a diagnosis of exclusion).

In all patients with third-trimester bleeding:

○ Start IV fluids, and give blood if necessary.

○ Give oxygen.

○ Order a complete blood count, coagulation profiles, and US.

○ Set up fetal and maternal monitoring.

○ Do an illicit drug screen if drug abuse is suspected (cocaine causes placental abruption).

○ Give Rh immune globulin if the mother is Rh negative.

○ The *Kleihauer-Betke* test can be used to quantify the amount of fetal blood in the maternal circulation and calculate the dose of RhoGAM.

Preeclampsia

Look for *hypertension* (if the woman has preexisting hypertension, look for >30/15-mm Hg increase in blood pressure over baseline); urinalysis with *proteinuria*, oliguria, *swelling or edema of the hands and/or face;* headache; visual disturbances; and HELLP syndrome (*h*emolysis, *e*levated *l*iver enzymes, *l*ow *p*latelets, often with right upper quadrant or epigastric pain). Preeclampsia usually occurs in the *third trimester.* The main risk factors are chronic renal disease, chronic hypertension, family history, multiple gestation, nulliparity, extremes of reproductive age (the classic case is a *young female with her first child*), diabetes, and black race.

Mild preeclampsia: BP greater than 140/90, 1-2+ proteinuria on urine dipstick testing. Severe preeclampsia: BP greater than 160/100 mm Hg and 3-4+ proteinuria on urine dipstick testing with severe symptoms. Treatment includes stabilization and delivery if the patient is at term. If the patient is premature and has mild disease, give *hydralazine* or *labetalol* for hypertension and *magnesium sulfate* for seizure prophylaxis, prescribe bed rest, and observe in the hospital. If the patient has severe disease (oliguria, mental status changes, headache, blurred vision, pulmonary edema, cyanosis, HELLP, BP >160/110 mm Hg, progression to eclampsia [seizures]), deliver regardless of gestational age, because both mother and infant may die. *Preeclampsia plus seizures equals eclampsia.*

Mild ankle edema is normal in pregnancy, but severe ankle edema or hand edema should make you suspect preeclampsia.

Hypertension plus proteinuria in a pregnant patient is preeclampsia until proved otherwise.

○ Do not wait to remeasure high blood pressure in a pregnant patient. Err on the safe side: Assume that it represents preeclampsia, and start treatment.

○ Do not try to deliver the infant until the mother is stable (e.g., do not perform a cesarean section while the mother has seizures).

○ Preeclampsia and eclampsia cause uteroplacental insufficiency, IUGR, fetal demise, and increased maternal morbidity and mortality rates.

○ Preeclampsia and eclampsia are generally not considered risk factors for future development of hypertension or end-organ effects of hypertension.

📋 **CASE SCENARIO:** Preeclampsia symptoms that develop before the third trimester should make you consider what disorder? Molar pregnancy.

📋 **CASE SCENARIO:** What is the best way to prevent eclampsia? Regular prenatal care, which allows you to detect the disorder in the preeclampsia stage and treat appropriately.

📋 **CASE SCENARIO:** What is the initial treatment of choice for eclamptic seizures? Magnesium sulfate, which also lowers blood pressure. Toxic effects include *hyporeflexia (first sign of toxicity), respiratory depression, central nervous system depression,* coma, and death. If toxicity occurs, the first step is to stop the magnesium infusion.

High-risk obstetrics/problem pregnancies

Hyperemesis gravidarum: Intractable nausea and vomiting leading to dehydration and possible electrolyte disturbances. The condition presents in the first trimester, usually in *younger women with their first pregnancy* and some *underlying social stressors* or psychiatric problems. Treat with supportive care including small, frequent meals and antiemetics (fairly safe in pregnancy). With severe dehydration and/or electrolyte disturbances, admit to the hospital for treatment with IV fluids and observation.

 With all high-risk pregnancies, consider a BPP once or even twice a week in the third trimester until delivery.

📋 **CASE SCENARIO:** A pregnant woman's last child had spina bifida, and she wants to know if her fetus has it. Should you do chorionic villus sampling? No, because chorionic villus sampling cannot detect neural tube defects. It is generally reserved for women with previously affected offspring with a known genetic disease, because it can be done at 9–12 weeks (earlier than amniocentesis), which gives women the advantage of a first-trimester abortion if a fetus is affected. Chorionic villus sampling carries a slightly higher miscarriage rate than with amniocentesis.

Maternal complications of gestational diabetes: Polyhydramnios, preeclampsia, and complications of diabetes. Problems in infants born to diabetic mothers include *macrosomia* (with gestational diabetes) or IUGR (with preexisting diabetes); *respiratory distress syndrome; cardiovascular, colon, craniofacial,* and *neural tube defects;* and *caudal regression syndrome* (the lower half of the body is incompletely formed).

Treat with diet, exercise, and/or insulin. Do not use oral hypoglycemics, which can cross the placenta. Tighter control results in better outcomes for mother and baby. Check HbA_{1c} to determine compliance and glucose fluctuations.

📋 **CASE SCENARIO:** What is the classic glucose problem after birth in an infant born to a diabetic mother? Postdelivery *hypoglycemia.* In utero, fetal islet-cell hypertrophy results from maternal and thus fetal hyperglycemia. After birth, when the infant is cut off from the mother's glucose supply, hyperglycemia resolves, but islet cells continue to overproduce insulin and cause hypoglycemia. Treat with IV glucose.

Maternal hypertension causes IUGR and is a risk factor for preeclampsia.

IgG is the only maternal antibody that crosses the placenta. An elevated neonatal IgM concentration is never normal, whereas an elevated neonatal IgG often represents maternal antibodies.

Multiple gestation: usually results in premature labor and delivery due to limitations of uterine size. If the sex or blood type is different, twins are *dizygotic.* If the placentas are monochorionic, the twins are *monozygotic.* These three simple factors differentiate monozygotic from dizygotic twins in 80% of cases. In the remaining 20%, HLA typing studies may be necessary.

Other complications of multiple gestations (the higher the number of fetuses, the higher the risk of most of these conditions)

❍ Maternal: anemia, hypertension/preeclampsia, postpartum uterine atony, postpartum hemorrhage.

❍ Fetal: polyhydramnios, malpresentation, placenta previa, abruptio placentae, velamentous cord insertion/vasa previa, umbilical cord prolapse, IUGR, congenital anomalies, increased perinatal morbidity and mortality.

 With vertex-vertex twin presentations, you can try vaginal delivery for both infants; with any other combination of presentations or more than two fetuses, do a cesarean section.

Rh incompatibility/hemolytic disease of the newborn occurs when the mother is Rh-negative and the infant is Rh-positive. If both mother and father are Rh-negative, there is nothing to worry about—the infant will be Rh-negative. If the mother is Rh-negative and the father is Rh-positive, the infant has a 50/50 chance of being Rh-positive. If there is a potential for hemolytic disease, check maternal Rh antibody titers.

Give Rh immune globulin automatically at 28 weeks and within 72 hours after delivery, as well as after any procedures that may cause transplacental hemorrhage (e.g., amniocentesis). There *must be previous sensitization* for disease to occur. In other words, if a nulliparous mother has never received blood products, her first Rh-positive infant most likely will not be affected by hemolytic disease. The second Rh-positive infant, however, will be affected (unless Rh immune globulin is administered at the right times during the first pregnancy). If you check maternal Rh antibodies and they are strongly positive, Rh immune globulin does not help because sensitization has already occurred. Rh immune globulin administration is a good example of *primary prevention.*

❍ If not detected or prevented, Rh incompatibility can lead to fetal hydrops (edema, ascites, pleural/pericardial effusions) and demise.

❍ Amniotic fluid spectrophotometry can gauge the severity of fetal hemolysis.

❍ Treatment of hemolytic disease involves delivery if the fetus is mature (check lung maturity with L-to-S ratio), *intrauterine blood transfusion,* and *phenobarbital,* which helps the fetal liver break down bilirubin by inducing enzymes.

❍ ABO blood group incompatibility (and other minor antigens) can also cause hemolytic disease of the newborn when the mother is type O and the infant is type A, B, or AB. Previous sensitization is not required because IgG antibodies (which can cross the placenta) occur naturally in people with blood type O. The disease is usually less severe than Rh incompatibility, but treatment is the same.

🔲 **CASE SCENARIO:** The mother is Rh-negative and has a high titer of Rh antibodies. The father is Rh-positive. Should you give Rh immune globulin? No—you are too late. Antibodies have already formed. Instead, monitor fetus closely.

Hydatiform mole: Look for *preeclampsia before the third trimester;* an *HCG level* that does not return to zero after a delivery/abortion or rapidly rises during pregnancy; first- or second-trimester bleeding with possible expulsion of *"grapelike vesicles"*; uterine size/dates discrepancy; and/or a *"snowstorm"* pattern on US (Table 4-5).

TABLE 4-5 Complete versus Incomplete Hydatidiform Mole

Complete moles	46, XX (90%) 46, XY (10%)	Fertilization of an oocyte with absent maternal chromosomes and duplication of paternal chromosomes or fertilization of an empty oocyte with 2 sperm. Contains no fetal tissue	Treat with uterine dilatation and curettage; then follow HCG levels until they fall to zero. Administer Rh immune globulin if Rh-negative
Incomplete moles	69, XXY	Fertilization of a normal oocyte with 2 sperm. Contains fetal tissue	

If the HCG does not fall to zero or rises, the patient has either an invasive mole or choriocarcinoma. Of complete moles, 15-20% will develop into trophoblastic neoplasia, and of partial moles the rate is 1-5%. In either case, the patient needs chemotherapy (usually with *methotrexate* or actinomycin D).

In women with antiphospholipid antibodies and previous problem pregnancies (e.g., recurrent abortions), low-dose *aspirin* with low-dose subcutaneous *heparin* may help in subsequent pregnancies (normally, aspirin and other NSAIDs should be avoided in pregnancy).

Pregnant women can have the same surgical conditions as nonpregnant women. In general, treat the disease, regardless of the pregnancy. This rule of thumb applies to all acute surgical conditions (e.g., appendicitis, cholecystitis). With semiurgent conditions (e.g., ovarian neoplasm), it is best to wait until the second trimester, when the patient and fetus are most stable. Purely elective cases are avoided. Appendicitis may manifest with right upper quadrant pain or tenderness due to the uterine displacement of the appendix. Do a laparoscopy if you are unsure and the patient has peritoneal signs.

If a woman develops tuberculosis (TB) during pregnancy (positive purified protein derivative [PPD] skin test and suspicious chest radiograph and/or positive sputum culture), treat as you would any other patient. If the woman is a known recent PPD converter or has additional risk factors (e.g., HIV infection or living with an active case of TB), treat with isoniazid prophylaxis just like a regular patient. Be sure to give the mother vitamin B$_6$ with isoniazid to prevent deficiency in her and the fetus. Avoid *streptomycin*, which may cause deafness and/or nephrotoxicity in the fetus.

Obstetric pharmacology and teratogenesis (Table 4-6)

TABLE 4-6 Teratogenic Agents

AGENT	DEFECT(S) CAUSED
Accutane (isotretinoin)	Facial-ear anomalies, heart disease, CNS anomalies
Alcohol	Fetal alcohol syndrome
Aminoglycosides	Deafness
Aminopterin	Intrauterine growth retardation, CNS defects, cleft lip, cleft palate
Amphetamines	Congenital heart disease, IUGR, withdrawal
Antineoplastics	Many
Birth control pills	VACTERL syndrome (vertebral, anal, cardiac, tracheoesophageal, renal, and limb malformations)
Carbamazepine	Fingernail hypoplasia, craniofacial defects, spina bifida
Cigarettes	Intrauterine growth retardation, LBW, prematurity
Cocaine	Cerebral infarcts, mental retardation, microcephaly, LBW, IUGR, behavioral disturbances
Diazepam	Cleft lip, cleft palate
Diethylstilbestrol	Clear cell vaginal cancer, adenosis, cervical incompetence
Iodine	Goiter, cretinism
Isotretinoin*	CNS, craniofacial, ear, and cardiovascular defects
Lithium	Cardiac (Ebstein) anomalies
Phenytoin†	Craniofacial and limb defects, mental retardation, cardiovascular defects
Progesterone	Masculinization of female fetus
Radiation	Intrauterine growth retardation, CNS and face defects, leukemia
Streptomycin	Deafness
Tetracycline	Yellow or brown teeth, retarded skeletal growth, cataract
Thalidomide	Phocomelia (limb deformities)
Trimethadione	Craniofacial and cardiovascular defects, mental retardation
Valproic acid	Spina bifida, hypospadias
Warfarin	Fetal bleeding and death, hypoplastic nasal structures, stillbirth

CNS, Central nervous system; *IUGR*, intrauterine growth retardation; *LBW*, low birth weight. *Note:* Marijuana and LSD (lysergic acid diethylamide) have not been confirmed as teratogens.
*Vitamin A in general is considered teratogenic when recommended intake levels are exceeded.
†Diphenylhydantoin.

Drugs that are generally safe in pregnancy: Acetaminophen, penicillin, cephalosporins, erythromycin, nitrofurantoin, histamine H$_2$ receptor blockers, antacids, heparin, hydralazine, methyldopa, labetalol, insulin, and docusate.

Postpartum period

For the first several days post partum, it is normal to have some discharge (lochia), which is red the first few days and gradually turns to a white/yellowish-white color by day 10.

▢ **CASE SCENARIO:** If lochia becomes foul-smelling, what condition should you suspect? Endometritis.

The major causes of maternal mortality are pulmonary embolism, pregnancy-induced hypertension (PIH), and hemorrhage.

▢ **CASE SCENARIO:** When a newly postpartum mother develops dyspnea, tachypnea, chest pain, and hypotension, what condition does she probably have? Amniotic fluid embolism.

Postpartum hemorrhage: Greater than 500 mL blood loss during a vaginal delivery or greater than 1000 mL during a cesarean section. The most common cause is *uterine atony* (75–80% of cases). Other causes include lacerations; retained placental tissue (*placenta accreta,* increta, or percreta); coagulation disorders (e.g., disseminated intravascular coagulation, von Willebrand disease); low placental implantation, and uterine inversion. Patients with severe hemorrhage may develop hypopituitarism *(Sheehan syndrome).* The major risk factors for retained placental tissue are previous uterine surgery and previous cesarean section.

Uterine atony is often caused by *overdistention of the uterus* (multiple gestation, polyhydramnios, macrosomia); *prolonged labor; oxytocin usage;* grand multiparity (history of five or more deliveries); and precipitous labor (<3 hours). Treat with bimanual compression and massage of the uterus while giving a dilute oxytocin infusion. If this approach fails, you can try ergonovine or another ergot drug (contraindicated with maternal hypertension) or prostaglandin $F_{2\alpha}$. If these also fail to stop bleeding, a hysterectomy may be necessary.

In patients with retained products of conception (which is probably the most common cause of delayed postpartum hemorrhage), remove the placenta manually to stop bleeding; then do curettage in the operating room under anesthesia. If the patient has placenta accreta, increta, or percreta (placental tissue grows into or through the myometrium), a hysterectomy is usually necessary to stop the bleeding.

With uterine inversion (the uterus inverts and can be seen outside the vagina), put the uterus back in place manually (anesthesia may be required) and give IV fluids and oxytocin. Uterine inversion is usually iatrogenic (due to *pulling too hard on the cord*).

Postpartum fever, defined as a fever for at least 2 consecutive days, is usually due to breast engorgement; urinary tract infection; or endometritis, endomyometritis, or puerperal sepsis. Important predisposing factors for endometritis are cesarean section, PROM or preterm PROM, prolonged labor, frequent vaginal exams during labor, and manual removal of the placenta or retained placental fragments. Look for *tender uterus* and/or *foul-smelling lochia.* Treat with broad-spectrum antibiotics after performing cultures of the endometrium, vagina, blood, and urine.

If a postpartum fever from endometritis fails to resolve with broad-spectrum antibiotics, there are two main possibilities: progression to pelvic abscess or pelvic thrombophlebitis. Order a CT scan, which will show an abscess (which needs to be drained). If there is no abscess on CT, think of pelvic thrombophlebitis, which manifests with persistent spiking fevers and lack of response to antibiotics. Give *heparin* for an easy cure (and diagnosis in retrospect).

If a postpartum patient goes into shock and no bleeding is seen, think of amniotic fluid embolism, uterine inversion, or concealed hemorrhage (e.g., uterine rupture with bleeding into the peritoneal cavity).

Postpartum blues and depression: A majority of women (85%) experience some degree of postpartum mood disturbance. Postpartum depressive disorders are typically divided into three categories: (1) postpartum blues, (2) nonpsychotic major depression, and (3) puerperal psychosis.

Postpartum blues is common and does not indicate psychopathology. Symptoms include mood disturbances, tearfulness, and irritability and are limited to 10 days post partum. Treat with reassurance.

Postpartum major depression symptoms usually appear over the first 2 to 3 months following delivery and include depressed mood, irritability, loss of interest in usual activities, insomnia, fatigue, and loss of appetite. Treatment can include SSRIs (e.g., fluoxetine).

Postpartum psychosis is a psychiatric emergency. Symptoms include restlessness, agitation, sleep disturbance, paranoia, delusions, disorganized thinking, impulsivity, and behaviors that place mother and infant at risk. Onset is typically within the first 2 weeks after delivery. Treatment may include hospitalization, mood stabilizers, antipsychotic medications, benzodiazepines, or electroconvulsive therapy.

Breast-feeding

If a woman does not want to breast-feed, prescribe tight-fitting bras, ice packs, and analgesia. Breast-feeding is generally encouraged because it is good for mother-child bonding and may protect the baby from infections.

If a woman breast-feeds, watch for mastitis, which usually develops in the first 3 months of breast-feeding. Breasts are red, indurated, and painful, and the patient has a fever. The most common pathogen is *Staphylococcus aureus,* and less common organisms are group A beta-hemolytic streptococci, *Streptococcus pneumoniae,* and *Escherichia coli.* The mainstay of therapy is effective milk removal through continued breast-feeding. Antibiotics (cephalexin, dicloxacillin) are often used, as well as pain relief with NSAIDs. If abscess formation occurs, surgical drainage is indicated.

Breast-feeding is contraindicated with maternal HIV infection and when the mother uses illicit drugs, prescription sedatives or stimulants, lithium, or chemotherapy.

5 PSYCHIATRY AND ETHICS

SCHIZOPHRENIA AND PSYCHOTIC DISORDERS

The diagnostic criteria for schizophrenia and related psychotic disorders (Table 5-1) include *positive symptoms* (delusions, hallucinations, disorganized speech, grossly disorganized or catatonic behavior) and *negative symptoms* (flat affect, alogia/refusal to talk, avolition/apathy). The typical age at onset is 15–25 years for men (look for a deteriorating college student) and 25–35 years for women. Roughly 1% of people in all cultures have schizophrenia. There is a 50% concordance rate among monozygotic twins. In the United States, most schizophrenic patients are born in the winter (reason unknown). Up to 10% of schizophrenics eventually commit suicide; a past attempt is the best predictor of eventual success. Treat with antipsychotic medications and psychosocial therapy and support. Medications are used first, but the best treatment (as in most psychiatric disorders) is medication plus therapy (Tables 5-2 through 5-4).

TABLE 5-1 Psychotic Disorders

DIAGNOSIS	TIME FRAME	SYMPTOMS	TREATMENT
Brief psychotic disorder	>1 day but <1 mo	Schizophrenia symptoms as a reaction to marked stress in persons with borderline or antisocial personality disorders	Control agitation, antipsychotics, hospitalization if needed
Schizophreniform disorder	<6 mo	Same symptoms as schizophrenia	Same as schizophrenia (see below)
Schizophrenia	>6 mo	Positive and negative symptoms; see below	Antipsychotics (see below) plus psychosocial therapy
Schizoaffective disorder	Schizophrenia symptoms for >2 wk	Schizophrenia symptoms plus meets criteria for major depression or mania	Antipsychotics plus mood stabilizers

TABLE 5-2 Schizophrenia Symptoms and Prognosis

POSITIVE SYMPTOMS	NEGATIVE SYMPTOMS	GOOD PROGNOSTIC FACTORS	POOR PROGNOSTIC FACTORS
Delusions	Flat affect	Good premorbid functioning	Poor premorbid functioning
Hallucinations	Alogia (no speech)	Late onset	Early onset
Bizarre behavior	Avolition (apathy)	Obvious precipitating factors	No precipitating factors
Thought disorder	Anhedonia	Married	Single, divorced, widowed
Poor attention		Family history of mood disorders	Family history of schizophrenia
		Positive symptoms	Negative symptoms
		Good support system	Poor support system

TABLE 5-3 Antipsychotic Medications

	HIGH POTENCY	LOW POTENCY	ATYPICAL*
Example(s)	Haloperidol, fluphenazine	Chlorpromazine	Risperidone, olanzapine, aripiprazole, quetiapine, paliperidone, ziprasidone
Extrapyramidal side effects	High incidence	Low incidence	Low incidence

Continued

TABLE 5-3 Antipsychotic Medications—cont'd

	HIGH POTENCY	LOW POTENCY	ATYPICAL*
Autonomic side effects†	Low incidence	High incidence	Medium incidence
Positive symptoms	Works well	Works well	Works well
Negative symptoms	Works poorly	Works poorly	Works somewhat

*Atypical, newer agents are the drugs of choice for maintenance therapy because of reduced extrapyramidal side effects and beneficial effect on negative symptoms.
†Autonomic side effects include anticholinergic (dry mouth, urinary retention, blurry vision, mydriasis), α₁ blockade (orthostatic hypotension), and antihistamine effects (sedation).

TABLE 5-4 Extrapyramidal Side Effects of Antipsychotic Medications

DISEASE	TIME COURSE	SYMPTOMS	TREATMENT
Acute dystonia	Within the first few hours or days of treatment	Muscle spasms or stiffness (e.g., torticollis, trismus), tongue protrusions or twisting, opisthotonos, and oculogyric crisis (forced sustained deviation of the head and eyes). Most common in young men	Treat with antihistamines (e.g., diphenhydramine) or anticholinergics (e.g., benztropine, trihexyphenidyl)
Serotonin syndrome	Within the first few hours of treatment	Triad of mental status changes, autonomic hyperactivity (diarrhea, tremor, hyperthermia, tachycardia) and neuromuscular abnormalities (muscular clonus, hyperkinesias)	Discontinue the offending drug, treat rhabdomyolysis if it develops, provide supportive care, resolves in 1-3 days
Akathisia	Within the first few days of treatment	Subjective feeling of restlessness; the patient may pace constantly, alternate sitting and standing positions, or be unable to sit still	Lower the dose, try β-blocker (e.g., propranolol) or switch to atypical antipsychotic
Parkinsonism	Within the first few months of treatment	Stiffness, cogwheel rigidity, shuffling gait, masklike facies, and drooling. Most common in older women.	Treat with antihistamines (e.g., diphenhydramine) or anticholinergics (e.g., benztropine, trihexyphenidyl)
Tardive dyskinesia	Occurs after years of treatment	Perioral movements (e.g., darting, protruding movements of the tongue, chewing, grimacing, puckering). Patients also may have involuntary, choreoathetoid movements of head, limbs, and trunk	No known treatment for tardive dyskinesia; discontinue the antipsychotic and consider switching to an atypical antipsychotic (e.g., risperidone, clozapine). Drug holidays may be helpful
Neuroleptic malignant syndrome	Can occur any time during treatment	Rigidity, mutism, obtundation, agitation, high fever (temperatures up to 107°F), high level of creatine phosphokinase (often >5000), sweating, and myoglobinuria. A life-threatening condition	Discontinue the antipsychotic, give supportive care for fever and renal failure due to myoglobinuria; discontinue the antipsychotic and administer benzodiazepines; consider dantrolene (as in malignant hyperthermia)

Other facts about antipsychotic medication are as follows:
❍ Antipsychotics can cause dopamine blockade. Dopamine is a *prolactin-inhibiting factor* in the tuberoinfundibular tract of the brain. Thus dopamine blockade causes an increase in prolactin, which may result in *high prolactin levels, galactorrhea* (typically bilateral), impotence, *menstrual dysfunction*, or decreased libido.
❍ Watch for anticholinergic symptoms (dry mouth, urinary retention, constipation, blurred vision), weight gain, and sedation.
❍ Individual antipsychotic side effects can occur: Thioridazine causes retinal pigment deposits, clozapine causes *agranulocytosis* (white blood cell counts must be monitored), and chlorpromazine causes jaundice and photosensitivity.

MOOD DISORDERS (Table 5-5)

DISEASE	TIME COURSE	SYMPTOMS	TREATMENT
Major depressive disorder (MDD)	>2 wk	Depressive mood, accompanied by at least physical, somatic, psychologic, cognitive, and behavioral symptoms, lasting for at least 2 wk	SSRI or SNRI: first-line agent
Adjustment disorder with depressed mood	<6 mo	Patient does not handle a stressful situation well and feels "bummed out" (for <6 mo) but does not meet criteria for full-blown depression (e.g., teenage girl who breaks up with her boyfriend and seems to cry a lot, skips a few days of school, and does not want to talk to her friends for a week)	Cognitive behavioral therapy first line. Antidepressants if patient meets criteria for MDD
Dysthymia	>2 yr	Presence of depressed mood (can be irritable mood in children/adolescents for longer than 1 yr), for more days than not, for at least 2 yr. No episodes of major depression, mania/hypomania, or psychosis	Antidepressants (SSRIs) plus psychotherapy
Seasonal affective disorder (SAD)	Several years	Symptoms during the winter and go away in the spring or when the patient is exposed to daylight. The cognitive, psychologic, and behavioral symptoms are similar to those in other types of depression, but the somatic symptoms are typically the opposite (e.g., increased sleep and increased appetite)	Light therapy

SNRI, Serotonin-norepinephrine reuptake inhibitors; *SSRI,* selective serotonin reuptake inhibitors.

Depression

DSM-IV criteria for major depressive disorder (MDD) includes depressive mood (irritable mood in children and adolescents), accompanied by at least physical, somatic, psychologic, cognitive, and behavioral symptoms, lasting for at least 2 weeks. Patients described on the boards usually do not come out and say, "I'm depressed." You have to watch for the clues: change in sleep habits (classically, *insomnia*); vague *somatic complaints;* anxiety; low energy level or *fatigue;* change in appetite (classically, *decreased appetite*); poor concentration; *psychomotor retardation; hallucinations;* and/or *anhedonia* (loss of pleasure; previously fun activities are no longer enjoyed). In children, depression often manifests as an irritable mood instead of a depressed mood, and in the elderly, it may manifest as *pseudodementia.*

Look for precipitating factors in the history such as loss of a loved one, divorce or separation, unemployment or retirement, or chronic disease. Depression is more common in women. "Pencil-and-paper" tests (e.g., Beck's depression inventory) are sometimes used for screening. Treat with both antidepressants and psychotherapy; the combination works better than either modality alone.

Antidepressants

❍ Selective serotonin reuptake inhibitors (SSRIs) (e.g., fluoxetine, paroxetine) prevent reuptake of serotonin only and have few serious side effects *(insomnia, anorexia, sexual dysfunction).* They are the first-line agents in all depressed patients due to their favorable side effect profile.
❍ Serotonin-norepinephrine reuptake inhibitors (SNRIs) (e.g., venlafaxine, duloxetine) inhibit the reuptake of both serotonin and norepinephrine. They are commonly used for first-line therapy and as a next step to SSRIs.
❍ Norepinephrine-dopamine reuptake inhibitors (NDRIs) (e.g., bupropion) are as effective as the SSRIs and SNRIs in the treatment of depressive and anxiety symptoms in depression, and they are more effective than the SSRIs in the treatment of sleepiness and fatigue in depression. Sometimes NDRIs are not used as first-line agents owing to their potential to lower the seizure threshold.
❍ Tricyclic antidepressants (TCAs) (e.g., nortriptyline, amitriptyline) prevent reuptake of norepinephrine and serotonin. They are not first line due to their side effects. They block α-adrenergic receptors (watch for orthostatic hypotension, dizziness, and falls). TCAs are dangerous in overdose, primarily because of *cardiac arrhythmias,* which may respond to *bicarbonate.*

○ Monoamine oxidase inhibitors (MAOIs) (e.g., phenelzine, tranylcypromine) are older medications and are not first-line agents. They may be good for *atypical depression* (look for hypersomnia and hyperphagia—the opposite of classic depression). When patients eat *tyramine-containing foods* (especially wine and cheese), they may have a *hypertensive crisis.*

Bipolar disorder

Mania lasting for at least 1 week is the only criterion required for a diagnosis. Depression commonly manifests before or after mania. Look for classic symptoms such as *decreased need for sleep, pressured speech, sexual promiscuity, shopping sprees,* and *exaggerated self-importance* or delusions of grandeur. The initial onset is classically between 16 and 30 years of age. There is a 75% concordance rate among monozygotic twins (highest among psychiatric disorders). *Lithium* and *valproic acid* are first-line treatment agents. Typical antipsychotics (e.g., haloperidol), atypical antipsychotics (e.g., risperidone, quetiapine, clozapine, ziprasidone, aripiprazole), carbamazepine, and gabapentin are second-line agents. Antidepressants can trigger mania or hypomania, especially in bipolar patients.

○ Bipolar II disorder is hypomania (mild mania without psychosis that does not cause occupational dysfunction) plus major depression.
○ Cyclothymia is defined as at least 2 years of hypomania alternating with depressed mood (with no full-blown episodes of mania or depression).
○ Lithium causes renal dysfunction *(diabetes insipidus),* thyroid dysfunction, *tremor,* and central nervous system (CNS) effects at toxic levels. Valproic acid causes *liver dysfunction,* and carbamazepine may cause bone marrow depression.

Suicide

The major risk factors are age *older than 45, alcohol or substance abuse, history of rage or violence, prior suicide attempts,* male sex (men commit suicide three times more often than women due to more lethal means [e.g., firearms], but women attempt it four times more often than men), *prior psychiatric history, depression,* recent loss or separation, loss of health, unemployment or retirement, and single, widowed, or divorced marital status.

▢ **CASE SCENARIO:** What is the best predictor of future suicide? A past attempt.

Consider hospitalizing an acutely suicidal patient (against the person's will, if necessary) for treatment. Patients who are just coming out of a deep depression are at increased risk for suicide: The antidepressant may begin to work, and the person has more energy—just enough to commit suicide. Suicide rates are rising most rapidly among 15- to 24-year-olds, but the greatest risk is in people older than age 65.

▢ **CASE SCENARIO:** True or false: Asking about suicide does not increase the risk of suicide. True. Always ask depressed patients about suicide to assess their risk.

Normal versus pathologic grief, mourning, and bereavement: Initial grief after a loss (e.g., death of a loved one) may include a state of shock, feeling of numbness or bewilderment, distress, crying, sleep disturbances, decreased appetite, difficulty in concentrating, weight loss, and survivor guilt for *up to 1 year*—in other words, the same symptoms as depression! Intense yearning (even years after the death) and even searching for the deceased are normal. *Feelings of worthlessness, psychomotor retardation,* and *suicidal ideation* are not signs of normal grief; they are signs of depression.

▢ **CASE SCENARIO:** A 68-year-old man comes to see you 2 weeks after his wife of 40 years died. He complains of poor appetite and crying spells and says that he keeps thinking he sees his wife, only to realize it is not her. He also feels guilty. He denies suicidal ideation. What does the patient have? Normal grief. It is normal to have an illusion or hallucination about the deceased. A normal grieving person knows that it was an illusion or hallucination, whereas a depressed person believes that the illusion or hallucination is real.

ANXIETY DISORDERS

Panic disorder: Look for a 20- to 40-year-old patient who thinks that he or she is dying or having a heart attack, even though the patient is healthy and has a negative workup for organic disease. Patients often hyperventilate and are extremely anxious. Remember the association with *agoraphobia* (fear of leaving the house). Treat long term with cognitive behavioral therapy and SSRIs (e.g., fluoxetine). Benzodiazipines (e.g., alprazolam) are effective in the acute setting.

Generalized anxiety disorder: Patient *constantly worries about everything* (e.g., career, family, future, relationships, money) at the same time; not as dramatic/acute as panic disorder. Treat with SSRIs, buspirone (nonaddictive, nonsedating), or benzodiazepines (addictive, sedating) short term.

Simple phobias: Fear of needles, blood products, animals, heights, or other specific triggers. Treat with behavioral therapy such as *flooding* (e.g., a patient afraid of dogs is locked in a room with many dogs); *systematic desensitization* (e.g., a patient with fear of dogs is asked to think about dogs and then listen to a dog bark, look at a live dog, etc.); biofeedback; and mental imagery. *Social phobia* is a specific subtype of simple phobia that is best treated with behavioral therapy. β-*Blockers* may be used before an unavoidable public appearance to reduce symptoms, and SSRIs may help.

Post-traumatic stress disorder: Symptoms exist for more than 6 months. It is called "acute stress disorder" if symptoms exist less than 6 months. Look for someone who has *been through a life-threatening event* (e.g., Gulf War veteran, survivor of severe accident or rape) who *recurrently experiences the event* (nightmares, flashbacks); *tries to avoid thinking about it;* and has *depression* or *poor concentration* as a result. Treat with cognitive behavioral therapy. Use SSRIs as first-line agents for chronic therapy and benzodiazepines for short-term acute therapy.

SOMATOFORM DISORDERS

Patients with somatoform disorders *do not intentionally create symptoms.* Treat with frequent return clinic visits and/or psychotherapy.
- **Somatization disorder**: Patients have multiple complaints in *multiple organ systems* over many years and have had extensive workups in the past. Symptoms include pain in more than four different sites, gastrointestinal symptoms, sexual dysfunction, and neurologic complaints.
- **Conversion disorder**: After an obvious precipitating factor (e.g., fight with boyfriend), patients have *unexplainable neurologic symptoms* (blindness, stocking-glove numbness).
- **Hypochondriasis**: Patients continue to believe that they have a certain disease despite extensive negative workup.
- **Body dysmorphic disorder**: Patients are preoccupied with an *imagined physical defect* (e.g., a teenager thinks that her nose is too big when its size is normal).

Somatoform disorder versus factitious disorder versus malingering:
- **Somatoform disorders**: Patients do not intentionally create symptoms.
- **Factitious disorders**: Patients intentionally create their illness or symptoms (e.g., they inject insulin to induce hypoglycemia) and subject themselves to procedures to *assume the role of a patient* (unique type of secondary gain) with no financial or other secondary gain.
- **Malingering**: Patients intentionally create their illness for secondary gain (e.g., money, release from work or prison).

PERSONALITY DISORDERS

Personality disorders are lifelong disorders with no real treatment (although psychotherapy can be tried):
- **Paranoid**: belief of patients that everyone is out to get them; they often start lawsuits.
- **Schizoid**: the classic loner; no friends and no interest in having friends.
- **Schizotypal**: bizarre beliefs (e.g., extrasensory perception, cults, superstition, illusions) and bizarre manner of speaking but no psychosis.
- **Avoidant**: lack of friends but desire to have them; fear of criticism or rejection causes patients to avoid others (inferiority complex).
- **Histrionic**: overly dramatic and attention-seeking and may be inappropriately seductive; patients must be the center of attention.
- **Narcissistic**: egocentric, lack empathy, use others for their own gain, and have a sense of entitlement.
- **Antisocial**: may have a *long criminal record* (con men) and may have tortured animals or set fires as children (a history of childhood *conduct disorder* is required for this diagnosis). Patients are

aggressive and do not pay bills or support children; they are also liars and *feel no remorse* (without conscience). The disorder has a strong association with alcoholism or drug abuse and *somatization* disorder. Most patients are male.

○ **Borderline**: instability of mood, behavior, relationships (many are bisexual), and self-image. Look for *splitting* (people and things are all good or all bad and may frequently change categories), suicide attempts, micropsychotic episodes (2 minutes of psychosis), impulsiveness, and constant crisis (e.g., Glenn Close's character in *Fatal Attraction*).

○ **Dependent**: cannot be (or do anything) alone; highly dependent on others (e.g., a wife may stay with an abusive husband).

○ **Obsessive-compulsive**: Patients are anal-retentive, stubborn, and cheap with restricted affect. Rules are more important than objectives. Different from obsessive-compulsive disorder (OCD)!

MISCELLANEOUS

Dissociative fugue/psychogenic fugue: A reversible amnesia for personal identity including the memories, personality, and other identifying characteristics of individuality. The classic patient develops amnesia, travels, and assumes a new identity but does not remember the event upon returning.

Dissociative identity disorder/multiple personality disorder: Most likely disorder to be associated with *childhood sexual abuse.*

Homosexuality and homosexual experimentation are not considered a disease at any age; they are normal variants.

🔲 **CASE SCENARIO:** A woman complains that her husband has mentioned a few "kinky" fantasies and occasionally wears her underwear. What disorder does the man have? None. His behavior is within the realm of normal.

Obsessive-compulsive disorder: Patients have recurrent *thoughts* or *impulses* (obsessions) and/or recurrent *behaviors* (compulsions) that cause marked dysfunction in their occupational or interpersonal lives. Look for washing (the patient may wash the hands 30 times a day) and checking rituals (the patient may check to see whether the door is locked 30 times a day). The onset is usually in adolescence or early adulthood. Treat with SSRIs (especially *fluvoxamine*) or clomipramine. Behavioral therapy (e.g., flooding) may also be effective.

Narcolepsy: Daytime sleepiness; *decreased rapid eye movement (REM) latency* (patients enter the REM stage as soon as they fall asleep); *cataplexy* (loss of muscle tone, falls); and *hypnopompic* (as the patient wakes up) or hypnagogic (as the patient falls asleep) hallucinations. Treat with *modafinil* (a nonamphetamine stimulant), methylphenidate, or amphetamines.

 Hospitalize patients (against their will, if necessary) who are a danger to themselves (suicidal or unable to take care of themselves) or others (homicidal).

DRUGS OF ABUSE

Marijuana is the most commonly abused illegal drug. Look for a teenager who is withdrawn and has a decline in school performance. Also look for *"amotivational syndrome"* (chronic use leads to laziness and lack of motivation), time distortion, and "munchies" (eating binge during intoxication). Patients have no physical withdrawal symptoms, although they may report psychologic cravings. Overdoses are not dangerous, although patients may experience temporary dysphoria and pulmonary symptoms with long-term use.

Cocaine is associated with sympathetic stimulation *(insomnia, tachycardia, mydriasis, hypertension, sweating),* hyperalertness, and possible paranoia, aggressiveness, delirium, psychosis, or *formications* (patients think that bugs are crawling on them). Overdoses can be fatal because of arrhythmia, myocardial infarction, seizure, or stroke. On withdrawal, patients become sleepy, hungry (vs. anorexic with intoxication), and irritable with possible severe depression. Withdrawal is not dangerous, but psychologic cravings are usually severe. Cocaine is *teratogenic* (vascular disruptions in the fetus).

Amphetamines are more classically associated with psychotic symptoms (patients may appear to be full-blown schizophrenics), but otherwise symptoms are similar to those with cocaine. Young adults may abuse prescribed medications such as methylphenidate and dextroamphetamine/ amphetamine.

Opioids include heroin and related agents. They cause *euphoria, analgesia, drowsiness, miosis, constipation,* and CNS/respiratory depression. Overdose can be fatal because of respiratory depression; treat with *naloxone.* Because the drug is usually taken intravenously, there are associated serious side effects as well as fatalities (e.g., endocarditis, HIV infection, cellulitis, talc damage to the lung). Withdrawal is not life-threatening, but patients act as though they are going to die. Signs and symptoms include *gooseflesh, diarrhea, insomnia,* and cramping or pain. *Methadone* treatment is sometimes given to opiate addicts through supervised clinics. Methadone or buprenorphine can be used to reduce acute withdrawal symptoms.

Lysergic acid diethylamide (LSD)/mushrooms causes symptoms of intoxication: *hallucinations* (usually visual vs. auditory in schizophrenia), *mydriasis,* tachycardia, diaphoresis, and perception and mood disturbances. Overdoses are not dangerous (unless the patient thinks that he or she can fly and jumps out a window), and there are no withdrawal symptoms. Patients may have *"flashbacks"* months to years later (brief feeling of being on the drug again, even though none was taken) or a "bad trip" (acute panic reaction or dysphoria). Treat bad trips with reassurance or a benzodiazepine/antipsychotic agent, if needed.

📁 **CASE SCENARIO:** What are the known teratogenic effects of LSD? None. Neither LSD nor marijuana has been definitely proved to be teratogenic, though smoke inhalation (marijuana) is thought to have ill effects on the fetus (as it is with cigarette smoking).

Phencyclidine (PCP) causes symptoms of LSD/mushroom intoxication plus confusion, agitation, and aggressive behavior. Also look for *vertical and/or horizontal nystagmus,* plus possible schizophrenic-type symptoms (e.g., paranoia, auditory hallucinations, disorganized behavior and speech). Overdose can be fatal (convulsions, coma, respiratory arrest); treat with supportive care and *urine acidification* to hasten elimination. There are no withdrawal symptoms.

Inhalants (e.g., gasoline, glue, varnish remover) cause euphoria, dizziness, slurred speech, a feeling of floating, ataxia, and/or a sense of heightened power. Inhalant use is usually seen in *younger teenagers* (11–15 years). Overdoses can be fatal (respiratory depression, cardiac arrhythmias, asphyxiation) or cause severe permanent sequelae (nervous system, liver, or kidney toxicity, peripheral neuropathy). There is no known withdrawal syndrome.

Benzodiazepines/barbiturates cause sedation and drowsiness, as well as reduced anxiety and disinhibition. Overdoses can be fatal (respiratory depression); treat overdoses of benzodiazepines with *flumazenil.* In addition, withdrawal can be fatal (as with alcohol) because of seizures and/or cardiovascular collapse. Treat withdrawal on an inpatient basis with benzodiazepines, and gradually taper the dose over several days. Benzodiazepines and barbiturates are dangerous when mixed with alcohol (all three are CNS depressants).

 Caffeine can cause **headaches, irritability,** *and* **fatigue** *in withdrawal.*

ETHICS

Do *not* force adult Jehovah's Witness patients to accept blood or other biologic products.

A physician is not obligated to provide treatment that he or she does not believe offers a benefit or may harm the patient. However, take the request seriously and formulate a plan that would be acceptable.

If a child has a life-threatening condition and the parents refuse a simple, curative treatment (e.g., antibiotics for meningitis), first try to persuade the parents. Then get a court order to give the treatment. Parents are allowed to refuse treatments that do not place the child at significant harm (e.g., vaccinations).

Let competent people die if they want to do so; never force treatments on adults of sound mind. It is important to evaluate these patients for underlying depression. On the other hand, do not commit active euthanasia. Respect the patient's wishes for passive euthanasia, although this issue is controversial.

Do not tell anyone how your patient is doing unless the patient has given authorization. If Mary has cancer and she asks you not to tell her husband, do not tell the husband if he asks. If a colleague asks about a friend who happens to be your patient, *refuse to answer.*

When it is permissible to break patient confidentiality:
○ At the patient's request
○ Suspected child abuse and elder abuse
○ Court mandate
○ Duty to warn and protect (if a patient says that he is going to kill Joe, you have to tell Joe, the proper authorities, or both)
○ Reportable disease
○ Danger to others. For example, if a driver is blind or has seizures, let the proper authorities know so that they can take away the patient's driver's license. If an airplane pilot is a paranoid, hallucinating schizophrenic, the proper authorities need to know.

Informed consent involves giving the patient information about the diagnosis (his or her condition and what it means), the prognosis (the natural course of the condition without treatment), the proposed treatment (description of the procedure and what the patient will experience), the potential risks and benefit of the treatment, and alternative treatments. Patients are then allowed to make their own choice. The documents that patients are made to sign on wards are not required or sufficient for informed consent; they are used for documentation and medicolegal purposes (i.e., lawsuit paranoia).

When a patient is incompetent, a surrogate decision maker or health care power of attorney must speak for him or her. If no appropriate surrogate decision maker is available, the physician is expected to act in the best interest of the patient until a surrogate is found or appointed.

Living wills and do-not-resuscitate (DNR) orders should be respected and followed if done correctly. For example, if John specifies in his living will that he does not want to be put on a ventilator, do not put him on a ventilator, even if a spouse, child, or significant other tells you to do so. Of course, be courteous and discuss it with those concerned in a caring, professional manner.

Depression should always be evaluated as a reason for "incompetence." A patient who is suicidal may refuse all treatment. This refusal should not be respected until the depression is treated.

Psychiatric patients can be hospitalized for a limited time against their will if they are a danger to self or others. After 1–3 days of hospitalization, most states require a formal hearing to determine whether the patient has to remain in custody. This practice is based on the principle of beneficence (doing good and avoiding harm).

Restraints can be used on an incompetent or violent (delirious, psychotic) patient if necessary, but their use should be brief and re-evaluated frequently. They should be used sparingly for board purposes.

📁 **CASE SCENARIO:** How effective are restraints in preventing falls in demented or delirious patients? Restraints generally do not reduce the risk of falls and can cause serious injury.

Patients younger than age 18 do not require parental consent if they are emancipated (married, living on their own and financially independent, raising children, serving in the armed forces); have a sexually transmitted disease; want contraception; are pregnant; want drug treatment or counseling; or have psychiatric illness. Some states have exceptions to these statements, but for the boards, let minors make their own decisions in such settings.

If a patient is comatose and no surrogate decision maker has been appointed, the wishes of the family should generally be respected. If there is a family disagreement or ulterior motives are suspected, talk to the hospital ethics committee. Use courts as a last resort.

📁 **CASE SCENARIO:** What should you do in a pediatric emergency when parents, caretakers, or family members are not available to give consent? Treat the child as you see fit.

Do not hide a diagnosis from patients (including children) if they want to know the diagnosis (even if the family asks you to do so). Do not lie to any patient because the family asks you to do so. The only times to withhold information are (1) when you have compelling evidence that disclosure will cause real and predictable harm (e.g., disclosure will make the patient suicidal) or (2) when the patient does not want to know the diagnosis.

📁 **CASE SCENARIO:** A family asks you not to tell Grandma the diagnosis. What should you do first? Ask the family about their concerns. If this approach does not resolve the issue, ask the patient whether she wants to know the diagnosis. If she does, tell the family that you are obligated to give her the information.

🗀 **CASE SCENARIO:** What should you do if a patient who needs treatment cannot communicate (e.g., comatose or unconscious patients)? Give all required care unless you know that the patient does not want it.

Withdrawing and withholding care are legal equivalents. The fact that a patient is on a ventilator does not mean that you can never turn it off.

In terminally ill patients, give enough pain medication to relieve pain. Do not be afraid to use narcotics, and do not worry about addiction in this setting.

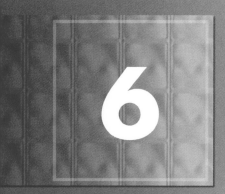

6 SURGERY AND SURGICAL SUBSPECIALTIES

TRAUMA

The ABCDEs are the key to the initial management of patients with trauma. Always do them in order. For example, if the patient is bleeding to death and has a blocked airway, you may have to choose which issue to address first. The first priority is airway management.

A = Airway maintenance and cervical spine care. Provide, protect, and maintain an adequate airway at all times and assume a cervical injury is present while doing so (i.e., place cervical collar, and do not hyperextend neck) until it is excluded. If the patient can answer questions, the airway is fine. You can use an oropharyngeal or nasopharyngeal airway in uncomplicated cases and give supplemental oxygen. When the airway is blocked or if the Glasgow Coma Scale (GCS) score is less than 8, intubate. If intubation fails, do a cricothyroidotomy.

B = Breathing and ventilation. Assess chest wall, lung expansion, lung function, and ventilation. If the airway is open and patient is not breathing, intubate. If intubation fails, do a cricothyroidotomy. Look for acute problems such as flail chest, tension pneumothorax, or massive hemothorax.

C = Circulation and control of hemorrhage. If the patient seems hypovolemic (tachycardia, bleeding, weak pulse, paleness, diaphoresis, capillary refill >2 seconds), give intravenous (IV) fluids and/or blood products. The initial procedure is to start two large-bore catheters and give a bolus of 10–20 mL/kg (roughly 1 L) of lactated Ringer's solution (IV fluid of choice in trauma) and blood. Then reassess the patient for improvement. Repeat the bolus if necessary.

D = Disability and neurologic status. Check neurologic function (using the Glasgow Coma Scale). Rule out hypoxia, hypovolemia, and hypoglycemia before considering central nervous system injury.

E = Exposure/Environment. Remove the patient's clothing and "put a finger in every orifice" so that you do not miss any occult injuries. Look for hypothermia.

In general, all trauma patients should have chest and pelvic radiographs, with computed tomography (CT) scans used as needed for further evaluation or persistent symptoms despite negative radiographs.

Evaluate head and cervical spine trauma with *noncontrast CT* (better than magnetic resonance imaging [MRI] for intracranial hemorrhage and fractures).

Abdominal trauma

Blunt abdominal trauma: Initial findings determine a course of action (Table 6-1):

TABLE 6-1 Evaluation of Abdominal Trauma

STUDY	FEATURES	ADVANTAGES	DISADVANTAGES
Plain radiographs	Limited value in most abdominal traumas because CT provides better detail	Useful for projectile penetrating abdominal trauma (gunshot trajectory)	Not useful for blunt or nonprojectile penetrating abdominal trauma
Diagnostic peritoneal lavage	Generally not used anymore and replaced by FAST and CT scans	Takes little time to perform	Invasive, does not detect retroperitoneal bleed, does not detect organ damage
FAST scan	Gaining widespread use for initial evaluation of blunt trauma	Portable, rapid, noninvasive, useful for detecting hemoperitoneum	Does not detect organ damage, operator-dependent, may miss small bleeds (<100 mL)

TABLE 6-1 Evaluation of Abdominal Trauma—cont'd

STUDY	FEATURES	ADVANTAGES	DISADVANTAGES
CT scan	Commonly used if time permits	Provides details on hemorrhage and organ damage	Time constraints limit use in hemodynamically unstable patients
Laparotomy	Used for hemodynamically unstable patients who do not have time to undergo other studies	Rapid assessment and correction of abnormalities	Invasive, may not detect some organ injuries

○ If the patient is awake and stable and your exam is benign, observe and repeat the abdominal exam later.

○ If the patient has significant trauma and does not require urgent surgery, order a focused assessment with sonography for trauma (FAST) ultrasound or CT scan of the abdomen and pelvis with IV contrast after the patient is stabilized (diagnostic peritoneal lavage is no longer used). Do not send an unstable patient to the CT scanner.

○ If the patient is hemodynamically unstable (from hypotension and/or shock that does not respond to a fluid challenge), proceed directly to laparotomy.

Penetrating abdominal trauma: Type of injury and initial findings determine the course of action:

○ With a gunshot wound in an unstable patient, proceed directly to laparotomy.

○ With a wound from a sharp instrument, management is more controversial. Either proceed directly to laparotomy (better choice if the patient is unstable) or do a CT scan. If the results are positive, consider laparotomy on the basis of the injury; if the results are negative, observe and repeat the exam later.

Chest trauma

Six thoracic injuries can be rapidly fatal and must be recognized immediately:

1. **Airway obstruction:** The patient has no audible breath sounds and cannot answer questions even though he or she may be awake and gurgling. Clear the airway if possible and treat with *endotracheal intubation.* If intubation fails, do a *cricothyroidotomy* (or tracheostomy in the operating room if there is time).

2. **Open pneumothorax:** An open defect in the chest wall causes poor ventilation and oxygenation. Treat with *endotracheal intubation, positive-pressure ventilation,* and *closure of the defect in the chest wall.* Gauze should be used and taped on only three sides to allow excessive pressure to escape so that you do not convert an open pneumothorax into a tension pneumothorax.

3. **Tension pneumothorax:** Usually seen after blunt trauma, tension pneumothorax occurs when air is forced into the pleural space and cannot escape. It collapses the affected lung and then *shifts the mediastinum and trachea to the opposite side* of the chest. The patient has *absent breath sounds* and a *hypertympanic or hyperresonant percussion sound* on the affected side. Impaired cardiac filling may result in hypotension and/or *distended neck veins.* Treat with *needle thoracentesis* (anterior second intercostal space usually preferred), followed by insertion of a chest/thoracostomy tube.

4. **Cardiac tamponade:** The classic history is one of penetrating trauma to the left chest. The patient has hypotension (due to impaired cardiac filling), *distended neck veins, muffled heart sounds, pulsus paradoxus* (exaggerated fall in blood pressure on inspiration), and *normal breath sounds.* Treat with *pericardiocentesis* if the patient is unstable: Put a catheter in the pericardial sac (via a subxiphoid approach) and aspirate the blood or fluid. If the patient is stable, you can do a Fast scan, an echocardiogram, or a chest CT scan to confirm the diagnosis.

5. **Massive hemothorax:** With loss of more than 1 L of blood into the thoracic cavity, the patient will have *decreased breath sounds* on the affected side, *dull note on percussion,* hypotension, *collapsed neck veins* (from blood leaving the vascular tree), and tachycardia. Placement of a chest tube allows the blood to come out. Give IV fluids and/or blood before you place the chest tube. If the bleeding stops after the initial outflow, order a radiograph and/or CT scan to check for remaining blood or pathology and treat supportively. Emergent thoracotomy is required if the bleeding does not stop or is massive.

6. **Flail chest:** When several adjacent ribs are broken in multiple places, the affected part of the chest wall can move paradoxically (inward during inspiration, outward during expiration) during respiration (Fig. 6-1). There is almost always an associated *pulmonary contusion,* which, combined with pain, may make respiration inadequate. When you are in doubt or if the patient is not doing well, *intubate* and give *positive-pressure ventilation.*

FRACTURED RIBS - FLAILING

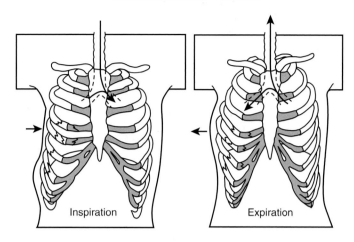

Inspiration

Expiration

FIGURE 6-1 Paradoxical respiration: inward motion with inspiration; outward motion with expiration. *(From James EC, Corry RJ, Perry JF: Principles of Basic Surgical Practice. Philadelphia, Hanley & Belfus, 1987.)*

Other injuries

Thoracic aortic injury/rupture: The most common cause of immediate death after an automobile accident or fall from great height. Usually occurs just beyond the takeoff of the subclavian artery (aortic isthmus, where the aorta is tethered in place by the ligamentum arteriosum). Thoracic aortic laceration with a contained rupture (i.e., intact adventitia) can allow survival, but in many cases with rupture (50%), the patient dies within 24 hours of reaching the hospital. Thus, treat with immediate surgical management after diagnosing with chest CT with IV contrast. Without treatment survival beyond 4 months is less than 5%.

📁 **CASE SCENARIO:** What is the classic chest x-ray finding with aortic laceration? Widened mediastinum. Order a CT chest with contrast (or CT angiogram) if you are suspicious (because of x-ray findings or due to trauma degree, location, and/or type). Treat with immediate surgical repair.

📁 **CASE SCENARIO:** On which side does a traumatic diaphragm rupture usually occur? The left. The liver is believed to protect the right side. The classic findings consist of bowel sounds auscultated in the chest or seeing bowel loops in the thorax on chest radiograph. Fix surgically.

Head trauma: See "Neurosurgery" later.
Neck trauma: The neck is divided into three zones for trauma:
○ **Zone I:** base of the neck (from 2 cm above the clavicles to the level of the clavicles)
○ **Zone II:** midcervical region (2 cm above the clavicle to the angle of the mandible)
○ **Zone III:** the angle of the mandible to the base of the skull
Management is dictated by location of the injury:
○ With symptomatic zone I and III injuries, do a CT angiogram before going to the operating room in a stable patient.
○ With zone II injuries, proceed to the operating room for surgical exploration in symptomatic patients; consider CT angiogram first if the patient is stable.
○ In patients with obvious bleeding or a rapidly expanding hematoma, proceed directly to the operating room no matter where the injury is.
Choking victim: Leave choking patients alone if they are speaking, coughing, or breathing. If they stop doing all of these things, perform the Heimlich maneuver.
If a tooth is knocked out, put it back in place with no cleaning (or rinse it only with saline or milk) and stabilize as soon as possible. The sooner this is done, the better the prognosis for salvage of the tooth.

Burns

Burns may be electrical, chemical, or thermal. Initial management of all burns includes plenty of IV fluids (use lactated Ringer solution or normal saline if lactated Ringer is not a choice), removal of all clothes and other smoldering items on the body, copious irrigation of chemical burns, and, of course, the ABCs. You should have a low threshold for intubation; use 100% oxygen until significant carboxyhemoglobin from carbon monoxide inhalation is ruled out.
○ **Electrical burns.** Because most of the destruction is internal, patients may have myoglobinuria, acidosis, and renal failure. Use aggressive IV fluids to prevent renal failure. The immediate,

life-threatening risk with electricity exposure and burns (including lightning and putting a finger in an electrical outlet) is cardiac arrhythmias. Order an electrocardiogram (ECG).

○ **Chemical burns.** Alkali burns are worse than acidic burns because alkali penetrates more deeply. Treat all chemical burns with copious irrigation from the nearest water source.

○ **Thermal burns.** Burned skin is much more prone to infection, usually by *Staphylococcus aureus* or *Pseudomonas* spp. Pseudomonal infection causes a *fruity smell* and/or *blue-green color.* Prophylactic antibiotics are given topically, not systemically. Severity is classified as shown Table 6-2.

TABLE 6-2 Burn Depth Classification

BURN DEPTH	APPEARANCE	SKIN LAYER(S)	SENSATION	HEALING
Superficial	Dry, pink or red	Epidermis	Painful	Days, keep clean
Superficial partial thickness	Moist, pink or red with blisters	Epidermis, less than ½ of dermis	Painful	7-14 days. Remove blister, apply antibiotic ointment, apply dressing
Deep partial thickness	Dry, white, brown, leathery, vesicles, blisters	Epidermis, more than ½ of dermis including nerves	Less painful than superficial burns	14-21 days. Keep clean and infection-free, apply antibiotic ointment, apply dressing, monitor fluid loss
Full thickness	Dry, brown, charred	Epidermis, full dermis including nerves	Dull	Excision, skin grafting, monitor fluid loss and metabolic effects

Many burns have a combination of degrees. Watch for compartment syndrome, which is treated with escharotomy.

▭ **CASE SCENARIO:** What is the major difference in symptoms between superficial and deep burns? Superficial burns are painful, whereas deep burns are classically *painless* initially because of nerve damage.

▭ **CASE SCENARIO:** What vaccine should burn victims receive? Tetanus.

Hypothermia and Hyperthermia

Hypothermia: Treatment varies depending on the degree of hypothermia and background health (Table 6-3).

TABLE 6-3 Overview of Hyperthermia

DEGREE	TEMPERATURE*	SYMPTOMS	WARMING THERAPY
Mild hypothermia	32.2-35°C	Arrhythmia, ataxia, shivering	Remove wet clothing, warm blankets
Moderate hypothermia	28-32.2°C	Decreased consciousness, decreased pulse and respiration, dysrhythmias, no shivering	Warm IV fluids, warm oxygen, warm bath water, extracorporeal blood warming with cardiopulmonary bypass
Severe hypothermia	<28°C	Absence of reflexes, no response to pain, risk of ventricular fibrillation	

*Measured core body temperatur.

In general, secure the airway, intubate if necessary, remove wet clothing, rewarm with blankets, and/or give warm IV fluids. The most important point is to monitor the ECG for arrhythmias, which are common with hypothermia. The rare but classic finding is the *J wave*, a small, positive deflection following the QRS complex (Fig. 6-2). Also monitor electrolytes, renal function, and acid-base status.

With frostnip (cold, painful areas of skin; mild injury) and frostbite (cold, anesthetic areas of skin; more severe injury), treat by rewarming affected areas with warm water (not scalding hot) and generalized warming (e.g., blankets).

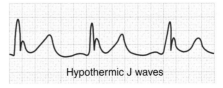

FIGURE 6-2 Hypothermic J waves. *(From Ferri FF: Practical Guide to the Care of the Medical Patient, 8th ed. Philadelphia, Mosby, 2011.)*

Hypothermic J waves

Hyperthermia may be due to heat exhaustion (38.7–40°C) and heat stroke (>40°C). Heat exhaustion symptoms include generalized malaise, weakness, cramps, nausea, and *sweating*. Heat stroke symptoms include neurologic abnormalities (seizures, psychosis, coma), dehydration, and the *absence of sweating*. Treat heat exhaustion with cooling in a dry area and oral replacement of fluids and salt. Treat heat stroke with airway support (ABCs), immediate cooling (wet blankets, ice packs, cold water), and IV fluids. The immediate threats to life are convulsions (treat with diazepam) and cardiovascular collapse. Rule out infection and other classic culprits:

1. Malignant hyperthermia: Look for succinylcholine or halothane exposure. Treat with supportive care and *dantrolene.*
2. Neuroleptic malignant syndrome: The classic patient is taking an antipsychotic. First, stop the medication. Second, treat with support (especially lots of IV fluids to prevent renal shutdown from rhabdomyolysis) and possibly dantrolene.

📁 **CASE SCENARIO:** What lab value is markedly elevated in patients with neuroleptic malignant syndrome? The *creatine kinase (CK)* level, because of muscle breakdown.

3. Drug fever: idiosyncratic reaction to a medication that usually was started within the past few weeks.

Near drowning

Fresh water is said by some to be worse than salt water because fresh water, if aspirated, can cause hypervolemia, electrolyte disturbances, and hemolysis. Others think this distinction is nonsense. Intubate patients if they are unconscious, and monitor arterial blood gases if they are conscious. Patients who almost drown in cold water often do better than those who almost drown in warm water (due to decreased metabolic needs). Death usually results from hypoxia and/or cardiac arrest.

GENERAL SURGERY

Acute abdomen:

An inflamed peritoneum often buys the patient a laparotomy because it signifies a potentially life-threatening condition; important exceptions are pancreatitis, most cases of diverticulitis, and spontaneous bacterial peritonitis. The best physical confirmation of peritonitis is rebound tenderness and involuntary guarding/abdominal muscular rigidity. Voluntary guarding is a softer sign, as is tenderness to palpation; both are often present in benign diseases. When you are in doubt and the patient is stable, withhold narcotics, which mask symptoms, until you have a diagnosis. Do serial abdominal exams. Perform CT scan with oral and IV contrast. If the patient is unstable, proceed to laparoscopy/laparotomy.

Acute abdomen localization:
1. Right upper quadrant (RUQ): Think of gallbladder (cholecystitis), bile ducts (cholangitis), or liver (abscess).
2. Left upper quadrant (LUQ): Think of spleen (rupture with blunt trauma or rarely, abscess).
3. Right lower quadrant (RLQ): Think of appendix (appendicitis) or obstetric/gynecologic problem.
4. Left lower quadrant (LLQ): Think of sigmoid colon (diverticulitis) or obstetric/gynecologic problem.
5. Epigastric: Think of stomach (penetrating ulcer) or pancreas (pancreatitis).

Cholecystitis: The four Fs summarize the classic patient with *cholesterol* stones: fat, forty, fertile, female, and a fifth F, febrile, suggests cholecystitis, especially if gallstones are seen on ultrasound scan or the patient has a history of gallstones and/or gallstone-type symptoms (e.g., postprandial right upper quadrant [RUQ] colicky pain with bloating and/or nausea and vomiting). Look for the *Murphy sign.* Ultrasound imaging is the preferred initial test. Do a hepato-iminodiacetic acid (HIDA) scan if ultrasound findings are equivocal. Do a cholecystectomy for most patients. Remember that *pigment gallstones* are seen in patients with hemolytic anemias, not "5-F" patients.

📁 **CASE SCENARIO:** What triad of findings is associated with cholangitis? *RUQ pain, fever* (usually with shaking chills), and *jaundice.* Patients often have a history of gallstones. Start antibiotics after getting blood cultures, and do a cholecystectomy once the patient is stable.

Splenic rupture: Patients have a history of blunt abdominal trauma, hypotension or tachycardia, shock, and *Kerr sign* (pain referred to the left shoulder). Ultrasound and CT can be used to evaluate the

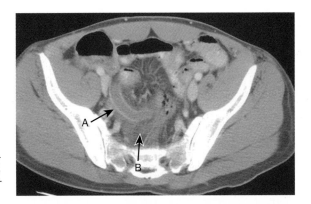

FIGURE 6-3 Appendicitis. Dilated thickened appendix (*A*), with adjacent hazy fat (**B**). *(From Rakel RE, Rakel D: Textbook of Family Medicine, 8th ed. Philadelphia, Saunders, 2011.)*

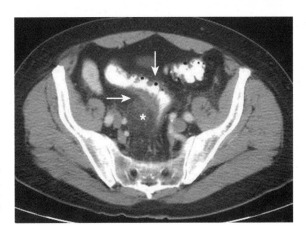

FIGURE 6-4 Diverticulitis. Computed tomography (CT) image demonstrates thickened wall of the sigmoid colon *(arrows)* with stranding in the adjacent fat (*). *(From McNally PR: GI/Liver Secrets Plus, 4th ed. Philadelphia, Mosby, 2010.)*

extent of injury. Consider splenectomy if the patient is unstable or if the spleen is extensively injured with continuous bleeding. Do not let patients with Epstein-Barr virus (EBV) infection play contact sports. Do not forget to immunize postsplenectomy patients (pneumococcal, meningococcal, *Haemophilus influenzae* type b vaccines).

Appendicitis: The incidence peaks in 10- to 30-year-olds. The classic history is crampy, poorly localized periumbilical pain followed by nausea and vomiting, then localization of pain to the RLQ and peritoneal signs with worsening of nausea and vomiting. Patients who are hungry and asking for food do not have appendicitis. Remember the Rovsing sign, as well as McBurney point tenderness. Use CT scan of the abdomen (or ultrasound in children or pregnant women) to help make the diagnosis when patients are stable (Fig. 6-3). Do an appendectomy even if the imaging is negative if the history and exam are indicative.

Diverticulitis: Localized LLQ pain in a patient older than 50 is diverticulitis unless you have a good reason to think otherwise. *CT scan* with oral, rectal, and/or IV contrast is the best test to confirm disease, rule out a complicating abscess, and exclude an alternative diagnosis (Fig. 6-4). Treat medically with broad-spectrum antibiotics (e.g., ciprofloxacin + metronidazole) and place the patient on NPO (nothing-by-mouth) status. If disease is recurrent or refractory to medical therapy, if there is an abscess, or if peritonitis is present, consider surgical resection. Diverticular abscesses can be treated with percutaneous drainage.

Acute pancreatitis: Look for epigastric pain in an alcohol abuser or a patient with a known history of gallstones. Pain may radiate to the back, and serum *amylase* and *lipase* are elevated (if these values are not given, order these tests). Other common symptoms include decreased bowel sounds, local ileus (sentinel loop of bowel on radiograph), nausea, vomiting, and anorexia. CT scan is the preferred imaging test (Fig. 6-5). Treat with pain medications, NPO status, nasogastric tube, IV fluids, and supportive care. Watch for complications of *pseudocyst* and *pancreatic abscess,* which may require surgical intervention.

▢ **CASE SCENARIO:** A patient has a history of ulcers, epigastric pain, peritoneal signs, mildly elevated amylase, and normal lipase. A small amount of free air is noted under the diaphragm on abdominal radiograph. What is the likely diagnosis? Perforated peptic ulcer, which can cause elevated amylase (but lipase is typically normal).

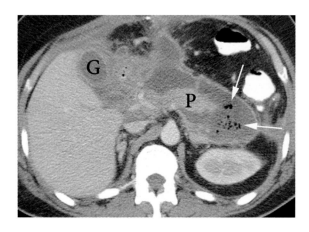

FIGURE 6-5 Acute necrotizing pancreatitis. On contrast-enhanced computed tomography scan, the pancreas (P) is surrounded by peripancreatic inflammation that contains bubbles of air *(arrows)* due to sterile necrosis. G, Gallbladder. *(From Feldman M, Friedman LS, Brandt LJ: Sleisenger and Fordtran's Gastrointestinal and Liver Disease, 8th ed. Philadelphia, Saunders, 2006.)*

Small bowel obstruction: Signs and symptoms include *bilious vomiting* (early symptom), *abdominal distention,* constipation, hyperactive bowel sounds (high-pitched, rushing sounds), and pain that is usually poorly localized. Radiograph shows multiple air-fluid levels in dilated small bowel loops. Patients often have a *history of previous surgery;* the most common cause of small bowel obstruction (SBO) in adults is *adhesions,* which usually develop from prior surgery. In children, think of *incarcerated inguinal hernia* or *Meckel diverticulum.* Start treatment with NPO status, nasogastric tube with suction, and IV fluids. Order CT scan with IV contrast to confirm the diagnosis and exclude a specific underlying disorder other than adhesions (e.g., hernia, tumor). If symptoms do not resolve or if the patient develops peritoneal signs, laparotomy is necessary to relieve the obstruction.

Large bowel obstruction: Signs and symptoms include gradually increasing abdominal pain, *abdominal distention,* constipation, and *feculent vomiting* (late symptom). This condition is seen more often in older patients as a result of *diverticulitis, colon cancer,* or *volvulus.* Treat early with NPO status and nasogastric tube. Sigmoid volvulus often can be decompressed with an endoscope. Other causes or refractory cases require surgery to relieve the obstruction. CT scan with IV contrast or barium enema can confirm the diagnosis and may suggest the etiology. In children, watch for *Hirschsprung disease.*

Hernias

The four common types (there are others) are treated with surgical repair if they are symptomatic. Now that bariatric surgery has become more common, internal hernias have also become more common:

1. **Indirect:** most common in both sexes and all age groups. The hernia sac travels through the inner and outer inguinal rings (protrusion begins lateral to the inferior epigastric vessels) and *into the scrotum (or labia)* due to a patent processus vaginalis (congenital defect).
2. **Direct:** the hernia (no sac) protrudes *medial to the inferior epigastric* vessels (and not into the scrotum or labia) due to weakness in the abdominal musculature (of Hesselbach triangle).
3. **Femoral:** more common in women. The hernia (no sac) goes through the femoral ring onto the *anterior thigh (located below the inguinal ring).* Femoral hernias are the most susceptible to incarceration and strangulation.
4. **Incisional:** after any wound (especially surgical), a hernia can occur through the site of the incision. There are two main complications associated with hernias:
❍ Incarceration is when herniated organs are trapped, cannot be reduced, and become swollen or edematous.
❍ Strangulation is when the entrapment/incarceration becomes so severe that the blood supply is cut off. *Strangulation can lead to necrosis and is a surgical emergency.* Patients may present with SBO symptoms and shock.

▢ **CASE SCENARIO:** What is the most common cause of small bowel obstruction in a person who has never had surgery before? Incarcerated hernia (which is the second most common cause in patients with prior abdominal surgery, after adhesions).

Preoperative and postoperative points

1. Preoperatively, keep the patient on NPO status for at least 8 hours (when possible) to reduce the chance of aspiration.

2. Spirometry (and, of course, a good history) is the best preoperative test to order for assessment of pulmonary function. It measures forced vital capacity (FVC), forced expiratory volume in 1 second (FEV_1), FEV_1/FVC ratio (%), and maximum voluntary ventilation.

3. Use compressive/elastic stockings, early ambulation, and/or prophylactic-dose low-molecular-weight heparin to help prevent deep venous thrombosis and pulmonary embolism.

4. The most common cause of postoperative fever in the first 24 hours is *atelectasis* (usually low-grade fever). Prevent or treat with early ambulation, chest physiotherapy/percussion, incentive spirometry, and proper pain control. Both too much pain and too many narcotics increase the risk of atelectasis.

5. The mnemonic *"water, wind, walk, wound, and wonder drugs"* will help you recall the causes of postoperative fever: water, urinary tract infection; wind, atelectasis/pneumonia; walk, deep venous thrombosis; wound, surgical wound infection; wonder drugs, drug fever. If daily fever spikes occur, think about an intraabdominal abscess; consider a CT scan to locate the abscess. Abscesses often need surgical or CT-guided catheter drainage.

6. Fascial/wound dehiscence typically occurs 5–10 days postoperatively. Look for leakage of serosanguineous fluid from the wound (often after the patient coughs or strains), which is especially associated with wound infection. Treat with antibiotics (if secondary to infection) and reclosure of the incision.

EAR, NOSE, AND THROAT SURGERY

Infections

Rhinitis: edematous, vasodilated nasal mucosa and turbinates with clear nasal discharge. Causes include the following:

1. **Viral infection** (common cold): due to rhinovirus (most common), influenza virus, parainfluenza virus, adenovirus, or others. Treatment is symptomatic with short-term use of vasoconstrictors such as phenylephrine. Vasoconstrictors may cause rebound congestion, however.

2. **Allergy** (hay fever): associated with *seasonal* flare-ups, *boggy* and *bluish* turbinates, onset before the age of 20 years, *nasal polyps,* sneezing, pruritus, conjunctivitis, wheezing, asthma, eczema, family history, *eosinophils in nasal mucus,* and elevated serum immunoglobulin E (IgE) levels. Skin tests may identify an allergen. Treat with avoidance of any known antigen (e.g., pollen), antihistamines, immunotherapy, and/or *intranasal steroid spray* for severe symptoms. Desensitization is also an option.

3. **Bacterial infection:** typically due to streptococci, pneumococci, or staphylococci. Do a streptococcal throat culture. Treat with antibiotics if appropriate (sore throat, fever, tonsillar exudate).

   Sinusitis is usually due to viral or bacterial causes (*Streptococcus pneumoniae, Haemophilus influenzae, Moraxella* spp., other streptococci, or staphylococci). Look for fever, *tenderness over the affected sinus, headache,* and *purulent nasal discharge* (yellow or green) generally for >10 days. The diagnosis is generally based on clinical signs. The gold standard for diagnosis is positive culture from the paranasal sinuses. Imaging helps support the diagnosis. A four-view sinus radiograph may show opacification or air-fluid levels. CT scan is more sensitive than radiographs (and is now the imaging modality of choice if imaging is necessary) and is used to evaluate chronic sinusitis or suspected extension of infection outside the sinus (in patients with high fever and chills) (Fig. 6-6). Acute viral sinusitis generally resolves in 2 weeks without antibiotics. For moderate or severe symptoms, treat with antibiotics (amoxicillin, macrolide, cephalosporin, or doxycycline) for 10–14 days. Surgical drainage is indicated for intracranial complications, frontal sinusitis, or sinusitis recalcitrant to medical therapy. Deviated nasal septum or other congenital defects causing recurrent sinusitis are treated with surgical correction.

   Otitis externa (swimmer's ear): most commonly due to *Pseudomonas aeruginosa. Manipulation of the auricle produces pain* (this sign is not present in otitis media), the skin of the auditory canal is erythematous and swollen, and patients may have a foul-smelling discharge and conductive hearing loss. CT scan (rarely needed) may help define bone involvement and extent of disease. Treat with 2% acetic acid to inhibit growth, topical antibiotics (neomycin/polymyxin B), and steroids to help reduce swelling and inflammation.

▢ **CASE SCENARIO:** What are the classic physical findings and bacterial cause for infectious myringitis? Otoscopy classically reveals vesicles on the tympanic membrane, and the classic cause is *Mycoplasma* spp. Other causes include *S. pneumoniae* and viruses. Treat with antibiotics.

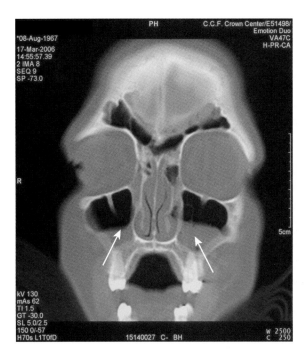

FIGURE 6-6 Computed tomography scan showing acute sinusitis. Note the fluid levels in the maxillary sinuses *(arrows)*. *(From Cleveland Clinic: Current Clinical Medicine, 2nd ed. Philadelphia, Saunders, 2010.)*

Causes of hearing loss

1. **Aging** (presbycusis): most common cause of *sensorineural hearing* loss in adults; a normal part of aging, not a disease. Patients can use hearing aids, if necessary.
2. **Environmental noise:** Prolonged or intense loud noise can permanently affect hearing. Advise earplugs for occupationally exposed patients.
3. **Otosclerosis:** most common cause of progressive *conductive hearing loss* in adults. Otic bones become fixed together, impeding hearing. Treat with hearing aids or surgery.
4. **Meningitis or recurrent otitis media:** the classic causes in children. Screen for hearing loss after meningitis.
5. **Congenital hearing loss:** toxoplasmosis, other (congenital syphilis and viruses), rubella, cytomegalovirus, and herpes simplex virus (TORCH) infection or inherited disability.
6. **Ménière disease:** usually occurs in middle-aged patients. The cause is unknown. Look for severe *vertigo, tinnitus, fluctuating hearing loss, fullness in the ear.* Treat with diuretics (hydrochlorothiazide), prochlorperazine, antihistamines (e.g., *meclizine*), diuretics (hydrochlorothiazide), or surgery (for refractory cases).
7. **Drugs:** aminoglycosides, aspirin (overdose causes tinnitus), quinine, loop diuretics, cisplatin.
8. **Tumor:** usually a vestibular schwannoma (schwannoma of the eighth cranial nerve, associated with neurofibromatosis 2).
9. **Labyrinthitis:** may have a viral etiology or follow or extend from meningitis or otitis media. Viral etiology often causes sudden deafness that develops over a few hours. Hearing usually returns within 2 weeks, but loss may be permanent. No treatment has proved effective. Reassurance and bed rest are preferred. Antiemetic (phenergan), vestibular suppressant (meclizine), and empirical steroids (methylprednisone) often are used.

Causes of vertigo

1. **Ménière disease:** accompanied by tinnitus, hearing loss, and nausea/vomiting. See earlier discussion.
2. **Benign positional/paroxysmal vertigo:** *induced by certain head positions* and may be accompanied by nystagmus without hearing loss. Cases often resolve spontaneously; the only treatment generally necessary is to avoid the position that provokes symptoms.
3. **Acoustic schwannoma**
4. **Stroke**
5. **Infection**
6. **Multiple sclerosis:** a possible cause of any weird neurologic symptoms, usually in women of reproductive age.

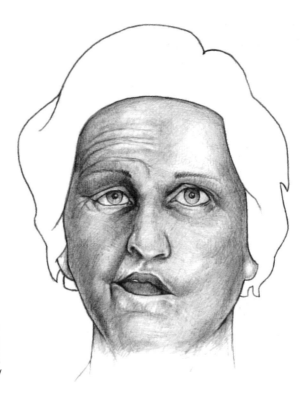

Figure 6-7 Bell palsy (facial nerve palsy). Note unwrinkled forehead, widely opened eyes (with weakness of eyelid color), flattening of the nasolabial fold, and a droop of the corner of the mouth. *(From Remmel KS, et al: Handbook of Symptom-Oriented Neurology, 3rd ed. St Louis, Mosby, 2002.)*

Causes of facial paralysis

Note Perform CT or MRI if stroke, tumor, or fracture is suspected.

1. **Stroke:** commonly associated with older age, other deficits, and stroke risk factors.
2. **Bell palsy:** acute facial (seventh) nerve palsy (Fig. 6-7). Characterized by sudden unilateral onset, usually after an upper respiratory infection. Peak incidence in persons older than 70 years and pregnant women. The cause is thought to be a reactivation of *herpes simplex* virus 1 in most cases. Patients may have *hyperacusis* (everything sounds loud because the stapedius muscle in the ear is paralyzed). In cases in which patients are unable to close the affected eye, use artificial tears and a patch to protect the eye. Glucocorticoids and antivirals have shown benefit. Most cases resolve spontaneously in about 1–3 months, but some patients have permanent sequelae. Remember that the patient will have a lower motor neuron deficit in this disorder, so the upper half of the affected side of the face is involved (whereas it should be spared with an upper motor neuron lesion such as stroke).
3. **Herpes zoster** (Ramsay Hunt syndrome): also causes ear pain. Look for *vesicles on the pinna and inside the ear.* Encephalitis or meningitis may be present.
4. **Lyme disease:** probably the most common cause of bilateral facial nerve palsy.
5. **Middle ear or mastoid infections/meningitis:** Look for other symptoms of the infection.
6. **Temporal bone fracture:** Patients may have Battle sign (bruising over the mastoid process), bleeding from the ear, and deafness.

Neck mass

75% benign in children, 75% malignant in patients older than 40 years. Causes include the following:
1. **Branchial cleft cysts:** seen in children; *lateral;* may become infected.
2. **Thyroglossal duct cysts:** seen in children; *midline;* elevates with tongue protrusion.
3. **Cystic hygroma:** lymphangioma seen in children, classically in patients with *Turner syndrome;* treat with surgical resection.
4. **Cervical lymphadenitis:** may occur in children or adults, usually as a result of streptococcal pharyngitis, Epstein-Barr virus (common in adolescents and young adults in their 20s), cat-scratch disease, or mycobacterial infection *(scrofula).*
5. **Neoplasm:** more common in adults than in children. The mass may be lymphadenopathy from primary (lymphoma) or metastatic neoplasm (usually a squamous cell carcinoma of the pharynx or larynx), or it may be the tumor itself.

📁 **CASE SCENARIO:** What is the classic workup for an "unknown cancer" (unknown site of primary malignancy) found in the neck? Random biopsy of the nasopharynx, palatine tonsils, and the base of the tongue, as well as laryngoscopy, bronchoscopy, and esophagoscopy (with biopsies of any suspicious lesions)—the so-called triple endoscopy with triple biopsy. CT/MRI or positron emission tomography (PET) scan also may help to detect lesions not apparent on physical exam.

Parotid swelling: Classically due to mumps. The best treatment for mumps and the complication of infertility is prevention through immunization. Provide supportive care for acute cases. Parotid swelling also may be due to alcoholism, human immunodeficiency virus (HIV) infection–related, neoplasm (the most common is benign pleomorphic adenoma), Sjögren syndrome, or sarcoidosis.

After a nasal fracture (seen on radiograph or CT scan), rule out a septal hematoma, which must be evacuated to prevent pressure-induced septal necrosis.

NEUROSURGERY

Intracranial bleed

Whenever an intracranial bleed is suspected, order a *CT scan without contrast.* Blood appears white and may cause a shift of midline structures to the opposite side (Fig. 6-8). Causes include the following:

1. **Subdural hematoma,** which is due to bleeding from veins that bridge the cortex and dural sinuses. On radiographs the hematoma is *crescent-shaped.* Subdural hematomas are common in alcoholics and after head trauma. They may manifest immediately after trauma or as long as 1–2 months later. If the question gives a history of head trauma, always consider the diagnosis of a subdural hematoma. Treat with surgical evacuation if significant or progressive symptoms are present.

2. **Epidural hematoma** is due to bleeding from meningeal arteries (classically, the middle meningeal artery). On CT scan the hematoma is *biconvex.* Almost all epidural hematomas are associated with a *temporal bone skull fracture,* and roughly 50% of patients develop an *ipsilateral "blown" pupil.* The classic history is one of head trauma with loss of consciousness, followed by a *lucid interval* of minutes to hours and then neurologic deterioration. Treat with surgical evacuation.

3. **Subarachnoid hemorrhage** is due to blood between the arachnoid and pia mater. The most common cause is *trauma,* followed by *ruptured intracranial* (typically berry) *aneurysm.* Blood can be seen in the cerebral cisterns, ventricles, and sulci. The classic patient has an aneurysm rupture and presents with the *"worst headache of my life,"* although many die before they reach the hospital or may be unconscious. If awake, patients have *signs of meningitis* (Kernig and Brudzinski signs) without significant fever. Remember the association between *polycystic kidney disease* and berry aneurysms. CT scan is the test of choice to diagnose subarachnoid hemorrhage. Lumbar puncture will demonstrate *grossly bloody cerebrospinal fluid* (but is not necessary if the CT scan is positive). Treat with support, anticonvulsants, and observation. Perform CT angiography or magnetic resonance angiography (MRA) to look for aneurysms and arteriovenous malformations (AVMs), which are usually treated with surgical clipping and ligation. Conventional catheter-based angiography may be necessary to diagnose more subtle aneurysms if MRI is negative, and some aneurysms can be treated using endovascular coils rather than open surgery.

4. **Intraparenchymal hemorrhage** describes bleeding directly into the brain parenchyma. The most common cause is hypertension; other causes include AVMs, coagulopathies, tumor, and trauma. Two-thirds of hypertensive bleeds occur in the basal ganglia, and patients often present in a coma; the other common locations for hypertensive bleeds are the brainstem and cerebellum. Awake patients may have contralateral hemiplegia and hemisensory deficits. Blood (white) is seen in the brain parenchyma and also may be seen in the ventricles. Surgery is reserved for large bleeds that are accessible.

Intraparenchymal bleeds from trauma are most commonly in the inferior frontal lobes and anteroinferior temporal lobes, where the brain rubs on the irregular surface of the skull base.

After a history of trauma, a dilated, unreactive pupil (i.e., "blown" pupil) on only one side most likely represents impingement of the ipsilateral third cranial nerve and impending uncal herniation due to increased intracranial pressure. Of the different intracranial bleeds, this is most commonly seen with epidural bleeds.

📁 **CASE SCENARIO:** Why should you not do a lumbar puncture in the setting of trauma or evidence of increased intracranial pressure? You may cause uncal herniation and death. First do a CT scan without contrast. If it is negative and the diagnosis remains unclear, then consider lumbar puncture (rarely indicated to detect blood products).

Fractures and trauma

Basilar (skull base) fractures are usually only treated when contaminated or persistent bleeding or cerebrospinal leaking occurs and have four classic signs:

1. Raccoon eyes: periorbital ecchymosis
2. Battle sign: postauricular ecchymosis
3. Hemotympanum: blood behind the eardrum
4. Cerebrospinal fluid otorrhea/rhinorrhea: clear fluid drains from ears or nose

Skull fractures of the calvaria (top of skull) are seen on CT scan (test of choice), generally as a linear or depressed fracture. Surgical repair is done only for contaminated fractures (cleaning and débridement), impingement on the brain parenchyma, or an open fracture with cerebrospinal fluid leak. Otherwise, such fractures can be observed and generally heal on their own.

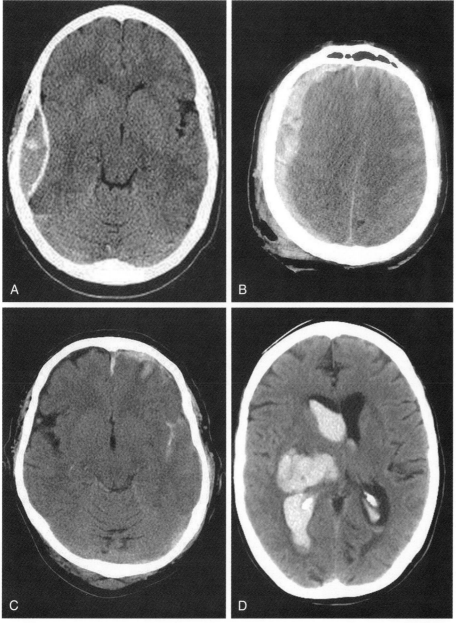

Figure 6-8 Computed tomography scans of intracranial hemorrhage. **A,** Epidural hematoma; **B,** subdural hematoma; **C,** subarachnoid hematoma; **D,** intracerebral hematoma. *(From DeLee JC, Drez D, Miller MD: DeLee and Drez's Orthopaedic Sports Medicine, 3rd ed. Philadelphia, Saunders, 2009.)*

Head trauma also may cause cerebral contusion or shear injury (i.e., *diffuse axonal injury*) of the brain parenchyma, both of which may not show up on a CT scan but may cause temporary or permanent neurologic deficits. They can be detected with MRI, but there is no treatment. MRI is used only for prognostic information in this setting.

Spinal cord trauma often manifests with "spinal shock" (loss of reflexes and motor function, hypotension). Order standard trauma radiographs (cervical spine, thorax, pelvis), as well as additional CT scans based on physical exam. Give IV corticosteroids immediately, which may improve outcome. Surgery is done for incomplete neurologic injury (with some residual function) with external bony compression of the cord (e.g., subluxation, bone chip).

Miscellaneous

Increased intracranial pressure (ICP), also known as intracranial hypertension (normal ICP = 5–15 mm Hg), should be suspected in patients with *bilaterally dilated and fixed pupils*. Other signs and symptoms include headache, *papilledema*, nausea and vomiting, and *mental status changes*. Look also for the classic *Cushing triad* (increasing blood pressure, bradycardia, and respiratory irregularity), which indicates very high ICP. The first step is to put the patient in reverse Trendelenburg position (head up) and intubate. Once intubated, the patient can be hyperventilated to lower the ICP rapidly. Hyperventilation decreases intracranial blood volume by causing cerebral vasoconstriction. If this maneuver does not lower ICP, *mannitol* diuresis can be tried to lessen cerebral edema. Furosemide is also used, but it is less effective. Decompressive craniotomy (burr holes) is a last resort. Prophylactic anticonvulsants are controversial.

🖿 **CASE SCENARIO:** How should hypertension be treated in the setting of increased intracranial pressure? It generally should not be treated! Cerebral perfusion pressure = blood pressure – ICP. The body, therefore, reflexively causes hypertension in the setting of increased ICP to maintain cerebral perfusion.

Subacute spinal cord compression is often due to metastatic cancer but also may result from a primary neoplasm, subdural, or epidural abscess or hematoma (especially after a lumbar tap or epidural/spinal anesthesia in patients with a bleeding disorder or taking anticoagulation). Patients present with local spinal pain (especially with bone metastases) and neurologic deficits below the lesion (e.g., hyperreflexia, Babinski sign, weakness, sensory loss). The first step is to give high-dose IV *corticosteroids*. Then order MRI of the appropriate spinal level. Give radiotherapy if radiosensitive metastases are present. Alternatively, surgical decompression can be done for radioresistant tumors. For hematoma or subdural/epidural abscess (seen especially in diabetics, usually due to *S. aureus*), surgery is indicated for decompression and drainage.

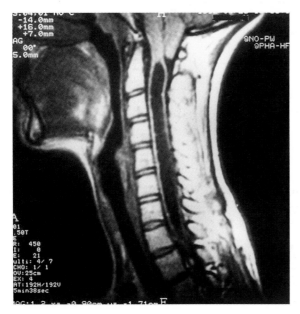

FIGURE 6-9 Magnetic resonance image demonstrates a large syringomyelic cavity in the cervical cord. *(From Bradley WG, Daroff RB, Fenichel G, Jankovic J: Neurology in Clinical Practice, 5th ed. Philadelphia, Butterworth-Heinemann, 2008.)*

Syringomyelia is a central pathologic cavitation of the spinal cord, usually in the cervical or upper thoracic region. It may be idiopathic, the result of trauma, or congenital cranial base malformations (e.g., *Arnold-Chiari malformation* or Dandy-Walker syndrome). The classic presentation is a *bilateral loss of pain and temperature sensation below the lesion in the distribution of a "cape"* secondary to involvement of the lateral spinothalamic tracts. The cavitation in the cord gradually widens to involve other tracts, causing motor and sensory deficits. MRI is the diagnostic study of choice (Fig. 6-9), and treatment is typically surgical (creation of a shunt).

📁 **CASE SCENARIO:** In what condition of the elderly is the classic triad of ataxia, dementia, and urinary incontinence seen? Normal-pressure hydrocephalus, which is a type of communicating hydrocephalus that sometimes requires treatment with ventricular shunt tube placement.

OPHTHALMOLOGY

Conjunctivitis

Conjunctivitis causes conjunctival vessel hyperemia and eye irritation. If vision loss occurs, think of more serious conditions. Classic causes are listed below Table 6-4.

TABLE 6-4 Overview of Conjunctivitis		
ETIOLOGIC CATEGORY	**UNIQUE SIGNS/SYMPTOMS**	**TREATMENT**
Allergic	Itching; bilateral, seasonal, long duration	Topical antihistamine (e.g., cetirizine) or mast cell inhibitors (cromolyn)
Viral (especially adenovirus)	Preauricular adenopathy; highly contagious (history of infected contacts); one eye affected and then the other, clear, watery discharge	Supportive treatment; hand washing (prevents spread)
Bacterial	Purulent discharge; look for its presentation in a neonate	Topical antibiotics (e.g., fluoroquinolone); *Chlamydia* or gonorrheal infections necessitate systemic antibiotics as well

Glaucoma

Glaucoma is best thought of as ocular hypertension with corresponding optic nerve damage and loss of visual field. Two types exist:

1. **Open-angle glaucoma** accounts for 90% of the cases of glaucoma. Risk factors include increased intraocular pressure, thin central corneal thickness, positive family history, increased age, and African-American ancestry. It is *painless* and has no acute attacks. The only signs are elevation of intraocular pressure (usually 20–30 mm Hg), a *gradually progressive visual field loss* (starts in the periphery), and *optic nerve changes* (increased cup-to-disc ratio on funduscopic exam, with possible disc hemorrhage). Treat with several different types of medications, including β-blockers (timolol), prostaglandins (latanoprost), acetazolamide, and mannitol, and/or surgery.
2. **Closed-angle glaucoma** can be either chronic or acute. Acute angle closure is the rare type that everyone worries about. It manifests with *sudden ocular pain,* seeing *haloes around lights, red eye,* very high intraocular pressure (>30 mm Hg), nausea and vomiting, headache, sudden decrease in vision, and a *fixed, middilated pupil.* Treat immediately with IV mannitol or topical pressure-lowering drops (pilocarpine, β-blockers, acetazolamide) to break the attack. Then use laser or surgery to prevent further attacks *(peripheral iridotomy).* Very rarely, anticholinergic medications can cause an attack of closed-angle glaucoma in a susceptible, previously untreated patient. Medications do not cause attacks in patients with open-angle glaucoma or surgically treated closed-angle glaucoma.

Steroids, whether topical or systemic, used long term can cause glaucoma and cataracts. Topical steroids can worsen fungal infections. For board purposes, do not give steroid eye drops. Refer the patient to an ophthalmologist if you think that it is indicated.

📁 **CASE SCENARIO:** A patient complains of eye pain and has a branching dendritiform ulcer over his cornea with terminal bulbs that stain green with fluorescein. What condition does the patient have? Herpes simplex keratitis. Refer to an ophthalmologist promptly for antiviral treatment (e.g., oral acyclovir, topical ganciclovir, topical trifluridine).

Vision Loss

Sudden unilateral, *painless* vision loss includes the following differential diagnoses:

1. **Central retinal artery occlusion.** The funduscopic appearance is classic, with retinal whitening and a cherry-red spot in the macula (Fig. 6-10). The most common cause is emboli (from carotid plaque or heart); treatment is generally supportive unless the cause is temporal arteritis (in which case you should give high-dose corticosteroids immediately to decrease risk of vision loss in the other eye).

2. **Central retinal vein occlusion.** The funduscopic appearance is classic "blood and thunder," with tortuous veins and retinal hemorrhages (Fig. 6-11). No satisfactory treatment is available. The most common causes are hypertension, diabetes, glaucoma, and increased blood viscosity (e.g., leukemia). Complications (vision loss, glaucoma) are related to ischemia and neovascularization.

3. **Retinal detachment.** The history usually includes seeing *"floaters"* and *flashes of light.* Patients often describe the presentation as a *"curtain or veil coming down in front of my eye."* This history should prompt immediate referral to an ophthalmologist, as prompt surgery (reattachment of the retina) may save the patient's vision.

4. **Vitreous hemorrhage.** The most common cause is bleeding from areas of neovascularization, classically in *diabetics.* The condition sometimes resolves or may improve after surgical vitrectomy.

5. **Optic neuritis/papillitis.** This condition takes at least a few hours to develop and is usually painful, but it may occur quickly and without pain. Sometimes symptoms are bilateral. Presentation in a 20–40-year-old woman should raise suspicion for multiple sclerosis, particularly if there is history of prior neurologic deficits (or Lyme disease with the appropriate history). Worry about a tumor in male patients with bilateral optic nerve edema and signs of intracranial hypertension or other neurologic deficits. Disc margins are typically blurred on funduscopic exam, as in papilledema.

6. **Stroke or transient ischemic attack:** see Table 6-5 for visual pathway lesions.

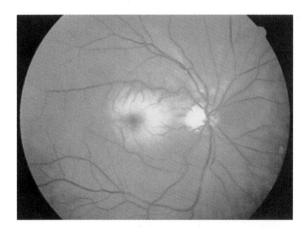

FIGURE 6-10 Central retinal artery occlusion. Note the cherry-red spot in the center of the macula, with surrounding whitening of the retina. *(From Bradley WG, Daroff RB, Fenichel G, Jankovic J: Neurology in Clinical Practice, 5th ed. Philadelphia, Butterworth-Heinemann, 2008.)*

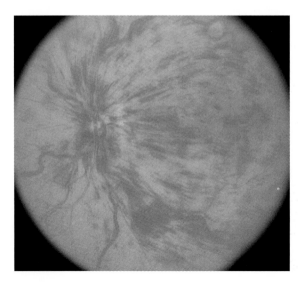

FIGURE 6-11 Central retinal vein occlusion. Note the dramatic retinal hemorrhages in all four quadrants. The veins are dilated and tortuous. The optic disc is blurred with blood from peripapillary hemorrhage. *(From Palay DA, Krachmer JH: Primary Care Ophthalmology, 2nd ed. Philadelphia, Mosby, 2005.)*

TABLE 6-5 Visual Pathway Lesions	
VISUAL FIELD DEFECT	**LOCATION OF LESION**
Right anopsia (monocular blindness)	Right optic nerve
Bitemporal hemianopsia	Optic chiasm (classically due to pituitary tumor)
Left homonymous hemianopsia	Right optic tract
Left upper quadrant anopsia	Right optic radiations in the right temporal lobe
Left lower quadrant anopsia	Right optic radiations in the right parietal lobe
Left homonymous hemianopsia with macular sparing	Right occipital lobe (from posterior cerebral artery occlusion)

Sudden unilateral, *painful vision loss*:

1. **Trauma:** The history gives it away. Encourage use of goggles or safety glasses during athletics and work. With chemical burns to the eye (acid or alkaline), the key to management is *copious irrigation with the closest source of water* (tap water is fine). Check pH again after irrigation. The longer you wait, the worse the prognosis; do not get additional history in this instance. *Alkali burns have a worse prognosis* because they tend to penetrate more deeply into the eye.
2. **Closed-angle glaucoma:** See previous discussion for presenting signs and symptoms and treatment.
3. **Optic neuritis:** Usually painful, as described earlier.
4. **Migraine headache:** Common! Look for nausea, vomiting, and aura.

Sudden bilateral loss of vision is rare, but consider the following possible causes:

1. **Toxins:** The classic example is *methanol poisoning*, usually seen in alcoholics.
2. **Exposure to ultraviolet light** can cause keratitis (corneal inflammation) with resultant pain, foreign body sensation, red eyes, tearing, and decreased vision (usually some vision remains). Patients have a history of *welding, using a tanning bed or sunlamp,* or *snow-skiing* ("snow-blindness"). Treat with a topical antibiotic, possibly also with an anticholinergic (cycloplegic) agent to reduce pain.
3. **Conversion reaction/hysteria/nonorganic**

Gradual-onset loss of vision, unilateral or bilateral, has a longer list for the differential diagnosis but is more common than sudden-onset vision loss:

1. **Cataracts** are the most common cause of a painless, slowly progressive loss of vision. Often bilateral, but one side may be worse than the other. Look for an opacified lens and the patient complaining of *"looking through a dirty windshield"* (Fig. 6-12). Treatment is surgical.
2. **Open-angle glaucoma:** See earlier discussion for specifics. Screen people older than 40, especially if they are Black or have a positive family history. This is the most common cause of irreversible blindness in African-Americans.
3. **Macular degeneration** is the most common cause of blindness in adults older than 60 years of age. Blindness is often bilateral, but one side may be worse than the other. The appearance of the fundus (the yellow-white deposits of drusen in the macular area) makes the diagnosis. No good treatment is available for the most common (dry-type) form, but high doses of vitamins A, C, and E and the minerals zinc and copper may delay progression. The less common wet-type form (10% of cases) of macular degeneration can be treated with antiangiogenic therapies.

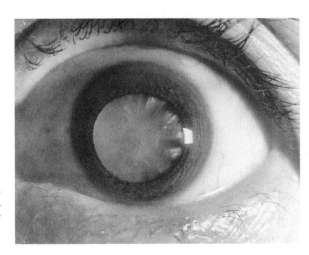

FIGURE 6-12 "Senile"-type cataract, which can occur at an earlier age in diabetic patients than in the normal population. *(From Forbes CD, Jackson WF: Endocrine, metabolic, and nutritional disorders. In Forbes CD, Jackson WF [eds]: Color Atlas and Text of Clinical Medicine. St. Louis, Mosby, 1993, pp 303-352.)*

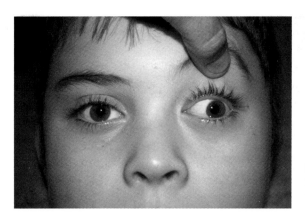

FIGURE 6-13 Third cranial nerve palsy of the left eye. *(From Kliegman RM, Stanton BMD, St. Geme J, et al: Nelson Textbook of Pediatrics, 19th ed. Philadelphia, Saunders, 2011.)*

4. **Diabetes** is the most common cause of blindness in adults overall. Retinal/fundus changes include *dot-blot hemorrhages, cotton-wool spots, microaneurysms,* and *neovascularization.* Proliferative diabetic retinopathy (with neovascularization) is treated by a laser applied to the periphery of the whole retina (*panretinal photocoagulation*). Focal laser treatment is often done for diabetic macular edema (the laser is applied only to the affected area).
5. **Uveitis:** Look for association with autoimmune-type diseases. Screen children with *juvenile rheumatoid arthritis* regularly to detect uveitis. The usual treatment is topical steroids (treated by an ophthalmologist).
6. **Papilledema** by definition is optic nerve edema due to increased intracranial pressure (e.g., brain tumor, idiopathic intracranial hypertension [IIH]/*pseudotumor cerebri*).
7. **Optic neuritis** classically results from autoimmune-type conditions (most often multiple sclerosis), infections (viral, Lyme disease), or drugs (*ethambutol*).
8. **Infection of the cornea** (herpes keratitis, corneal ulcer, especially with contact lens wear) or retina (cytomegalovirus retinitis in AIDS), or orbital cellulitis.
9. **Direct insult to brain:** stroke, tumor, meningitis (see Table 6-5 for visual pathway information).
10. **Presbyopia:** between ages 40 and 50 years, the lens gradually *loses its ability to accommodate.* People need bifocals or reading glasses for near vision. This is a normal part of aging, not a disease.

Miscellaneous conditions

Effects of hypertension on the fundus include arteriolar narrowing, copper/silver wiring, cotton-wool spots, and optic nerve edema (with severe hypertension).

Hordeolum (stye) is a painful, red lump near the lid margin. Treat with warm compresses, lid scrubs.

Chalazion is a chronic, painless lump near the lid margin. Treat with warm compresses and lid scrubs; if this approach fails, treat with steroid injection or incision and drainage.

Ophthalmic herpes zoster infection should be suspected with involvement of the tip of the nose (Hutchinson sign) and/or medial eyelid with a typical zoster dermatomal pattern. Check the cornea with fluorescein dye. Treat with oral acyclovir, topical ganciclovir, or topical trifluridine and ophthalmologic referral.

Ophthalmologic cranial nerve (CN) palsies are usually due to *vascular complications of diabetes or hypertension* and resolve gradually in 3–6 months. In patients younger than 40, those without diabetes or hypertension, patients with multiple cranial nerve palsies, other neurologic deficits or severe pain, and patients who fail to improve within 8 weeks, order MRI and MRA of the brain. Look for a tumor or aneurysm in this setting.

1. **Oculomotor (CN3):** Eye is *"down and out"* and cannot do anything but move laterally (Fig. 6-13). Patients can have complete ptosis (lower eye lid) on the same side.

▭ **CASE SCENARIO:** How can the pupil help you to decide between a serious and a benign cause of a third cranial nerve palsy? If the palsy is due to hypertension or diabetes, the pupil is usually normal. A "blown" (dilated, nonreactive) pupil is a medical emergency. The most likely cause is an aneurysm or tumor. Order MRI and MRA of the head.

2. **Trochlear (CN4):** When the gaze is medial, the patient *cannot look down* (vertical diplopia).
3. **Abducens (CN6):** The patient *cannot look laterally* with the affected eye (horizontal diplopia) (Fig. 6-14).

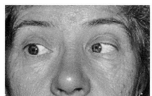 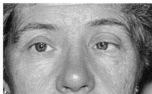 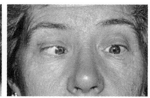

FIGURE 6-14 Left sixth cranial nerve paresis. Note the poor movement of the left eye in left gaze. *(From Palay DA, Krachmer JH: Primary Care Ophthalmology, 2nd ed. Philadelphia, Mosby, 2005.)*

4. **CN5 and CN7** palsies also affect the eye due to corneal drying (loss of corneal blink reflex). Use artificial tears/ointment and address the underlying cause, if possible.

ORTHOPEDIC SURGERY

Fractures

With any fracture, do a neurologic and vascular exam distal to the fracture site to determine whether there is any compromise of nerves or blood vessels (either may be an emergency). With a suspected or obvious fracture, get *two x-ray views* (usually anteroposterior and lateral) of the site, and include the joints above and below the suspected fracture site.

When a fracture is suspected clinically (severe pain, point tenderness, swelling) but the radiographs are negative, *treat conservatively as if the patient has a fracture.* Radiographs can be negative at first with smaller, nondisplaced fractures. Put the limb in a splint or even a cast, and tell the patient not to use it (no weight bearing) if symptoms are significant. If the suspected fracture is in the leg, the patient can use crutches. Repeat the radiograph in 1 week; evidence of a fracture is usually apparent by this time.

📁 **CASE SCENARIO:** What fractures are associated with the highest mortality rate? Pelvic fractures. Most pelvic fractures occur in elderly people who fall down and have many coexisting health problems. Young people, in whom pelvic fractures usually are due to severe trauma, may bleed to death. If a patient is unstable, consider heroic measures such as military antishock trousers and external fixator. Consider bladder or urethral injury from pelvic fractures in the setting of hematuria or blood at the meatus. Cystogram or retrograde urethrogram can be performed for further evaluation (see urology section later).

In an open (compound) fracture, the skin is broken over the fracture site. In a closed fracture, the skin is intact. For open fractures, give broad-spectrum antibiotics, do surgical débridement, give tetanus vaccine, lavage fresh wounds (<8 hours old), and do an *open reduction with internal fixation* (i.e., cut open the skin in the operating room to align the fracture fragments under more direct visualization). The main risk in open fractures is infection. Closed fractures often can be treated with *closed reduction and casting* (i.e., pull on the limb to align the fracture fragments without cutting open the skin).

Compartment syndrome usually occurs after fracture, crush injury, burn, or other trauma or as a reperfusion injury (e.g., after revascularization procedure). The most common site is in the *calf.* Symptoms and signs include *pain at rest; pain on passive movement* (out of proportion to the injury); *paresthesias;* cyanosis or pallor; a *firm-feeling muscle compartment;* hypesthesia or numbness (decreased sensation and two-point discrimination); paralysis (late, ominous sign); and *elevated compartment pressure* (>30–40 mm Hg). The diagnosis is usually made clinically without the need to measure compartment pressure, though this is fairly accurate and confirmatory. Compartment syndrome is an emergency, and quick action can save an otherwise doomed limb. *Pulses are usually palpable* (or detectable with Doppler ultrasound) at the time of diagnosis. Treatment is prompt *fasciotomy* (incising the fascial compartment relieves the pressure). Untreated, this condition progresses to permanent nerve damage and muscle necrosis.

The classic clinical scenarios for compartment syndrome include supracondylar elbow fracture in children, proximal or midshaft tibial fractures, electrical burns, arterial or venous disruption, and revascularization procedures.

Reasons to do an open surgical reduction (closed reduction should be done for all other fractures) are intraarticular fractures or articular surface malalignment, open (compound) fractures, nonunion or failed closed reduction, compromise of blood supply or nerves (Table 6-6), multiple trauma (to allow mobilization at earliest possible point), and extremity function requiring perfect reduction (e.g., professional athlete).

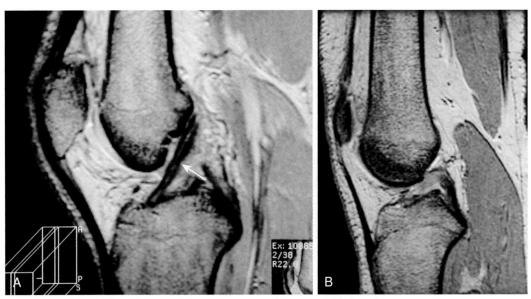

FIGURE 6-15 **A,** Normal anterior cruciate ligament (ACL) composed of separate anteromedial and posterolateral bundles. **B,** Sagittal image through the intercondylar region fails to demonstrate any normal anterior cruciate ligament indicating a chronic complete ACL rupture. *(From Adam A, Dixon AK, Grainger RG, Allison DJ: Grainger & Allison's Diagnostic Radiology, 5th ed. Philadelphia, Churchill Livingstone, 2008.)*

TABLE 6-6 Nerves Commonly Involved in Traumatic Injury			
NERVE	**MOTOR**	**SENSORY**	**WHEN CLINICALLY DAMAGED**
Radial	Wrist extension	Back of forearm, back of hand (first 3 digits)	Humeral fracture (wrist-drop)
Ulnar	Finger abduction	Front and back of last 2 fingers on hand	Elbow dislocation (claw-hand)
Median	Pronation, thumb opposition	Palmar surface of hand (first 3 digits)	Carpal tunnel syndrome, humeral fracture
Axillary	Abduction/lateral rotation	Lateral shoulder	Upper humeral dislocation/fracture
Peroneal	Dorsiflexion/eversion	Dorsal foot and lateral leg	Knee dislocation (foot-drop)

Ligament injuries in the knee

Ligament injuries in the knee commonly cause pain, joint effusions, instability of the joint, and history of the joint's *"popping," "buckling," or "locking up."*

1. **Anterior cruciate ligament (ACL).** ACL tears are the most common. Perform the *anterior drawer test.* The knee is placed in 90 degrees of flexion and pulled forward (like opening a drawer). If the tibia pulls forward more than normal (e.g., more than the unaffected side), the test is positive and you have an ACL tear (Fig. 6-15).
2. **Posterior cruciate ligament (PCL).** Perform the *posterior drawer test.* Push the tibia back with the knee in 90 degrees of flexion. If the tibia pushes back more than normal, the test is positive and a PCL tear is present (Fig. 6-16).
3. **Medial collateral ligament (MCL).** Perform the *abduction or valgus stress test.* With the knee in 30 degrees of flexion, abduct the ankle while holding the knee. If the knee joint abducts to an abnormal degree, the test is positive and a medical compartment injury is present (Fig. 6-17).
4. **Lateral collateral ligament.** Perform the *adduction* or *varus stress test.* Adduct the ankle while holding the knee. If the knee joint adducts to an abnormal degree, the test is positive and lateral compartment injury is present.
❍ MRI or arthroscopy can be used to look for other injuries or confirm a diagnosis in doubt.
❍ Treatment may be nonsurgical (older patient, nonathlete, minor injury) or surgical (young patient, athlete, severe injury).

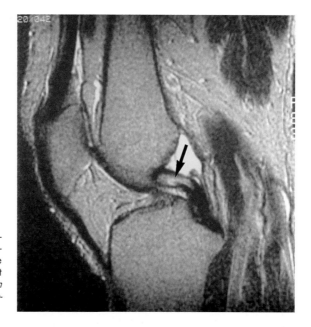

Figure 6-16 Posterior cruciate ligament tear. Sagittal T_2-weighted image shows abnormal bright signal *(arrow)* within normally dark posterior cruciate ligament. Fluid is also seen around proximal extent of partially torn posterior cruciate ligament. *(From Canale ST, Beaty JH: Campbell's Operative Orthopaedics, 11th ed. Philadelphia, Mosby, 2008.)*

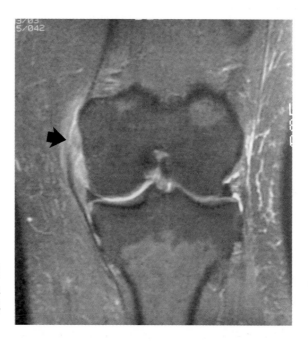

Figure 6-17 Medial collateral ligament tear. Complete disruption of proximal medial collateral ligament *(arrow)* is shown in coronal fat-suppressed, proton density–weighted image. *(From Canale ST, Beaty JH: Campbell's Operative Orthopaedics, 11th ed. Philadelphia, Mosby, 2008.)*

📋 **CASE SCENARIO:** What is the "unhappy triad" knee injury? Damage to *ACL, MCL, and medial meniscus.* Classically this triad occurs when an extended knee joint is hit from the side and the knee is pushed medially while the foot is planted.

Pain in the anatomic snuffbox after trauma (e.g., fall on an outstretched hand, especially in young adults) is usually a scaphoid bone fracture.

After a fall on an outstretched hand, the most likely fracture in older adults is a Colles fracture (distal end of radius).

Disk herniation

Lumbar disk herniation is a common correctable cause of low back pain. Look for sciatica (not just back pain) with the straight leg raise test. The most common site is the L5-1 disk; the second most common site is the L4-L5 disk.

1. **L5-S1 disk herniation** usually affects the S1 nerve root: decreased ankle jerk, weakness of plantar flexors in the foot, pain from the midgluteal area to the posterior calf (i.e., sciatica).

2. **L4-L5 disk herniation** usually affects the L5 nerve root: decreased biceps femoris reflex, weakness of foot extensors, and pain in the hip or groin.
   ○ Diagnosis is confirmed with MRI or CT myelogram.
   ○ Conservative treatment works in 90% of cases and includes rest and analgesics, followed by physical therapy. Surgical treatment (diskectomy) is an option if conservative treatment fails.
   ○ Cervical disk disease (classic symptoms include neck pain and cervical radiculopathy) is less common than lumbar disk diseases. Diagnosis can be confirmed with MRI. The C6-C7 disk is most commonly affected, typically with C7 nerve root involvement. Look for *decreased triceps reflex/strength* and *weakness of forearm extension.*

Miscellaneous conditions

Spinal stenosis is another cause of back pain that usually manifests in the elderly and is due to degenerative changes in the spine. Patients may complain of pain with activity that is relieved by rest (sometimes called *"neurogenic" claudication*). Diagnosis is confirmed with MRI or CT. Treatment is conservative with physical therapy and nonsteroidal antiinflammatory drugs (NSAIDs). Surgery (spinal decompression with laminectomy) is reserved for cases that fail conservative management.

Charcot joints and neuropathic joints are most commonly seen in *diabetes* and sometimes by other conditions causing peripheral neuropathy (e.g., tertiary syphilis). Lack of proprioception causes gradual arthritis/arthropathy and joint deformity. Order radiographs for any (even minor) trauma in neuropathic patients who may not feel even a severe fracture. MRI may be necessary for evaluation secondary to complex joint derangement on radiograph.

With a posterior knee dislocation, worry about vascular injury. Perform CT or magnetic resonance angiography (MRA) if pulses are asymmetric.

The most common type of bone tumor is metastatic (most commonly from the breast, lung, or prostate).

The most common cause of a pathologic fracture is *osteoporosis* (especially in elderly, thin women).

The most common pathogenic organism in osteomyelitis is *S. aureus*, but think of gram-negative organisms in immunocompromised patients and IV drug abusers, as well as *Salmonella* spp. in sickle cell disease. Aspirate the bone and do a Gram stain and culture and sensitivity of the sample, as well as blood cultures and complete blood cell count with differential if you are suspicious.

Septic arthritis is also most commonly due to *S. aureus*, but in a sexually active younger adult, suspect *Neisseria gonorrhoeae*. Aspirate the joint (arthrocentesis) and do a Gram stain and culture and sensitivity testing of the joint fluid, as well as blood cultures, complete blood cell count with differential, and urethral cultures when appropriate if you are suspicious.

UROLOGY

Testicular torsion versus epididymitis (Table 6-7)

TABLE 6-7 Overview of Testicular Torsion versus Epididymitis

	TESTICULAR TORSION	EPIDIDYMITIS
Age	<30 yr (classically, adolescent)	>30 yr
Appearance	Testis may be elevated into inguinal canal; swelling	Swollen testis, overlying erythema, positive urinalysis, urethral discharge/urethritis, prostatitis
Prehn sign	Pain stays the same or worsens	Pain decreases with testicular elevation
Ultrasound findings	No testicular blood flow	Normal testicular blood flow
Treatment	Immediate surgery to salvage the testicle; orchioplexy for both testes	Antibiotics*

*In men <50 yr, commonly due to chlamydial infection or gonorrhea; treat accordingly. In men >50 yr, commonly due to urinary tract infection; treat with trimethoprim-sulfamethoxazole or ciprofloxacin.

Testicular cancer

Testicular cancer usually manifests as a *painless mass in a young man* (age 20–40 years). The main risk factor is *cryptorchidism* (40-fold higher risk). Roughly 90% are germ cell tumors; the most common type is *seminoma*. Testicular cancer is generally treated with orchiectomy and radiation; if the disease is widespread, use chemotherapy. α-Fetoprotein is a tumor marker for yolk sac tumors, and human chorionic gonadotropin is a marker for choriocarcinoma. Leydig cell tumors may secrete androgens and leading onset of precocious puberty. The first site of metastasis is often *retroperitoneal lymph nodes,* as the testicular veins (and accompanying lymphatics) drain to the inferior vena cava (right) or renal vein (left).

Mumps

Remember mumps as a cause of orchitis (painful, swollen testis, usually unilateral, in a postpubertal male). The best treatment is *prophylaxis* (immunization). Orchitis rarely causes sterility, because it is usually unilateral.

Benign prostatic hyperplasia

Symptoms include urinary hesitancy, intermittency, terminal dribbling, decreased size and force of stream, sensation of incomplete emptying, nocturia, urgency, dysuria, and frequency of urination. Benign prostatic hyperplasia (BPH) may result in *urinary retention, urinary tract infections, hydronephrosis,* and even permanent kidney damage and/or failure in severe cases. PSA is elevated in 30–50% of patients. Drug therapy for BPH is started when the patient becomes symptomatic and includes α_1-blockade (e.g., *tamsulosin, prazosin*) and antiandrogens (e.g., *finasteride*). Saw palmetto is a dietary supplement that may help relieve symptoms. Transurethral resection of the prostate (TURP) is used for more advanced cases, especially those associated with recurrent urinary tract infections, acute urinary retention, and hydronephrosis or kidney damage from reflux. Prostatectomy may also be used, but it carries a higher risk of morbidity and is usually not the preferred treatment.

With acute urinary retention (pain, palpation of full bladder on abdominal exam, history of BPH, no urination in past 24 hours), the first step is to *empty the bladder.* If you cannot pass a regular Foley catheter, use a firm-tipped catheter (coudé catheter) or do a suprapubic tap/place a *suprapubic Foley catheter.* Then address the underlying cause.

Erectile dysfunction

Erectile dysfunction (impotence) is most commonly caused by *vascular disease.* Medications are also a common culprit (especially *antihypertensives* and *antidepressants*). Diabetes can be a vascular (increased atherosclerosis) or neurogenic cause of erectile dysfunction. Patients undergoing dialysis and patients with spinal cord injury also commonly have erectile dysfunction. Remember "point and shoot": Parasympathetic nerves mediate erection, sympathetic nerves mediate ejaculation.

History often gives you a clue if the cause of erectile dysfunction is psychogenic. Look for *selective dysfunction* (e.g., the patient has normal erections when masturbating, but not with his wife) and stress, anxiety, or fear.

▢ **CASE SCENARIO:** What does a normal pattern of nocturnal erections mean in a patient with erectile dysfunction? This finding essentially rules out a physical cause for the erectile dysfunction.

In all trauma patients, look for signs of *urethral injury* (high-riding ballottable prostate, blood at the urethral meatus, severe pelvic fracture, scrotal or perineal ecchymosis) before trying to pass a Foley catheter. If any of these signs are present, do not try to pass a Foley catheter until you have ruled out a urethral injury, which is a contraindication to a Foley catheter.

▢ **CASE SCENARIO:** What test should be ordered in the setting of possible urethral injury? A *retrograde urethrogram.* A contrast agent is injected backward through the urethra to look for a leak or tear.

Hydrocele versus varicocele

Hydrocele represents a remnant of the processus vaginalis and *transilluminates.* It generally causes no symptoms and requires no treatment. A varicocele is a *dilatation of the pampiniform venous plexus* (described as a "bag of worms" on physical exam, usually on the *left*), does not transilluminate, *disappears in the supine position,* and may be a cause of *male infertility* or pain (in which case it is surgically treated). Diagnosis of either can be confirmed using ultrasound, which can also help exclude other causes of palpable mass.

Renal stones

Renal stones (nephrolithiasis): The risk is increased with dehydration. Patients present with *severe, intermittent, colicky, unilateral flank and/or groin pain,* and, in most cases, nausea and vomiting. Patients with "renal colic" classically cannot get comfortable and often move about while trying to, whereas patients with peritonitis often lie still. Look for *hematuria* on urinalysis; 85% of stones show up on abdominal radiograph, but CT scan of the abdomen without contrast (or IV pyelogram) is generally performed to confirm the presence of a stone. Most cases are idiopathic and should be treated with hydration and pain control (to see if the stone will pass). If the stone does not pass, the patient needs shock wave lithotripsy or surgery (preferably endoscopic). Whenever possible, check stone composition, which can give a clue to the cause:

1. **Calcium stones** (75%): usually idiopathic but look for *hypercalcemia* (typically due to hyperparathyroidism or malignancy) or history of small bowel bypass (calcium oxalate stones).
2. **Struvite/magnesium-ammonium-phosphate stones** (10%): due to urinary tract infection (more common in women) with ammonia-producing bugs (*Proteus* spp., staphylococci). Look for staghorn calculi, which are large stones that fill up the renal pelvis and/or collecting system and form a "cast" of these structures.
3. **Uric acid stones** (10%): due to *hyperuricemia* and therefore associated with gout and leukemia treatment (allopurinol and IV fluids are often given before chemotherapy in leukemia to prevent stone formation). Uric acid stones usually dissolve with *alkalinization of the urine*.
4. **Cystine stones:** nearly diagnostic of *cystinuria*/aminoaciduria. Alkalinization of urine (i.e., getting to a pH of >7.5 with the use of penicillamine) is useful for patients with recurrent cystine stones.

▢ **CASE SCENARIO:** Which type of stone classically cannot be seen on radiographs? Uric acid stones. These can be seen on CT scans, however.

▢ **CASE SCENARIO:** A 32-year-old man has acute flank pain. An IV pyelogram reveals a 2-mm stone in the right ureter. How should you manage this patient? IV fluids and pain control. Let the patient pass the stone on his own. Do not be overly aggressive, because most small stones (<4–5 mm) pass spontaneously within 48 hours.

TRANSPLANT MEDICINE (Tables 6-8 and 6-9.)

TABLE 6-8 Indications for Organ Transplantation

ORGAN	MAJOR DISEASES
Heart	Coronary artery disease; cardiomyopathy (dilated, restrictive, hypertrophic); valvular heart disease; congenital heart disease
Lung	Congenital disease, emphysema, COPD, cystic fibrosis, idiopathic pulmonary fibrosis, primary pulmonary hypertension, α_1-antitrypsin deficiency
Liver	Chronic hepatitis B or C infection, alcohol-related liver disease, cryptogenic cirrhosis including NASH,* cholestatic liver disease, hepatocellular carcinoma, metabolic diseases, acute liver failure
Kidney	Glomerular diseases, diabetes mellitus, polycystic kidney disease, hypertensive nephrosclerosis, tubular and interstitial diseases, congenital and metabolic diseases
Pancreas	Diabetes mellitus, pancreatic cancer
Small bowel	Intestinal failure in which TPN can no longer be maintained

COPD, Chronic obstructive pulmonary disease; *NASH,* nonalcoholic steatohepatitis; *TPN,* total parenteral nutrition.

TABLE 6-9 Immunosuppressive Agents Following Transplantation

CLASS OF DRUG	MECHANISM OF ACTION	SIDE EFFECTS
Calcineurin inhibitors (cyclosporine, tacrolimus)	Inhibition of cytokine production from T cells	Nephrotoxicity, dyslipidemia, hypertension, hirsutism, hyperkalemia, gingival hyperplasia
Corticosteroids	Inhibition of cytokine production from T cells and antigen-presenting cells	Hypertension, mental status changes, dyslipidemia, impaired wound healing, hyperglycemia, Cushing syndrome, myopathy, osteoporosis, fluid retention
Antimetabolites (azathioprine, mycophenolate)	Antagonizes purine metabolism and/or synthesis	Nausea, vomiting, diarrhea, cytopenias, pancreatitis

TABLE 6-9 Immunosuppressive Agents Following Transplantation—cont'd

CLASS OF DRUG	MECHANISM OF ACTION	SIDE EFFECTS
Antibody induction (antithymocyte globulin, OKT-3, basiliximab, alemtuzumab)	Depletes and/or modulates T-cell function	Cytokine release syndrome, abdominal pain, cytopenias, dyspnea, hypertension, sepsis
Sirolimus	Blocks T- and B-cell activation by cytokines	Cytopenias, dyslipidemia, interstitial lung disease, peripheral edema, impaired wound healing

Renal transplantation

Renal transplantation is an option for many patients with end-stage renal disease. Living, related donors are best (siblings or parents), especially when human leukocyte antigen (HLA)-similar, but cadaveric kidneys are more common because of availability. Before the transplant, perform ABO blood typing and lymphocytotoxic (HLA) cross-matching.

○ A transplanted kidney is placed in the iliac fossa (for easy biopsy access in case of a problem, as well as for technical reasons). Usually the recipient's kidneys are left in place to reduce morbidity.

○ Unacceptable kidney donors: newborns, people older than 70, and people with a history of certain infections (e.g., AIDS, hepatitis), any disease with possible renal involvement (e.g., diabetes, hypertension, lupus erythematosus), or malignancy.

Transplant rejection

1. **Hyperacute rejection:** Occurs within minutes to hours and is due to *preformed cytotoxic antibodies* against donor kidney (occurs with ABO mismatch and other preformed antibodies). Classic description: Surgery is completed, vascular clamps are released, and the kidney quickly turns bluish-black. Treat by removing the kidney. Repeat transplant procedure new kidney.

2. **Acute rejection:** *T cell–mediated* rejection that presents within *days to weeks* with fever, oliguria, weight gain, tenderness and enlargement of the graft, hypertension, and/or renal function lab derangement. Treat by increasing steroids or using antithymocyte globulin (ATG) or other immunosuppressants. Accelerated rejection occurs over the *first few days* and is felt to reflect *reactivation of previously sensitized T cells.*

3. **Chronic rejection:** Occurs over *months to years* and is believed to be *T cell– and/or antibody-mediated.* Late cause of renal deterioration presenting with *gradual decline in kidney function, proteinuria, and hypertension.* Treatment is supportive and not effective, but the graft may survive for several years before it gives out completely. If possible, retransplant with a new kidney.

○ Follow serum creatinine to assess asymptomatic rejection.

○ Cyclosporine causes nephrotoxicity, which can be difficult to distinguish from graft rejection clinically. When in doubt, drug levels are checked and a biopsy and/or ultrasound scan of the graft should be done. Practically speaking, if you increase the immunosuppressive dose, acute rejection should decrease, whereas cyclosporine toxicity will stay the same or get worse.

○ The risks of immunosuppression include infection (with common and strange organisms seen in patients with AIDS) and cancer (especially lymphomas).

VASCULAR SURGERY

Carotid artery stenosis

The classic presentation is that of a transient ischemic attack (TIA), typically *amaurosis fugax* or sudden onset of transient, unilateral blindness, sometimes described as a "shade being pulled over one eye." Patients may have a *carotid bruit.* If a bruit is heard or the patient has a TIA, ultrasound imaging of the carotid arteries should be done to determine whether carotid stenosis is present. Cerebral angiography is the gold standard, but it is invasive, costly, and associated with complications.

▢ **CASE SCENARIO:** What is the best treatment for a patient with a TIA and carotid stenosis with <50% blockage? Aspirin and medical management of atherosclerosis risk factors.

The management of carotid stenosis depends on degree of stenosis, whether the patient is symptomatic, gender, and age (Table 6-10). In asymptomatic patients, carotid endarterectomy (CEA) is recommended in men younger than age 75 if the extent of blockage is >60%. CEA is not recommended for asymptomatic women. For symptomatic patients, CEA is recommended if blockage due to stenosis is >50% in men and >70% in women.

TABLE 6-10 Carotid Stenosis Management

CLINICAL CATEGORY	DEGREE OF STENOSIS		
	<50%	50-69%	70-99%
Asymptomatic	Medical management	Men: CEA if stenosis >60% and age <75 yr; otherwise, medical management Women: medical management	Men <75 yr: CEA Women: medical management
Symptomatic	Medical management	Men: CEA Women: medical management	Men: CEA Women: CEA

Data from Ferri FF: Ferri's Clinical Advisor 2012. Philadelphia, Mosby, 2012.
CEA, Carotid endarterectomy.

◯ Patients should not undergo CEA after a stroke that leaves them severely disabled because they will receive no benefit; the damage is already done. Nor should patients undergo CEA during a TIA or stroke in evolution; CEA is an elective, not emergent, procedure.
◯ Carotid stenosis and peripheral vascular disease (PVD) are generalized markers for atherosclerosis. Almost all patients have significant coronary artery disease (CAD). In fact, perioperative myocardial infarction (MI) is the most common cause of death in patients undergoing vascular surgery. Make sure to evaluate and medically manage risk factors for atherosclerosis in all "vasculopaths."

Aortic abnormalities

Abdominal aortic aneurysm: Look for a *pulsatile abdominal mass*, which may cause abdominal pain. If pain is present, suspect possible rupture of the AAA, although an unruptured AAA may cause some pain. CT scan is usually used for initial evaluation. Management of AAA depends on the size.
◯ AAA <4 cm: monitor by ultrasound imaging or CT every 2–3 years
◯ AAA 4–5.4 cm: monitor by ultrasound or CT every 6–12 months
◯ AAA ≥5.5 cm surgical repair should be performed. Some patients with AAA <5.5 cm may also benefit if it is rapidly enlarging. Surgical correction is generally advised, with either stent-graft placement or open surgical repair.

🗋 **CASE SCENARIO:** What should you do with a patient who has a pulsatile abdominal mass and hypotension? Prepare the patient for emergent laparotomy (get CT scan or US to confirm the diagnosis if patient is stable). This combination of findings suggests a ruptured AAA (mortality rate = roughly 90%).

Aortic dissection: Aortic wall splits and blood dissects in between layers of the media in the arterial wall. Classically causes a "tearing" or "ripping" type of chest pain that may radiate to the back and is generally seen in the setting of *hypertension* (e.g., whether essential or induced by cocaine) or *Marfan syndrome*. When this entity is suspected clinically, a CT scan of the chest (and possibly abdomen and pelvis) with IV contrast should be ordered. Treatment depends on the clinical classification. A dissection involving the ascending aorta and/or aortic arch (Stanford type A and DeBakey types I and II) is treated with immediate surgery (≤5% of patients survive 1 year without surgery). A dissection that spares the ascending aorta and arch (Stanford type B and DeBakey type III) typically begins just beyond the origin of the left subclavian artery in the isthmus of the aorta/proximal descending thoracic aorta and extends over a variable distance (may stop in the thoracic aorta or extend into the abdominal aorta and its branches). These types of dissections that spare the aortic arch and ascending aorta are managed medically with antihypertensives (>70% of patients survive more than 1 year without surgery), in the absence of any signs of impending rupture or end-organ ischemia from vascular compromise (which would indicate the need for surgical intervention). An aortic dissection may or may not be associated with an aneurysm (the term "dissecting aneurysm" is often misused, because many aortic dissections do not have aneurysmal dilatation associated with them).

Miscellaneous conditions

Claudication: Pain in the lower extremity (usually) brought on by exercise and relieved by rest. Claudication is an indicator of severe atherosclerotic disease. Associated physical findings include *cyanosis* (with dependent rubor); atrophic changes (*thickened nails, loss of hair, shiny skin*); *decreased temperature;* and *decreased (or absent) distal pulses.* The best treatment is conservative (smoking cessation, exercise, control of cholesterol, diabetes, and hypertension). β-Blockers may theoretically worsen claudication (due to β_2 receptor blockade), but affected patients (who almost always have associated coronary artery disease) may benefit from the cardioprotection of β-blockers due to prior myocardial infarction.

○ If claudication progresses to rest pain (forefoot pain, generally at night, relieved by hanging the foot over the edge of the bed) or the patient cannot continue current lifestyle or work obligations, advise a revascularization procedure (angioplasty and/or bypass graft).

○ Severe pain in the foot of sudden onset with no previous history of foot pain, trauma, or any associated chronic physical findings is generally more serious and may represent an embolus. Look for atrial fibrillation.

CASE SCENARIO: What is Leriche syndrome? Claudication in the buttocks, buttock atrophy, and impotence in men. It is a classic marker for aortoiliac occlusive disease. Patients usually benefit from an aortoiliac bypass graft.

Chronic mesenteric ischemia: The classic patient has a long history of postprandial abdominal pain (i.e., *"intestinal angina"*), which causes a "fear" of food that results in weight loss. This is a difficult diagnosis because the disorder classically manifests in patients older than 50 who have other problems that may cause similar symptoms (e.g., ulcers, pancreatic or stomach cancer). Look for a history of extensive atherosclerosis (previous MI or stroke, known coronary artery disease or peripheral vascular disease with several risk factors), *abdominal bruit,* and no jaundice (the presence of jaundice should steer you toward pancreatic cancer). Most patients get a CT scan of the abdomen, which is negative for tumor and will demonstrate atherosclerotic disease. The diagnosis is confirmed with CT/MRA. Patients should be treated surgically with revascularization (angioplasty with stent and/or surgical bypass) because of the risks of bowel infarction and malnutrition.

After penetrating trauma in an extremity (or iatrogenic damage), patients may develop an arteriovenous fistula. An important clue to this entity is a *bruit* over the area or a *palpable pulsatile mass* (pseudoaneurysm). Diagnosis can be confirmed with ultrasound or MRA/CT. Arteriovenous fistulas can be left alone if they are small, but surgical correction is often necessary.

Venous insufficiency: Generally refers to the lower extremities. Look for a history of deep venous thrombosis; chronic swelling in the extremity; pain, fatigability, and heaviness, all of which are *relieved by elevating the leg;* and/or *varicose veins.* Patients may have increased skin pigmentation around the ankles with skin breakdown and ulceration (venous stasis ulcer, classically over the *medial malleolus*) (Fig. 6-18). Ultrasound can help define whether the disease involves the superficial or the deep venous system (or both). The initial treatment is conservative: elastic compression stockings, elevation with minimal standing, and treatment of any ulcers with cleansing, wet-to-dry dressings, and antibiotics (if cellulitis is present).

Superficial thrombophlebitis: Patients have *localized leg pain with superficial, cordlike induration, reddish discoloration,* and mild fever. This should not be confused with deep venous thrombosis, because superficial thrombophlebitis generally does not cause pulmonary emboli and patients do not need anticoagulation. Many patients have associated varicose veins. Diagnosis can be confirmed with ultrasound imaging, if necessary. Medical therapy is used if the pain is mild or the patient does not want surgery; use *NSAIDs.* The pain generally subsides in a few days on its own. Surgical thrombectomy under local anesthesia is necessary for more severe cases that fail to respond to nonsurgical treatment.

Subclavian steal syndrome: Usually due to left subclavian artery obstruction/stenosis proximal to the left vertebral artery origin (85% of cases are left-sided). To get blood to an exercising arm, blood is "stolen" from the vertebrobasilar system. Blood flows retrograde through the vertebral artery into the distal subclavian artery instead of forward into the brainstem. The patient develops *central nervous system symptoms* (syncope, vertigo, confusion, ataxia, dysarthria) and unilateral *upper extremity claudication.* Treat with surgical bypass and/or stent placement.

Thoracic outlet syndrome: May be due to a cervical rib (a normal variant) or muscular hypertrophy that compromises subclavian vessel blood flow. Patients have unilateral *upper extremity claudication.* Confirm the diagnosis with angiography. Treat with surgery (e.g., rib resection).

CASE SCENARIO: What is the easy way to tell the difference between thoracic outlet syndrome and subclavian steal syndrome using only the patient history? Subclavian steal causes central nervous system symptoms; thoracic outlet syndrome does not. Both can cause unilateral upper extremity claudication.

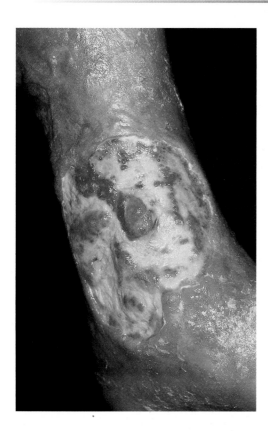

FIGURE 6-18 Venous stasis ulcer. Increased skin thickening and pigmentation with skin breakdown and ulceration are typically seen over the medial or lateral malleolus. The lesion is typically not nearly as painful as it looks and can be asymptomatic. *(From Bolognia JL, Jorizzo JL, Rapini RP, et al: Dermatology, 2nd ed. Philadelphia, Mosby, 2008.)*

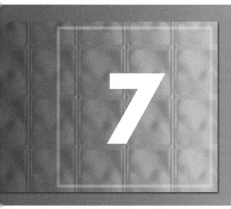

7 RADIOLOGY, LABORATORY MEDICINE, AND PHARMACOLOGY

RADIOLOGY

Screening and/or confirmatory radiologic tests for different diseases: see table 7-1.

TABLE 7-1 Screening and/or Confirmatory Radiologic Tests for Different Diseases

CONDITION	SCREENING (OR ONLY) TEST TO ORDER	CONFIRMATORY TEST	COMMENTS
Cardiovascular			
Aortic aneurysm	Abdominal US	CT with contrast	Screening US recommended for male smokers aged 65-75
Aortic dissection	CT with contrast	MRA or TEE	
Aortic tear (trauma)	CT with contrast	MRA or TEE	Laparotomy if patient is unstable
Carotid stenosis	Duplex US	MRA	
Gastrointestinal			
Abdominal abscess	CT scan with contrast		
Abdominal trauma	FAST scan to assess for hemoperitoneum	CT with contrast	Laparotomy is gold standard
Appendicitis	US (pediatrics and pregnant) or CT with contrast	CT with contrast	Never truly confirmed until surgery
Bowel perforation	Upright abdominal radiograph and chest radiograph	CT with contrast	
Cholecystitis	US	Nuclear hepatobiliary study (HIDA scan)	
Choledocholithiasis	US	ERCP or MRCP	
Cholelithiasis	US		
Diverticulitis	CT scan with contrast		No endoscopy or barium enema acutely due to perforation risk
Esophageal obstruction	Barium radiograph or endoscopy	Endoscopy	
Esophageal tear	Chest radiograph followed by meglumine diatrizoate (Gastrografin) radiograph	Endoscopy or surgery	
Hematemesis	Endoscopy		
Intestinal obstruction	Abdominal radiograph	CT scan with contrast	
Lower GI bleeding*	Radionuclide GI bleeding scan	Endoscopy	
Meckel diverticulum	Meckel scan (nuclear medicine)		
Peptic ulcer disease	Upper GI series or endoscopy	Endoscopy	
Pyloric stenosis	US	Barium radiograph	
Unknown GI bleeding*	Radionuclide medicine bleeding study		For brisk bleed, angiography or laparotomy

Continued

181

TABLE 7-1 Screening and/or Confirmatory Radiologic Tests for Different Diseases—cont'd

CONDITION	SCREENING (OR ONLY) TEST TO ORDER	CONFIRMATORY TEST	COMMENTS
Upper GI bleeding*	Upper GI series or endoscopy	Endoscopy	
Gynecologic			
Fibroid uterus	US	MRI	
Ovarian pathology	US	MRI or laparoscopy (CT helpful for staging if malignancy suspected)	
Pelvic mass (female)	US	MRI or CT with contrast or laparoscopy	
Pregnancy evaluation	US (transvaginal detects sooner than transabdominal)		First get β-hCG
Neurologic			
Acute stroke	CT without contrast	MRI of brain without contrast	
Brain tumor	MRI with contrast is most sensitive for masses. CT with contrast if contraindication for MRI		
Head trauma/skull fracture	CT without contrast		
Intracranial hemorrhage	CT without contrast		
Multiple sclerosis	MRI of brain with contrast		
Orthopedic			
Arthritis	Radiograph	MRI if more detailed evaluation is necessary	
Bone metastases	Bone scan	PET scan	Plain radiographs (skeletal surgery) for multiple myeloma
Fracture	Radiograph	Noncontrast CT	CT scan without contrast can help evaluate complex fractures, before ORIF
Osteomyelitis	Radiograph	Bone scan, tagged white blood cell nuclear scan, or MRI with contrast	
Respiratory			
Chest mass	Chest radiograph	CT scan with contrast	
Chest trauma	Chest radiograph	CT scan with contrast (indicated as first test if concern for vascular injury)	Some acute diagnoses (tension pneumothorax) based on physical exam
Hemoptysis	Chest radiograph	Bronchoscopy and/or CT scan with contrast	
Pneumonia	Chest radiograph	CT with contrast if needed	
Pulmonary embolism	CT with contrast	Conventional pulmonary arteriogram (rarely indicated)	Ventilation-perfusion radionuclide scan if unable to give contrast or radiation
Pulmonary nodule	Chest radiograph	CT with contrast	PET scan may be necessary to assess for malignancy
Urologic			
Hematuria (persistent)	CT scan with contrast (without contrast if suspicious for renal or ureteral calculi)	Cystoscopy	
Hydronephrosis	US	CT with contrast	
Nephrolithiasis	CT scan without contrast	Intravenous pyelography rarely indicated or used	

*For brisk bleeds, endoscopy is preferred. For occult bleeding, barium study or endoscopy may be used. An "unknown" GI bleed means that initial tests failed to localize the bleed and that the patient is still actively bleeding.

CT, Computed tomography; *CTA,* computed tomography angiogram; *ERCP,* endoscopic retrograde cholangiopancreatography; *GI,* gastrointestinal; *HCG,* human chorionic gonadotropin; *HIDA,* hepato-iminodiacetic acid; *MRA,* magnetic resonance angiogram (an *MRI* test); *MRCP,* magnetic resonance cholangiopancreatography; *MRI,* magnetic resonance imaging; *ORIF,* open reduction with internal fixation; *PET,* positron emission tomography; *US,* ultrasonography; *TEE,* transesophageal echocardiogram.

Note: With suspected *GI* perforation, do not use barium (it can cause a chemical peritonitis); use water-soluble contrast (e.g., Gastrografin).

LABORATORY MEDICINE

Common laboratory tests for Diagnosis of various diseases: see Table 7-2.

TABLE 7-2 Common Lab Tests for Various Diseases

DISEASE	DIAGNOSTIC TEST
Acromegaly	IGF-I level
Autoimmune hemolytic anemia	Direct antiglobulin (direct Coombs)
Antiphospholipid antibody syndrome	Anticardiolipin antibody (ACA), dRVVT, anti-β_2 glycoprotein 1 antibody
Autoimmune hepatitis type 2	Liver-kidney microsome type 1 antibodies (LKM1)
Celiac disease	Tissue transglutaminase antibody
Colorectal carcinoma	Carcinoembryonic antigen (CEA)
Congestive heart failure	B-type natriuretic peptide (BNP)
CREST syndrome	Anticentromere antibody
Cushing syndrome	Dexamethasone suppression
Disseminated intravascular coagulation (DIC)	D-dimer, fibrin degradation products (FDP)
Diabetes mellitus	Fasting glucose, glucose tolerance test, HbA$_{1C}$
Gestational trophoblastic disease, choriocarcinoma	Human chorionic gonadotropin (hCG)
Goodpasture syndrome	Glomerular basement membrane antibody
Hepatic encephalopathy	Ammonia level
Hepatocellular carcinoma	Alpha-fetoprotein
Hereditary spherocytosis	Osmotic fragility
Insulinoma	C-peptide
Iron deficiency anemia	Ferritin
ITP	Platelet antibodies
Lupus drug-induced	Antihistone antibodies
Lupus, systemic erythematosus	Anti-dsDNA, anti-Sm antibody
Medullary carcinoma of the thyroid	Calcitonin
Multiple myeloma	Serum protein electrophoresis, urine protein electrophoresis
Myasthenia gravis	Acetylcholine receptor (AChR) antibody
Myocardial infarction	Troponin
Paroxysmal cold hemoglobinuria	Donath-Landsteiner (D-L) test
Polymyositis	Anti Jo-1 antibody
Primary biliary cirrhosis	Antimitochondrial antibody (AMA)
Pernicious anemia	Schilling test, intrinsic factor and parietal cell antibodies
Pheochromocytoma	Plasma metanephrines
Primary aldosteronism	Plasma renin–aldosterone ratio
Rhabdomyolysis	Creatine kinase
Sarcoidosis	Angiotensin-converting enzyme (nonspecific)
Scleroderma (systemic sclerosis)	Anti–Scl-70
Sjögren syndrome	Anti-SSA (Ro)/SSB(La) antibodies
Syphilis	RPR, VDRL
Vitamin B$_{12}$ deficiency	Vitamin B$_{12}$ level, methylmalonic acid
Wegener's granulomatosis	Cytoplasmic ANCA pattern (cANCA)
Wilson's disease	Ceruloplasmin
Zollinger-Ellison syndrome	Gastrin level

CREST, Calcinosis, Raynaud phenomenon, esophageal involvement, sclerodactyly, and telangiectasia (syndrome); *dRVVT,* dilute Russell's Viper Venom test; *IGF-1,* insulin-like growth factor-1; *ITP,* idiopathic thrombocytopenic purpura; *RPR,* rapid plasmin reagin (test); *VDRL,* Venereal Disease Research Laboratory (test).

Isosthenuria/hyposthenuria is the inability to concentrate urine. Think of *diabetes insipidus* or *sickle cell disease/trait.*

High amylase may result from sources besides the pancreas *(salivary glands, gastrointestinal [GI] tract, renal failure, ruptured tubal pregnancy),* but elevation of both amylase and lipase in a patient with abdominal pain is almost always due to pancreatitis.

Elevated creatine kinase (CK), formerly measured as creatine phosphokinase (CPK), is typically due to *muscle injury* (striated or myocardial). Differential considerations include myocardial infarction (check the CK-MB fraction or cardiac troponin levels to confirm a cardiac source), rhabdomyolysis from drugs *(HMG-CoA reductase inhibitors), extreme exercise, trauma, neuroleptic malignant syndrome, alcoholism,* or *burns.*

▢ **CASE SCENARIO:** What can cause spurious (i.e., false) hyperkalemia? Hemolysis of the sample (repeat test on a new blood draw if suspicious).

▢ **CASE SCENARIO:** What do you have to remember if hyponatremia is present in a diabetic patient? The sodium level is artificially low in the setting of significant hyperglycemia. Chlorpropamide (rarely used) can cause the syndrome of inappropriate antidiuretic hormone secretion (SIADH).

▭ **CASE SCENARIO:** What is the relationship between pH and potassium and calcium? Alkalosis may cause hypokalemia and symptoms of hypocalcemia due to cellular shift—and acidosis may cause hyperkalemia by the same mechanism. Thus bicarbonate helps to treat severe hyperkalemia.

▭ **CASE SCENARIO:** What electrolyte disturbance can make hypokalemia and hypocalcemia almost impossible to correct? Hypomagnesemia. You usually cannot correct low potassium or calcium levels until you correct magnesium.

▭ **CASE SCENARIO:** How can the BUN-to-serum creatinine ratio help you to determine whether a patient is dehydrated or has prerenal renal insufficiency? A BUN-to-creatinine ratio >15 usually implies dehydration.

PHARMACOLOGY

Side effects: Bizarre, unique, and fatal side effects are typically tested, as well as common side effects of common drugs (Table 7-3).

TABLE 7-3 Side Effects of Commonly Used Drugs

DRUG	SIDE EFFECT(S)
Anesthesia and Pain Management	
Acetaminophen	Liver toxicity (in high doses)
Aspirin	GI bleeding, hypersensitivity
Halogen anesthetics	Malignant hyperthermia
Halothane	Liver necrosis
Local anesthetics	Seizures
Methoxyflurane	Diabetes insipidus
Morphine	Sphincter of Oddi spasm
Opiates	SIADH, respiratory depression, pinpoint pupils, decreased GI motility, nausea, itching
Succinylcholine	Malignant hyperthermia, increased intracranial pressure, hyperkalemia
Infectious Disease	
Aminoglycosides	Hearing loss, renal toxicity
Chloramphenicol	Aplastic anemia, gray baby syndrome
Clindamycin	Pseudomembranous colitis (may be caused by any broad-spectrum antibiotic)
Dideoxyinosine (DDI)	Pancreatitis, peripheral neuropathy
Ethambutol	Optic neuritis
Isoniazid	Vitamin B_6 deficiency, lupus-like syndrome, liver toxicity
Metronidazole	Disulfiram-like reaction with alcohol
Penicillins	Anaphylaxis, rash with Epstein-Barr virus
Quinolones	Teratogens (cartilage damage), Achilles tendon rupture in adults
Rifampin	Hepatotoxicity
Tetracyclines	Photosensitivity, teeth staining in children
Vancomycin	Red man syndrome
Zidovudine (AZT)	Bone marrow suppression (will always produce macrocytic anemia)
Internal Medicine	
Acetazolamide	Metabolic acidosis
Amiodarone	Thyroid dysfunction, pulmonary fibrosis, skin discoloration
Angiotensin-converting enzyme inhibitors	Cough, angioedema, hyperkalemia; teratogenic to fetal kidneys
Chlorpropamide	SIADH
Clofibrate	Increased GI neoplasms
Demeclocycline	Diabetes insipidus
Digitalis	GI disorders, vision changes, arrhythmias
Heparin	Thrombocytopenia, thrombosis
HMG-CoA reductase inhibitors	Liver and muscle toxicity
Hydralazine	Lupus-like syndrome
Methyldopa	Hemolytic anemia (Coombs-positive)
Niacin	Skin flushing, pruritus

TABLE 7-3 Side Effects of Commonly Used Drugs—cont'd

DRUG	SIDE EFFECT(S)
Phenytoin	Folate deficiency, teratogen, hirsutism, gingival hyperplasia
Procainamide	Lupus-like syndrome
Quinine	Cinchonism (e.g., tinnitus, vertigo)
Trimethadione	Terrible teratogen
Valproic acid	Neural tube defects in offspring
Warfarin	Necrosis, teratogen, bleeding
Oncology	
Bleomycin	Pulmonary fibrosis
Busulfan	Pulmonary fibrosis, adrenal failure
Cisplatin	Nephrotoxicity
Cyclophosphamide	Hemorrhage cystitis
Doxorubicin	Cardiomyopathy
Vincristine	Peripheral neuropathy
Psychiatry	
Bupropion	Seizures
Clozapine	Agranulocytosis
Lithium	Diabetes insipidus, thyroid dysfunction
Monoamine oxidase inhibitors	Tyramine crisis (cheese, wine)
Selective serotonin reuptake inhibitors (SSRIs)	Anxiety, agitation, insomnia, suicidality, sexual dysfunction
Thioridazine	Retinal deposits, cardiac toxicity
Trazodone	Priapism
Miscellaneous	
Cyclosporine	Renal toxicity
Isotretinoin	Terrible teratogen
Minoxidil	Hirsutism
Oxytocin	SIADH
Sulfa drugs	Allergies, kernicterus in neonates

GI, Gastrointestinal; HMG-CoA, 3-hydroxy-3-methylglutaryl-coenzyme A; SIADH, syndrome of inappropriate antidiuretic hormone.

Antidotes for acute poisoning or overdose: see Table 7-4.

TABLE 7-4 Agents Commonly Implicated in Poisoning/Overdose, with Antidotes

AGENT	ANTIDOTE(S)
Acetaminophen	N-acetylcysteine
Benzodiazepines	Flumazenil
β-Blockers	Glucagon
Carbon monoxide	Oxygen (hyperbaric if severe)
Cholinesterase inhibitors	Atropine, pralidoxime
Copper or gold	Penicillamine
Cyanide	Sodium nitrite, thiosulfate
Digoxin	Normalize potassium and other electrolytes, digoxin antibodies
Heparin	Protamine sulfate
Iron	Deferoxamine
Lead	Ethylenediaminetetraacetic acid, dimercaprol
Methanol or ethylene glycol	Fomepizole
Muscarinic receptor blockers (anticholinergics)	Physostigmine
Nitrites	Methylene blue
Opioids	Naloxone
Organophosphates	Atropine, pralidoxime
Phenothiazines	Diphenhydramine
Tricyclic antidepressants or quinidine	Sodium bicarbonate
Warfarin	Fresh frozen plasma (for immediate reversal), vitamin K

Combinations of drugs to avoid:
- Monoamine oxidase (MAO) inhibitors and opioids (can cause coma)
- MAO inhibitors and selective serotonin reuptake inhibitors (can cause serotonin syndrome: hyperthermia, rigidity, myoclonus, autonomic instability)
- Aminoglycosides and loop diuretics (enhanced ototoxicity)
- Thiazides and lithium (lithium toxicity)

Barbiturates, antiepileptics, and rifampin are classic inducers of hepatic enzymes; cimetidine and ketoconazole are classic inhibitors of hepatic enzymes (important for drug–drug interactions).

Herbal medicines and supplements

Herbal products are classified as dietary supplements and are not regulated as medications. Safety, quality, and efficacy for medicines are the responsibility of manufacturers.

The most frequently used herbal supplements include *Echinacea, Ginkgo biloba,* garlic, ginseng, saw palmetto, St. John's wort, ephedra (ma huang), and kava (Table 7-5).

TABLE 7-5 Common Herbal Supplements with Uses/Adverse Effects

HERBAL NAME	BOTANICAL NAME	USES	SIDE EFFECTS, DRUG INTERACTION
Betel nut	*Areca catechu*	Stimulant	Bronchospasm
Black cohosh	*Cimicifuga racemosa*	Premenstrual syndrome and menopause	Aspirin-like antiinflammation, estrogen effect-contraindicated in pregnancy, endometrial and breast cancer
Blue cohosh	*Caulophyllum thalictroides*	Menstrual cramps	Nicotinic effects
Dong quai	*Angelica polymorpha*	Hypertension, menopause, blood purifier	Anticoagulation, increases INR in patients on warfarin, dermatitis
Echinacea	*Echinacea purpurea*	Common cold	Fever, nausea, and vomiting. CYP3A4 inhibitor—contraindicated with immunosuppressive agents
Garlic	*Allium sativum*	Infection, hypertension, cholesterol, diabetes	Dermatitis, inhibits platelet aggregation, increases INR in patients on warfarin
Ginkgo	*Ginkgo biloba*	Depression, anxiety, memory, Alzheimer disease, claudication	GI effects, fibrinolytic—potentiates bleeding with aspirin, increases INR in patients on warfarin
Ginseng	*Panax ginseng*	Depression, stress, anxiety, fatigue	Can be abused, decreases INR in patients on warfarin
Gordolobo yerba	*Senecio longiloba*	URI, fever	Budd-Chiari syndrome
Kava kava	*Piper methysticum*	Aphrodisiac, fibromyalgia, ADHD	Hepatitis; do not give in pregnancy or Parkinson disease
Licorice	*Glycyrrhiza glabra*	Cough, GI illnesses, adrenal insufficiency	Hypokalemia in patients on digoxin
Ma huang (ephedra)	*Ephedra sinica*	Stimulant, common cold, asthma, COPD	Sympathomimetic—do not use with MAO inhibitors, do not use in patients with hypertension, myocardial infarction, arrhythmias
St. John's wort	*Hypericum perforatum*	Depression, anxiety	Serotonin syndrome in patients on SSRIs, decreased INR in patients on warfarin, interacts with cytochrome p450 causing decreased concentrations of oral contraceptives, digoxin, and many other drugs
Saw palmetto	*Serenoa repens*	Benign prostatic hypertrophy	Decreases prostate size, but does not affect PSA levels, GI effects
Valerian	*Valeriana officinalis*	Sleep, anxiety, general tonic	Hepatotoxicity
Yohimbine	*Pausinystalia yohimbe*	Sexual disorders, aphrodisiac	Hypertension, agitation, CNS effects

ADHD, Attention deficit-hyperactivity disorder; *CNS,* central nervous system; *COPD,* chronic obstructive pulmonary disease; *GI,* gastrointestinal; *INR,* international normalized ratio; *MA,* monoamine oxidase; *PSA,* prostate-specific antigen; *URI,* upper respiratory infection.

The lack of manufacturing quality control accounts for most toxicologic problems. Problems associated with herbal supplements arise from (1) misidentification of a herbal plant by the manufacturer, (2) contamination with other toxic material, (3) direct toxicity or overdose and (4) drug-herbal interaction, predominantly with warfarin, blood thinners, and MAO inhibitors.

Antihypertensive medications

Side effects of diuretics

❍ Thiazides (e.g., hydrochlorothiazide) cause hyperglycemia, hyperuricemia, hyperlipidemia, hyponatremia, hypokalemic metabolic alkalosis, and hypovolemia; thiazides are sulfa drugs (be careful with sulfa allergy).

❍ Loop diuretics (e.g., furosemide) cause *hypokalemic metabolic alkalosis,* hypovolemia, and ototoxicity. All are also sulfa drugs except ethacrynic acid.

❍ Carbonic anhydrase inhibitors cause *metabolic acidosis.*

▭ **CASE SCENARIO:** What is the difference between loop diuretics and thiazides in terms of their effects on calcium? Thiazides cause calcium retention and should be avoided in patients with hypercalcemia, whereas loop diuretics cause calcium excretion and are used as one of the treatments for hypercalcemia.

Side effects of antihypertensive drugs: sedation/fatigue (classic with β-blockers), depression (worst is methyldopa), and sexual dysfunction. β-Blockers, verapamil, and diltiazem can cause bradycardia or heart block in susceptible patients. β-Blockers can also precipitate attacks in *asthmatics* (who should not take them) and *mask the symptoms of hypoglycemia* in diabetic patients (though the benefits may outweigh the risks, such as in a person with a prior myocardial infarction). α_1-Antagonists classically cause *first-dose orthostatic hypotension.*

Estrogen/hormone replacement therapy

Hormone replacement therapy (HRT) is no longer thought to be beneficial for women other than for symptom relief. The patient must decide whether she wants HRT after you discuss with her the risks and benefits, the risks now thought to outweigh the benefits. Observation during therapy is necessary because estrogen and progesterone are far from harmless. The main reason to give progesterone with estrogen is to eliminate the increased risk of endometrial cancer. If a woman has no uterus, give estrogen only (without progesterone).

Known benefits of estrogen therapy: Decreased osteoporosis and fractures (especially hip fractures); reduced hot flashes; reduced genitourinary symptoms (helps with dryness, urgency, atrophy-induced incontinence, urinary frequency); decreased risk of colorectal cancer (according to the Women's Health Initiative, with combined estrogen and progesterone therapy).

Known risks of estrogen therapy: Increased risk of endometrial cancer (decreased by the coadministration of progesterones); a small increase in the risk of coronary heart disease with combined estrogen and progesterone therapy (though the risk is not increased in women who are <10 years postmenopausal or 50–59 years of age); increased risk of venous thromboembolism; increased risk of breast cancer (according to the Women's Health Initiative when combined estrogen and progesterone therapy is used; there was a slightly decreased risk of breast cancer with estrogen only, though this decrease was not statistically significant); increased risk of stroke; and increased risk of gallbladder disease.

Other side effects of estrogen therapy: Endometrial bleeding, breast tenderness, nausea, bloating, and headaches.

Absolute contraindications to estrogen therapy: Unexplained vaginal bleeding, active liver disease, history of thrombophlebitis or thromboembolism, history of endometrial or breast cancer.

Relative contraindications to estrogen therapy: Seizure disorder, hypertension, uterine leiomyomas, familial hyperlipidemia, migraines, thrombophlebitis, endometriosis, gallbladder disease.

Consider endometrial biopsy and dilatation and curettage at the onset of treatment to rule out hyperplasia and/or cancer and an evaluation of any unexplained bleeding while the patient is on therapy unless the patient has had a normal evaluation in the past 6 months.

Birth control pills/oral contraceptive pills

Oral contraceptive pills (OCPs) are the most common cause of secondary hypertension in women. Any woman taking OCPs who is noted have increased blood pressure should stop the OCPs and then have her blood pressure rechecked at a later date.

Absolute contraindications to OCPs: Smoking 15 or more cigarettes per day after age 35, past or current venous thromboembolism, cerebrovascular disease, coronary artery disease, complicated valvular heart disease, diabetes with complications, breast cancer, active pregnancy, lactation

(<6 weeks post partum), liver disease, headaches with focal neurologic symptoms, major surgery with prolonged immobilization, and hypertension (blood pressure >160/100 mm Hg or with concomitant vascular disease.

Relative contraindications to OCPs: Age >35 years and smoking <15 cigarettes per day; postpartum <21 days; lactation (6 weeks to 6 months); undiagnosed vaginal or uterine bleeding, history of breast cancer but no recurrence in the past 5 years; interacting drugs (e.g., certain anticonvulsants, rifampin); gallbladder disease; headaches without aura in patients age 35 or greater; and hypertension (well-controlled or blood pressure 140–159/90–99 mm Hg).

Side effects of OCPs: Glucose intolerance (check for diabetes mellitus annually in women at high risk), depression, edema (bloating), weight gain, cholelithiasis, benign *liver adenomas,* melasma ("mask of pregnancy"), nausea and vomiting, headache, *hypertension,* and drug interactions (drugs such as rifampin and antiepileptics may induce metabolism of OCPs and reduce their effectiveness).

Benefits of OCPs: Reduce ovarian cancer by up to 50%; decrease the risk of endometrial cancer; decrease the incidence of the following: menorrhagia, dysmenorrhea, benign breast disease, functional ovarian cysts (often prescribed for the previous four effects), premenstrual tension, iron deficiency anemia, salpingitis, and ectopic pregnancy.

Risks associated with OCPs: Because of the risks of thromboembolism, OCPs should be stopped 1 month before elective surgery and not restarted until 1 month after surgery.

Oral contraceptive pills have little, if any, effect on the risk of developing breast cancer. Cervical neoplasia may be increased (perhaps due to the confounding factor of increased sexual relations or number of partners). OCP users should have regular Pap smears.

Aspirin, NSAIDs, COX-2 inhibitors, acetaminophen

Effects: Aspirin and NSAIDs inhibit cyclo oxygenase (COX) centrally and peripherally, giving them *antiinflammatory, antipyretic, analgesic,* and *antiplatelet effects.* Aspirin inhibits COX irreversibly and thus for the life of the platelet, whereas other NSAIDs reversibly inhibit COX, both nonselectively. COX-2 inhibitors (e.g., celecoxib) only block COX-2 and therefore do not have an antiplatelet effect. Acetaminophen is mostly central-acting; thus, it is only an analgesic and antipyretic with no platelet or antiinflammatory effects.

Toxicity: Aspirin may cause GI upset, *GI bleeding, gastric ulcers,* and gout; very high doses cause *tinnitus,* vertigo, *respiratory alkalosis and metabolic acidosis,* hyperthermia, coma, and death. Aspirin can be removed by dialysis in severe overdose. Aspirin and other NSAIDs also may cause temporary and/or permanent *renal insufficiency/failure or damage* (e.g., interstitial nephritis, papillary necrosis or acute tubular necrosis), especially in patients who take high doses chronically and have preexisting renal disease.

 COX-2 specific inhibitors (e.g., celecoxib) or an NSAID–prostaglandin E_1 combination may help prevent GI toxicity, though the COX-2 inhibitors may not be as protective against GI bleeding as was initially thought.

Do not give aspirin to the following patients:

❍ Patients with allergies or asthma and *nasal polyps* (hypersensitivity reactions are extremely common in this group). Even in the absence of nasal polyps, patients with asthma may have an attack after taking aspirin.

❍ Children younger than 15 years of age. Aspirin may cause *Reye syndrome,* typically in the setting of a viral infection or fever; look for *encephalopathy* and *liver dysfunction* in affected children.

Low-dose aspirin has been proved to be of benefit in reducing the risk of myocardial infarction both in patients who have had a previous myocardial infarction and in patients with stable or unstable angina who have not had an infarction. The 2008 American College of Physicians (ACCP) clinical practice guidelines on antithrombotic and thrombolytic therapy recommend that all patients with chronic stable angina or other clinical or laboratory evidence of coronary artery disease receive aspirin indefinitely.

The data on the use of aspirin for primary prevention of myocardial infarction are inconclusive. However, aspirin is recommended in all diabetics with cardiovascular disease and for primary prevention in diabetics with one or more risk factors (e.g., age >40, cigarette smoking, hypertension, hyperlipidemia, obesity, albuminuria, or family history of cardiovascular disease). The risks associated with aspirin prophylaxis may outweigh the benefits in patients with a history of liver disease, kidney disease, peptic ulcer disease, or GI bleeding, poorly controlled hypertension, or a bleeding disorder.

Aspirin has been proved to reduce the risk of stroke in patients with a transient ischemic attack (TIA), previous stroke, and/or known carotid artery stenosis. However, the risks may outweigh the benefits, especially in patients with uncontrolled hypertension, in whom the risk of hemorrhagic stroke is increased with the use of aspirin.

Always weigh the risk and benefits of aspirin therapy. If the patient has a history of liver or kidney disease, peptic ulcers, GI bleeding, poorly controlled hypertension, or bleeding disorder, the risks of aspirin therapy may outweigh the benefits.

Stop aspirin 1 week before elective surgery; other NSAIDs should be stopped on the day before surgery.

Acetaminophen can cause liver toxicity and failure in high doses due to depletion of glutathione and hepatic necrosis. Treat with *acetylcysteine.*

Monoclonal antibody–based drugs: see Table 7-6.

TABLE 7-6 Summary of Monoclonal Antibody–Based Drugs

AGENT	ANTIBODY BINDS TO	CONDITION(S) USED FOR
Abatacept	CD80 and CD86 on APCs	Rheumatoid arthritis (RA)
Abciximab	Integrin GPIIb/IIIa receptor	Acute coronary syndrome
Adalimumab	TNF-α	RA
Alefacept	CD2 (thus blocks T-cell activation)	Psoriasis
Alemtuzumab	CD52 on white blood cells	Chronic B-cell leukemia
Basiliximab	CD25 on activated lymphocytes	Renal transplant rejection prevention/ treatment
Bevacizumab	Vascular endothelial growth factor	Colorectal carcinoma
Cetuximab	Epidermal growth factor receptor	Colorectal carcinoma
Daclizumab	IL-2 receptor	Renal transplant rejection prevention/ treatment
Eculizumab	Complement protein C5	Paroxysmal nocturnal hemoglobinuria
Efalizumab	CD11a	Psoriasis
Epratuzumab	CD22 on B lymphocytes	B-cell non-Hodgkin lymphoma
Etanercept	TNF-α and TNF-β	RA, psoriatic arthritis
Gemtuzumab*	CD33 on leukemic blast cells	Acute myelogenous leukemia (AML)
Ibritumomab tiuxetan*	CD20 on lymphocytes	B-cell non-Hodgkin lymphoma
Infliximab	TNF-α	RA, Crohn disease, ulcerative colitis, others
Labetuzumab	CEA	Colorectal cancer
Muromonab-CD3 (OKT3)	CD3 on T cells	Renal transplant rejection prevention/ treatment
Natalizumab	T-cell VLA4 receptor	Multiple sclerosis
Omalizumab	Immunoglobulin E (IgE)	Asthma
Palivizumab	Fusion protein of RSV	RSV (respiratory syncytial virus) prophylaxis
Panitumumab	Epidermal growth factor receptor	Colorectal carcinoma
Pemtumomab	MUC-1	Ovarian cancer
Ranibizumab	Vascular endothelial growth factor	Macular degeneration
Rituximab	CD20 on lymphocytes	B-cell non-Hodgkin lymphoma
Tositumomab*	CD20 on lymphocytes	B-cell non-Hodgkin lymphoma
Trastuzumab	HER-2/neu growth factor receptor	Breast cancer

*These agents are complexed to other agents that perform much of the therapeutic function. With ibritumomab and tositumomab, radioactive isotopes are attached (local radiation to cancer cells), and with gemtuzumab, ozogamicin is attached (synthetic antibiotic with antitumor activity).

APCs, Antigen-presenting cells; *CD,* cluster of differentiation (cell surface marker); *IL,* interleukin; *TNF,* tumor necrosis factor.

8 IMAGES

The most common types of images encountered on USMLE Step 3 are:
- Dermatology images
- Electrocardiogram (ECG) tracings
- Radiology images, including radiographs, computed tomography (CT) scans, and magnetic resonance imaging (MRI) scans
- Microscopy images, particularly infectious disease images
- Gross photographs of patients

DERMATOLOGY IMAGES

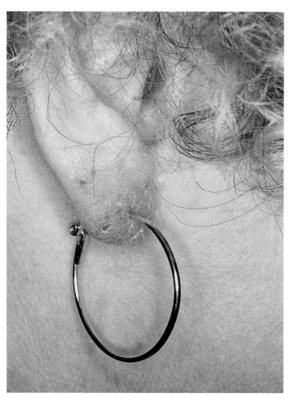

FIGURE 8-1 **Nickel dermatitis,** the most common form of contact dermatitis in women, from nickel earrings. See Plate 1. *(From Habif TP: Clinical Dermatology, 5th ed. Philadelphia, Mosby, 2010.)*

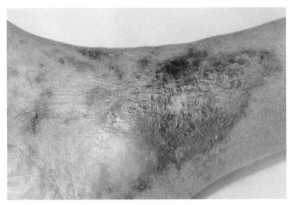

FIGURE **8-2 Stasis dermatitis** typically occurs on the lateral aspects of the shins. See Plate 2. *(From Cleveland Clinic: Current Clinical Medicine, 2nd ed. Philadelphia, Saunders, 2010.)*

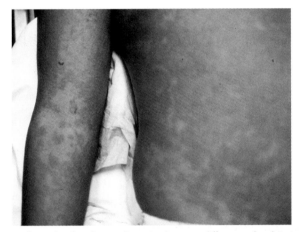

FIGURE **8-3 Staphylococcal toxic shock syndrome** showing diffuse erythrodermic rash. See Plate 3. *(From Baren JM, Rothrock SG, Brennan J, Brown L: Pediatric Emergency Medicine. Philadelphia, Saunders, 2008.)*

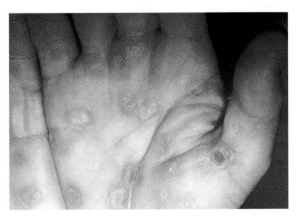

FIGURE **8-4 Secondary syphilis:** palmar lesions of secondary syphilis. See Plate 4. *(From Mandell GL, Bennett JE, Dolin R: Mandell, Douglas, and Bennett's Principles and Practice of Infectious Diseases, 7th ed. Philadelphia, Churchill Livingstone, 2010.)*

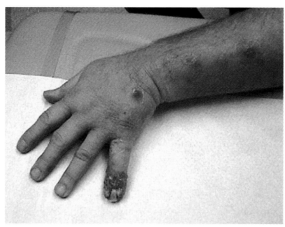

Figure 8-5 Sporotrichosis of the fifth finger in a gardener. Three nodular lesions are visible on the hand and arm. See Plate 5. *(From Mandell GL, Bennett JE, Dolin R: Mandell, Douglas, and Bennett's Principles and Practice of Infectious Diseases, 7th ed. Philadelphia, Churchill Livingstone, 2010.)*

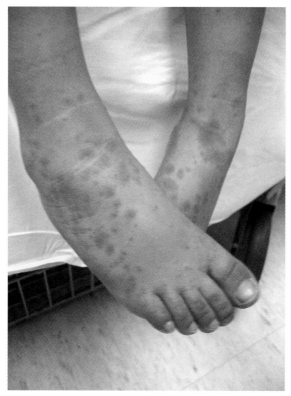

Figure 8-6 Henoch-Schönlein purpura in a 7-year-old child. Note typical red-purple rash on the lower extremities. See Plate 6. *(From Marx J, Hockberger R, Walls R: Rosen's Emergency Medicine, 7th ed. Philadelphia, Mosby, 2010.)*

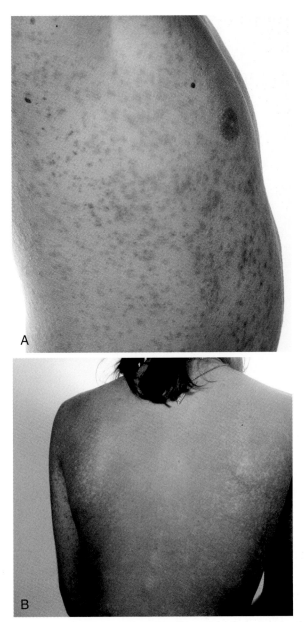

FIGURE 8-7 Morbilliform drug rash secondary to amoxicillin. Adolescents (**A**, **B**) with Epstein-Barr virus mononucleosis who received amoxicillin and developed diffuse erythematous raised rashes. Note predominance on trunk and coalescence (**B**). See Plate 7. *(From Long SS, Pickering LK, Prober CG: Principles and Practice of Pediatric Infectious Diseases Revised Reprint, 3rd ed. Philadelphia, Saunders, 2009.)*

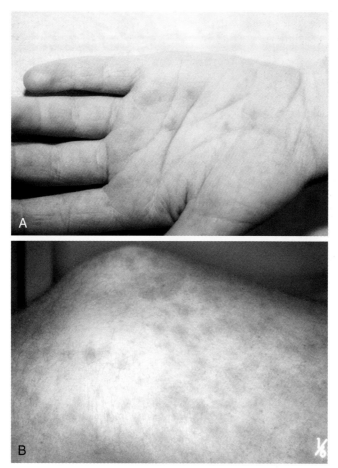

FIGURE 8-8 Rocky Mountain spotted fever rash. A, The wrist and palm manifest the rash of Rocky Mountain spotted fever with central petechiae in some of the maculopapules. **B,** Early petechial rash on arm. See Plate 8. *(From Mandell GL, Bennett JE, Dolin R: Mandell, Douglas, and Bennett's Principles and Practice of Infectious Diseases, 7th ed. Philadelphia, Churchill Livingstone, 2010.)*

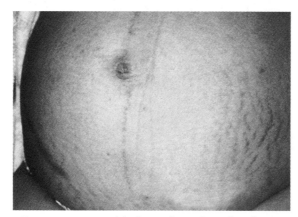

FIGURE 8-9 Linea nigra. Hyperpigmentation of the linea alba and stretchmarks (striae gravidarum) on the lateral aspects of the abdomen. See Plate 9. *(From James DK, Steer PJ, Weiner CP, Gonik B: High Risk Pregnancy, 4th ed. Philadelphia, Saunders, 2011.)*

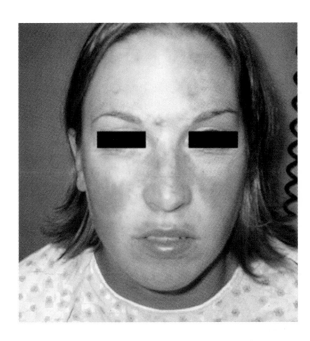

FIGURE 8-10 Melasma involving the cheeks, nose, upper lip, and forehead. See Plate 10. *(From Gabbe SG, Simpson JL, Niebyl JR, et al: Obstetrics: Normal and Problem Pregnancies, 5th ed. Philadelphia, Churchill Livingstone, 2007.)*

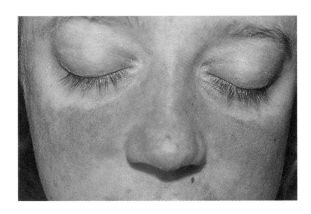

FIGURE 8-11 Malar rash of systemic lupus erythematous. See Plate 11. *(From Stern TA, Rosengaum AF, Fava M, et al: Massachusetts General Hospital Comprehensive Clinical Psychiatry. Philadelphia, Mosby, 2008.)*

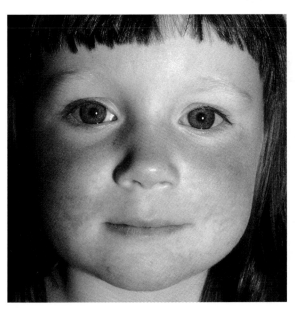

FIGURE 8-12 Erythema infectiosum. Facial erythema "slapped cheek." The red plaque covers the cheek and spares the nasolabial fold and the circumoral region. See Plate 12. *(From Habif TP: Clinical Dermatology, 5th ed. Philadelphia, Mosby, 2010.)*

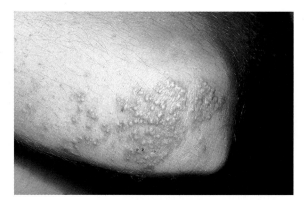

FIGURE 8-13 Cutaneous xanthomata on the extensor surface of the elbow. Other classic and common locations include the knee and over the Achilles tendon. Most are located along tendons and extensor surfaces of joints. See Plate 13. *(From Kanski J: Clinical Diagnosis in Ophthalmology. Philadelphia, Mosby, 2006.)*

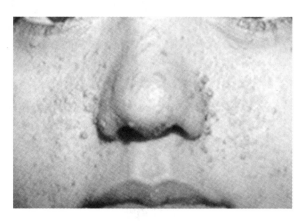

FIGURE 8-14 Mucocutaneous pigmentation in a patient with **Peutz-Jeghers syndrome.** See Plate 14. *(From Feldman M, Friedman LS, Brandt LJ: Sleisenger and Fordtran's Gastrointestinal and Liver Disease, 9th ed. Philadelphia, Saunders, 2011.)*

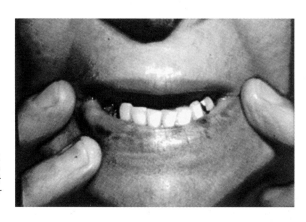

FIGURE 8-15 Adenoma sebaceum of face in a patient with tuberous sclerosis. See Plate 15. *(From Yanoff M, Duker JS: Ophthalmology, 3rd ed. Philadelphia, Mosby, 2009.)*

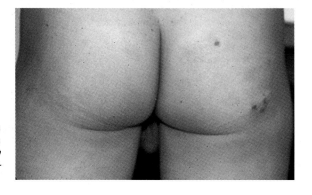

FIGURE 8-16 Patches of **mycosis fungoides** often arise on double-clothed areas, and the lesions may recede with light exposure. See Plate 16. *(From Jaffe ES, Harris NL, Vardiman JW, et al: Hematopathology. Philadelphia, Saunders, 2011.)*

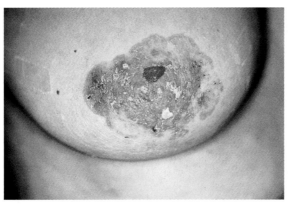

FIGURE 8-17 Paget's disease of the breast. Note the erythematous plaques around the nipple. See Plate 17. *(From Callen JP: Dermatologic signs of systemic disease. In Bolognia JL, Jorizzo JL, Rapini RP [eds]: Dermatology. Edinburgh, Mosby, 2003, p 714.)*

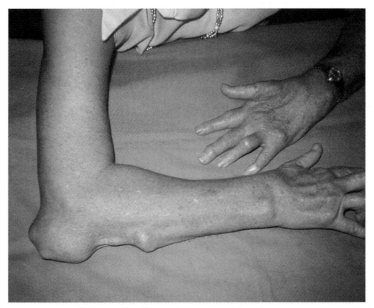

FIGURE 8-18 Rheumatoid nodules in the olecranon bursa and on subcutaneous surface of ulna. See Plate 18. *(From Canale ST, Beaty JH: Campbell's Operative Orthopaedics, 11th ed. Philadelphia, Mosby, 2008.)*

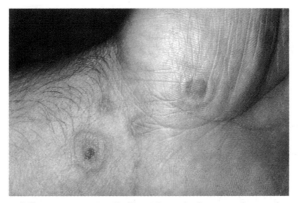

FIGURE 8-19 Erythema multiforme—target or "bull's-eye" annular lesions with central vesicles and bullae are characteristic. See Plate 19. *(From Goldman L, Schafer AI: Goldman's Cecil Medicine, 24th ed. Philadelphia, Saunders, 2012.)*

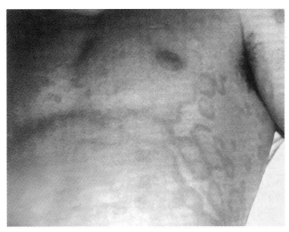

Figure 8-20 Rash of **erythema marginatum** in an adolescent boy with acute rheumatic fever occurred with its characteristic serpiginous and erythematous margins are evident. See Plate 20. *(From Cassidy JT, Petty RE, Laxer R, Lindsley C: Textbook of Pediatric Rheumatology, 6th ed. Philadelphia, Saunders, 2011.)*

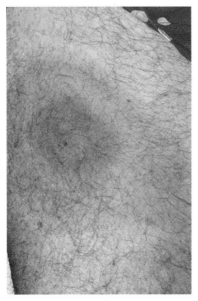

Figure 8-21 The pathognomonic bull's eye rash of **erythema migrans**. This is the characteristic rash of Lyme disease. See Plate 21. *(From Cleveland Clinic: Current Clinical Medicine, 2nd ed. Philadelphia, Saunders, 2010.)*

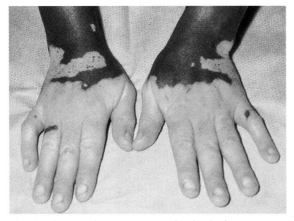

Figure 8-22 Vitiligo on the hands. See Plate 22. *(From Cleveland Clinic: Current Clinical Medicine, 2nd ed. Philadelphia, Saunders, 2010.)*

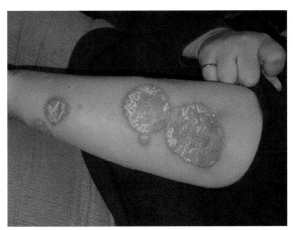

FIGURE 8-23 Psoriasis demonstrating typical well-demarcated, red plaques with silvery scales. See Plate 23. *(From Rakel RE, Rakel D: Textbook of Family Medicine, 8th ed. Philadelphia, Saunders, 2011.)*

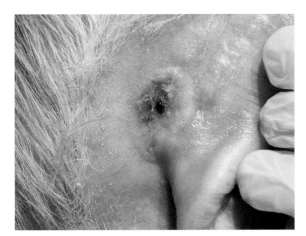

FIGURE 8-24 Ulcerated **basal cell carcinoma** with rolled borders on posterior ear. See Plate 24. *(From Abeloff MD, Armitage JO, Niederhuber JE, et al: Abeloff's Clinical Oncology, 4th ed. Philadelphia, Churchill Livingstone, 2008.)*

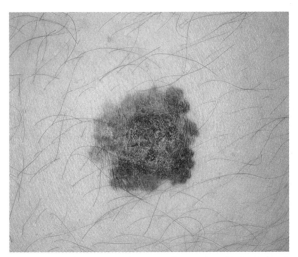

FIGURE 8-25 Superficial spreading **melanoma.** This 2-cm diameter melanoma developed over a 2-year period. See Plate 25. *(From Townsend CM, Beauchamp D, Evers BM, Mattox KL: Sabiston Textbook of Surgery, 18th ed. Philadelphia, Saunders, 2008.)*

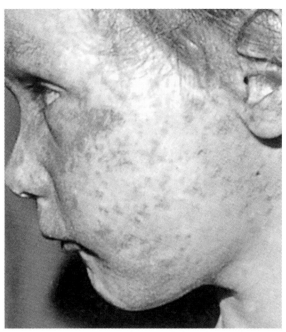

FIGURE 8-26 Rash of **rubella** typically begins on the face and neck as small, irregular pink macules that coalesce, and it spreads centrifugally to involve the torso and extremities. See Plate 26. *(From Kliegman RM, Stanton BMD, St. Geme J, et al: Nelson Textbook of Pediatrics, 19th ed. Philadelphia, Saunders, 2011.)*

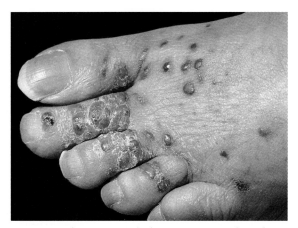

FIGURE 8-27 Kaposi sarcoma. Most lesions are on the lower extremities. Shown here are plaques and tumors. See Plate 27. *(From Habif TP: Clinical Dermatology, 5th ed. Philadelphia, Mosby, 2010.)*

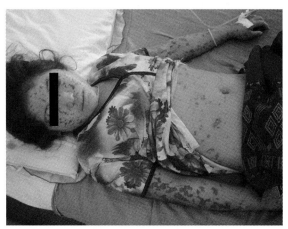

FIGURE 8-28 Classic rash of patient with **meningococcemia**. See Plate 28. *(From Cleveland Clinic: Current Clinical Medicine, 2nd ed. Philadelphia, Saunders, 2010.)*

ELECTROCARDIOGRAM TRACINGS

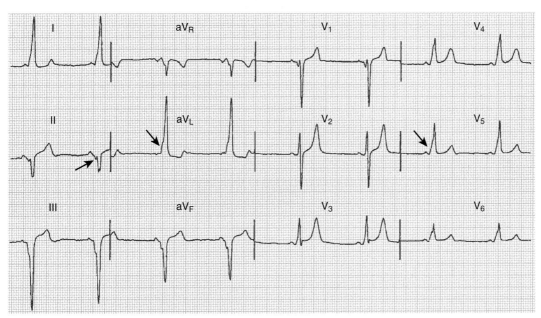

FIGURE 8-29 Wolff-Parkinson-White pattern. Triad of wide QRS complex, short PR interval, and delta waves *(arrows). (From Goldberger AL: Clinical Electrocardiography: A Simplified Approach, 7th ed. Philadelphia, Mosby, 2007.)*

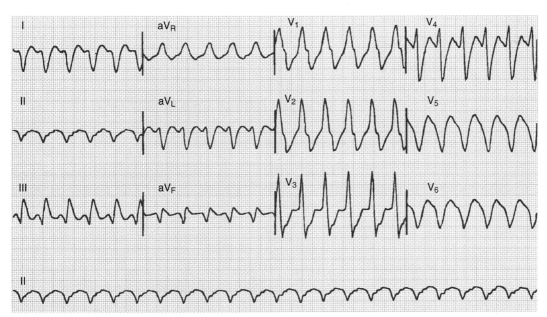

FIGURE 8-30 Ventricular tachycardia. Wide complex QRS tachycardia. *(From Goldberger AL: Clinical Electrocardiography: A Simplified Approach, 7th ed. Philadelphia, Mosby, 2007.)*

Ventricular fibrillation

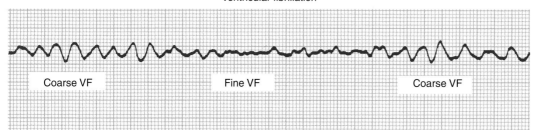

FIGURE 8-31 Ventricular fibrillation. Fibrillatory waves in an irregular pattern. *(From Goldberger AL: Clinical Electrocardiography: A Simplified Approach, 7th ed. Philadelphia, Mosby, 2007.)*

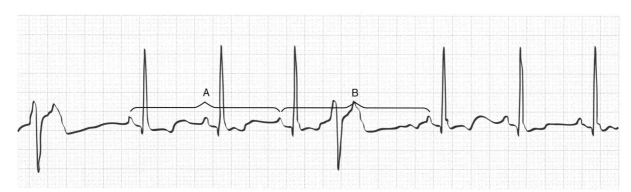

FIGURE 8-32 Premature ventricular contractions with compensatory pause. Note that a sinus P wave can be seen in the T wave of the extrasystolic beat. *(From Marx J, Hockberger R, Walls R: Rosen's Emergency Medicine, 7th ed. Philadelphia, Mosby, 2010.)*

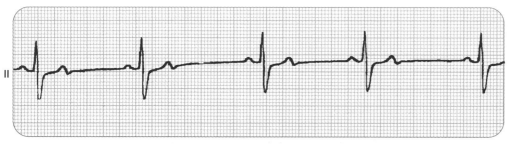

FIGURE 8-33 Sinus bradycardia with a slight sinus arrhythmia. *(From Goldberger AL: Clinical Electrocardiography: A Simplified Approach, 7th ed. Philadelphia, Mosby, 2007.)*

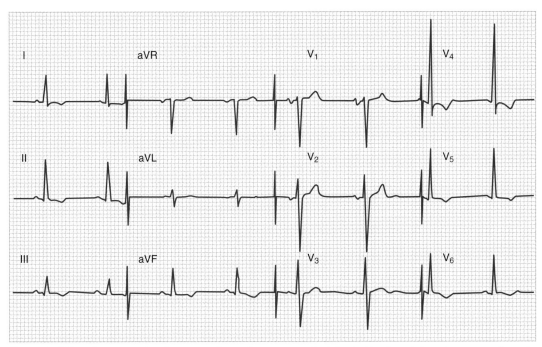

FIGURE 8-34 Left ventricular hypertrophy. Tall R waves on the left-sided leads and deep S waves on the right-sided ones, down-sloping ST-segment depression and T-wave inversion opposite the main R-wave axis. *(From Miller RD, Ericksson LI, Fleisher LA, et al: Miller's Anesthesia, 7th ed. Philadelphia, Churchill Livingstone, 2009.)*

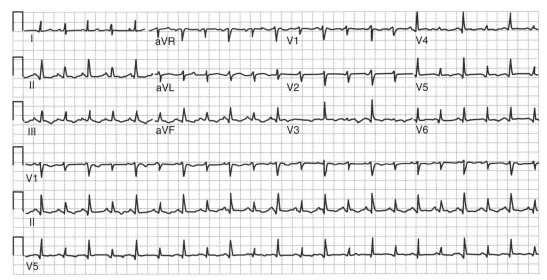

FIGURE 8-35 Electrical alternans in cardiac tamponade. Note changing QRS amplitudes, particularly in leads II, V4, and V5. *(From Bonow RO, Mann DL, Zipes DP, Libby P: Braunwald's Heart Disease—A Textbook of Cardiovascular Medicine, 9th ed. Philadelphia, Saunders, 2012.)*

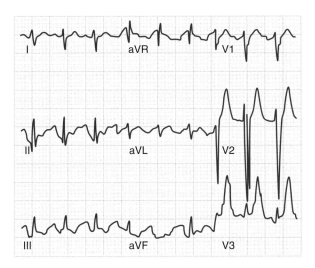

FIGURE 8-36 Tricyclic antidepressant poisoning. Sinus tachycardia with widened QRS complex and marked deviation of the terminal portion of the QRS complex in lead I (deep S wave) and aVR (large R wave). *(From Stern TA, Rosengaum AF, Fava M, et al: Massachusetts General Hospital Comprehensive Clinical Psychiatry. Philadelphia, Mosby, 2008.)*

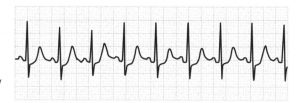

FIGURE 8-37 Sinus tachycardia at 120 beats/ min. *(From Goldman L, Schafer AI: Goldman's Cecil Medicine, 24th ed. Philadelphia, Saunders, 2012.)*

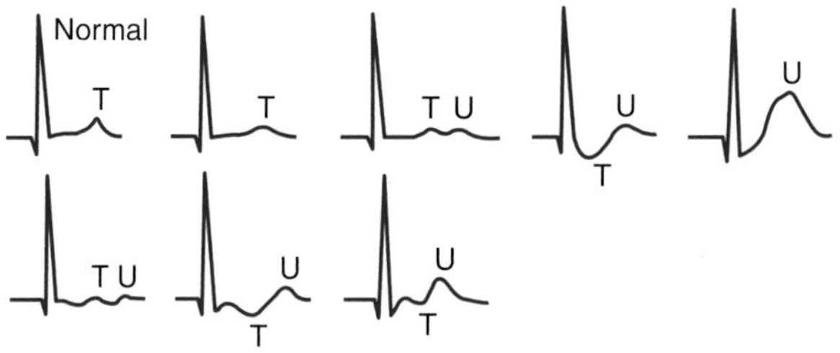

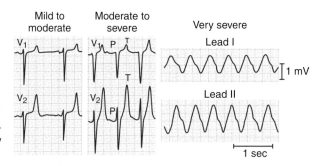

FIGURE 8-38 Hypokalemia. Variable ECG patterns can be seen, ranging from slight T wave flattening to the appearance of prominent U waves, sometimes with ST depressions or T wave inversions. *(From Ferri FF: Practical Guide to the Care of the Medical Patient, 8th ed. Philadelphia, Mosby, 2011.)*

FIGURE 8-39 Hyperkalemia. The earliest change with is peaking ("tenting") of the T waves. With progressive increases in serum potassium, the QRS complexes widen, the P waves decrease in amplitude and may disappear, and finally, a sine wave pattern leads to asystole. *(From Ferri FF: Practical Guide to the Care of the Medical Patient, 8th ed. Philadelphia, Mosby, 2011.)*

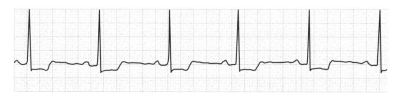

FIGURE 8-40 First-degree block (PR interval = 0.26 second). *(From Seelig CB: Simplified EKG Analysis. Philadelphia, Hanley & Belfus, 1992.)*

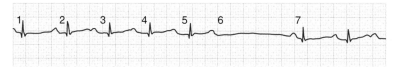

FIGURE 8-41 Mobitz type I second-degree AV block (Wenckebach). Note the gradual prolongation of the PR interval (1-5), the missing QRS complex after the sixth P wave, and the return of the PR interval to its shortest duration (7). *(From Seelig CB: Simplified EKG Analysis. Philadelphia, Hanley & Belfus, 1992.)*

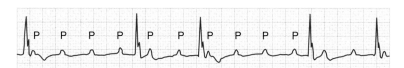

FIGURE 8-42 Mobitz type II second-degree AV block. Note that when beats are conducted, the PR interval is unvarying. *(From Seelig CB: Simplified EKG Analysis. Philadelphia, Hanley & Belfus, 1992.)*

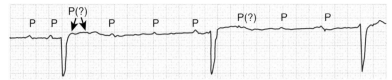

FIGURE 8-43 Third-degree AV block with a ventricular escape rhythm at 32 beats/min. P-wave activity is somewhat irregular. *(From Seelig CB: Simplified EKG Analysis. Philadelphia, Hanley & Belfus, 1992.)*

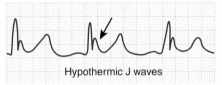

Hypothermic J waves

FIGURE 8-44 Hypothermia. Note the prominent J-waves which can sometimes be mistaken for ST-segment elevation. *(From Ferri FF: Practical Guide to the Care of the Medical Patient, 8th ed. Philadelphia, Mosby, 2011.)*

RADIOLOGY IMAGES

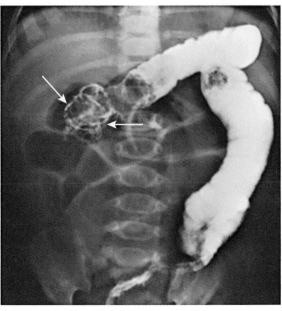

FIGURE 8-45 Intussusception in an infant. The obstruction is evident in the proximal transverse colon. Contrast material between the intussusceptum and the intussuscipiens is responsible for the coiled-spring appearance. *(From Kliegman RM, Behrman RE, Jenson HB, Stanton BMD: Nelson Textbook of Pediatrics, 18th ed. Philadelphia, Saunders, 2007.)*

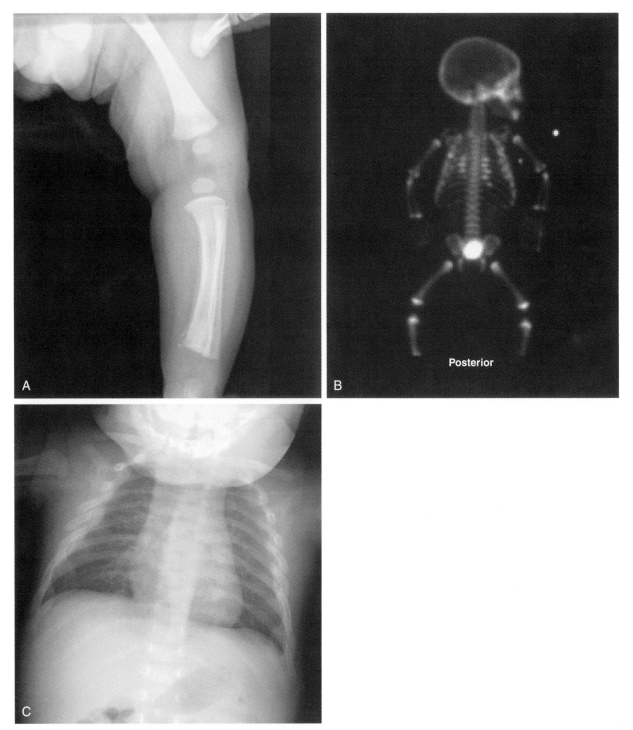

FIGURE **8-46 Child abuse. A,** Metaphyseal fracture of the distal tibia in a 3-month-old infant admitted to the hospital with severe head injury. **B,** Bone scan revealed multiple previously unrecognized fractures of the posterior and lateral ribs. **C,** Follow-up radiographs 2 weeks later showed multiple healing rib fractures. The mechanism of these injuries is usually violent squeezing of the chest. *(From Marcdante K, Kliegman R, Behrman R, Jenson H: Nelson Essentials of Pediatrics, 5th ed. Philadelphia, Saunders, 2005.)*

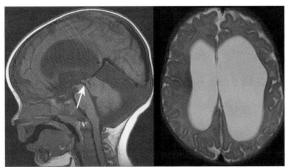

FIGURE **8-47 Hydrocephalus.** Child with aqueduct stenosis, the most common cause of hydrocephalus in children. There is dilatation of the lateral ventricles and proximal cerebral aqueduct *(arrow)*. The hydrocephalus is long-standing because there is white matter volume loss and the anterior recesses of the third ventricle are not bulging. There is more focal damage in the left frontal lobe, probably due to previous germinal matrix hemorrhage. A posterior fossa arachnoid cyst is also noted. *(From Adam A, Dixon AK, Grainger RG, Allison DJ: Grainger & Allison's Diagnostic Radiology, 5th ed. Philadelphia, Churchill Livingstone, 2008.)*

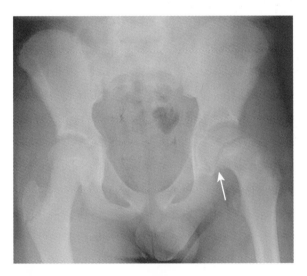

FIGURE **8-48** Anteroposterior radiograph of the hip showing **slipped capital femoral epiphysis** with arrow pointing to the site of slippage. *(From Slap GB: Adolescent Medicine: The Requisites in Pediatrics. Philadelphia, Mosby, 2008.)*

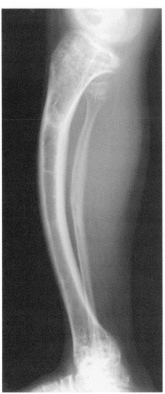

FIGURE **8-49** Lateral radiograph of the tibia of a boy with **rickets** demonstrates a bowing deformity. *(From Weissman BNW: Imaging of Arthritis and Metabolic Bone Disease. Philadelphia, Mosby, 2009, courtesy of Dr. Jeanne Chow, Children's Hospital, Boston.)*

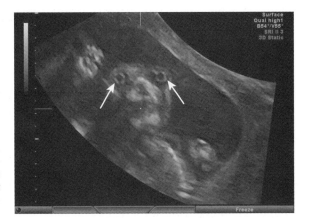

FIGURE 8-50 Two-dimensional image of **anencephaly** at 17 weeks' gestation. The cranial vault is absent above the orbits *(arrows)*. *(From Martin RJ, Fanaroff AA, Walsh MC: Fanaroff and Martin's Neonatal-Perinatal Medicine, 9th ed. Philadelphia, Mosby, 2011.)*

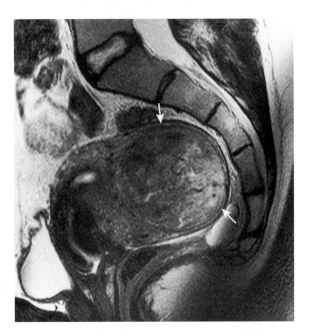

FIGURE 8-51 Leiomyoma, magnetic resonance image (MRI). T_2-weighted sagittal MRI. A subserosal leiomyoma *(arrows)* distends the posterior aspect of the uterus, displacing the endometrium. *(From Adam A, Dixon AK, Grainger RG, Allison DJ: Grainger & Allison's Diagnostic Radiology, 5th ed. Philadelphia, Churchill Livingstone, 2008.)*

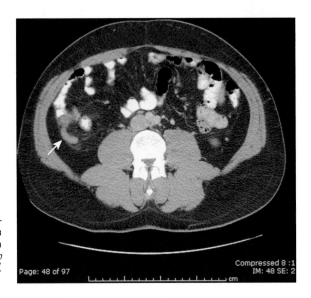

FIGURE 8-52 Appendicitis. A computed tomography scan shows an edematous appendix with a diameter greater than 1 cm *(arrow)*, consistent with acute, uncomplicated appendicitis. *(From Goldman L, Schafer AI: Goldman's Cecil Medicine, 24th ed. Philadelphia, Saunders, 2012.)*

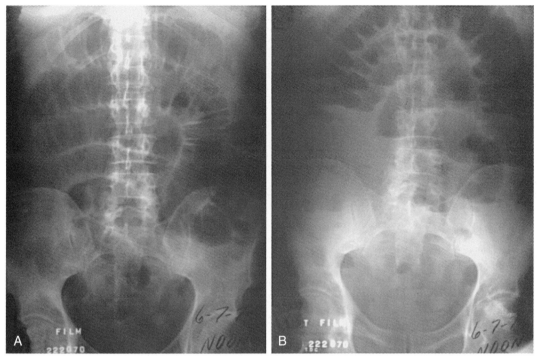

FIGURE 8-53 Plain abdominal radiographs of a patient with a complete **small bowel obstruction. A,** Supine film shows dilated loops of small bowel in an orderly arrangement, without evidence of colonic gas. **B,** Upright film shows multiple, short air-fluid levels arranged in a stepwise pattern. *(From Townsend CM, Beauchamp RD, Evers BM, Mattox KL: Sabiston Textbook of Surgery, 18th ed. Philadelphia, Saunders, 2008, courtesy of Melvyn H. Schreiber, MD, The University of Texas Medical Branch.)*

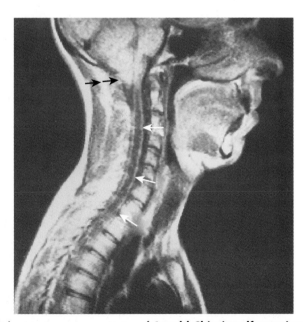

FIGURE 8-54 Midsagittal magnetic resonance image of **Arnold-Chiari malformation** *(small black arrows)* and **syringomyelia** *(three large white arrows)* in a 31-year-old man. Note the cerebellar tonsils extending below the posterior rim of the foramen magnum (dark structure immediately above the *black arrows*). The syrinx extends from the medulla well into the thoracic cord. *(From Andreoli TE [ed]: Cecil essentials of medicine, 4th ed. Philadelphia, WB Saunders, 1997.)*

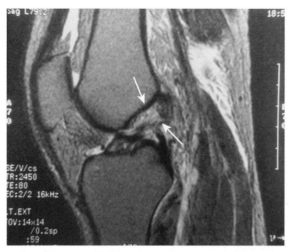

Figure 8-55 Anterior cruciate ligament (ACL) tear, magnetic resonance image. Disruption of ACL fibers at its femoral attachment *(arrows)* with waviness in contour of the middle third of the ligament and a large joint effusion. The patient sustained a complete acute ACL tear in a ski accident. *(From Scott WN: Insall & Scott Surgery of the Knee, 4th ed. Philadelphia, Churchill Livingston, 2006.)*

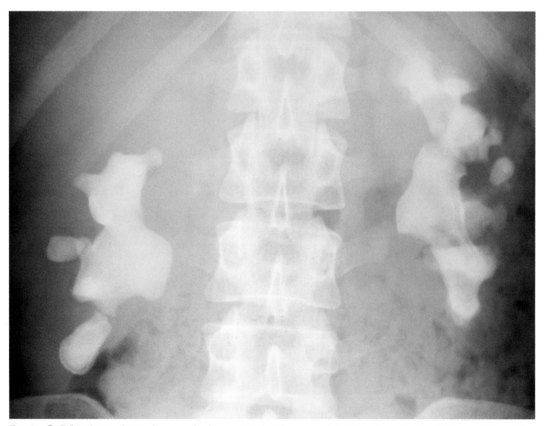

Figure 8-56 Bilateral staghorn calculi associated with recurrent *Proteus* urinary tract infections. *(From Adam A, Dixon AK, Grainger RG, Allison DJ: Grainger & Allison's Diagnostic Radiology, 5th ed. Philadelphia, Churchill Livingstone, 2008.)*

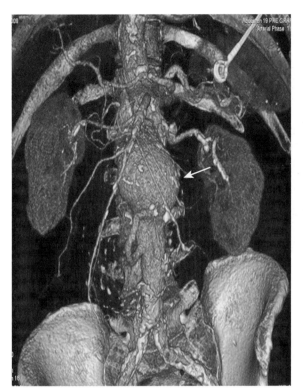

FIGURE 8-57 Three-dimensional reconstruction of a computed tomography (CT) scan in a patient with an infrarenal **abdominal aortic aneurysm** *(arrow)*. See Plate 29. *(From Bonow RO, Mann DL, Zipes DP, Libby P: Braunwald's Heart Disease—A Textbook of Cardiovascular Medicine, 9th ed. Philadelphia, Saunders, 2012.)*

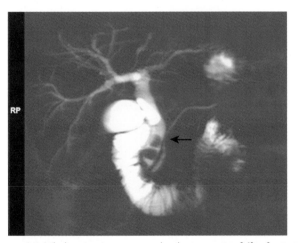

FIGURE 8-58 Magnetic resonance cholangiopancreatography demonstrating **bile duct stones** *(arrow)*. *(From Yeo CJ: Shackelford's Surgery of the Alimentary Tract, 6th ed. Philadelphia, Saunders, 2007.)*

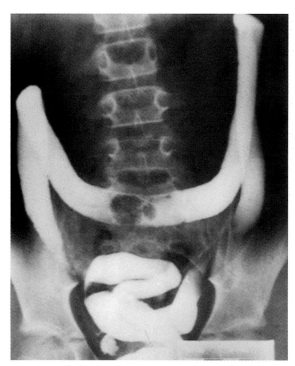

FIGURE 8-59 Barium enema radiograph from a 17-year-old girl with **chronic ulcerative colitis.** Note the shortening of the colon and loss of haustral markings, which give the colon a characteristic "lead pipe" appearance. *(From Grosfeld JL, O'Neill JA, Coran AG, Fonkalsrud EW: Pediatric Surgery, 6th ed. Philadelphia, Mosby, 2006.)*

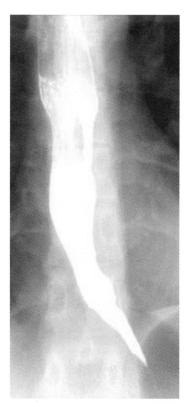

FIGURE 8-60 Characteristic upper gastrointestinal radiography in **achalasia,** with a distal tapered narrowing, the so-called "bird's beak" deformity. *(From Cameron JL, Cameron AM: Current Surgical Therapy, 10th ed. Philadelphia, Churchill Livingstone, 2011.)*

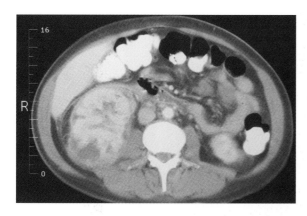

FIGURE 8-61 Acute pyelonephritis—contrast-enhanced CT scan. The heterogeneous CT nephrogram shows the diffuse involvement of the right kidney. There is stranding and some fluid seen in the perinephritic space with thickening of Gerota fascia. *(From Brenner BM: Brenner and Rector's The Kidney, 8th ed. Philadelphia, Saunders, 2008.)*

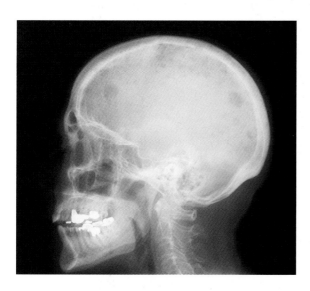

FIGURE 8-62 Osteolytic lesions in the skull on plain radiograph in a patient with **multiple myeloma.** *(From Abeloff MD, Armitage JO, Niederhuber JE, et al: Abeloff's Clinical Oncology, 4th ed. Philadelphia, Churchill Livingstone, 2008.)*

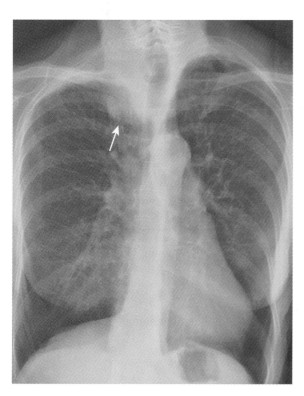

FIGURE 8-63 Pancoast tumor. This woman presented with deep shoulder pain. The PA radiograph of the chest, obtained after radiographs of the shoulder suggested an apical mass, confirmed a mass in the apex of the lung *(arrow)* with destruction of the underlying bone. *(From Weissman BNW: Imaging of Arthritis and Metabolic Bone Disease. Philadelphia, Mosby, 2009.)*

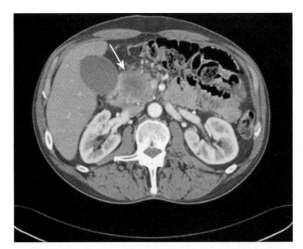

FIGURE 8-64 A 67-year-old woman with **pancreatic cancer.** Axial-view, contrast-enhanced CT shows a low-density mass *(arrow)* arising from pancreatic head and encasing or abutting the superior mesenteric vein. *(From Gunderson LL, Tepper JE: Clinical Radiation Oncology, 2nd ed. Philadelphia, Churchill Livingstone, 2007.)*

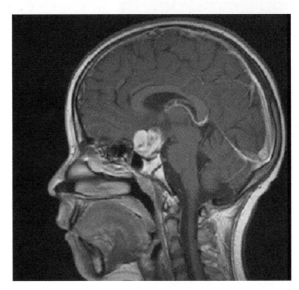

FIGURE 8-65 Sagittal view of a hypothalmic–optic pathway **glioma.** *(From Adam A, Dixon AK, Grainger RG, Allison DJ: Grainger & Allison's Diagnostic Radiology, 5th ed. Philadelphia, Churchill Livingstone, 2008.)*

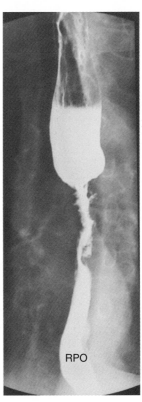

FIGURE 8-66 Barium contrast study showing a **midesophageal tumor.** Tumor stenosis with proximal dilatation of the esophagus is evident. *(From Yeo CJ: Shackelford's Surgery of the Alimentary Tract, 6th ed. Philadelphia, Saunders, 2007.)*

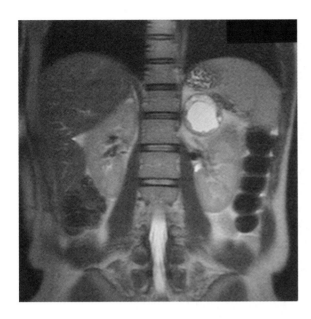

FIGURE 8-67 Appearance of **pheochromocytoma** on anatomic imaging. Coronal T$_2$-weighted magnetic resonance image (MRI) demonstrating a left adrenal pheochromocytoma with central cystic change. *(From Townsend CM, Beauchamp RD, Evers M, Mattox KL: Sabiston Textbook of Surgery, 18th ed. Philadelphia, Saunders, 2008.)*

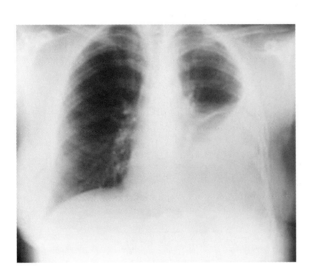

FIGURE 8-68 Posteroanterior chest radiograph showing **pleural effusion** in the left lung. The fluid fills about half of the left hemithorax. *(From Cleveland Clinic: Current Clinical Medicine, 2nd ed. Philadelphia, Saunders, 2010.)*

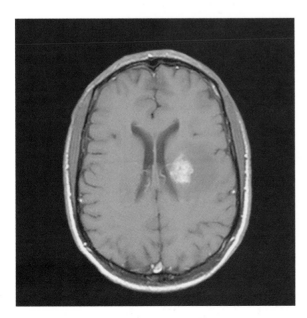

FIGURE 8-69 Brain magnetic resonance images of a 38-year-old man with **acquired immunodeficiency syndrome** and ***Toxoplasma* encephalitis.** The T$_1$-weighted image after gadolinium injection shows a large enhancing lesion in the left frontal lobe. *(From Mandell GL, Bennet JE, Dolin R: Mandell, Douglas, and Bennett's Principles and Practice of Infectious Diseases, 7th ed. Philadelphia, Churchill Livingstone, 2010.)*

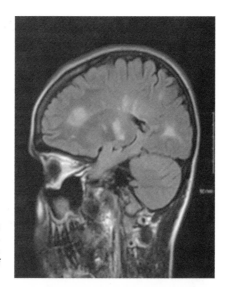

FIGURE 8-70 Multiple sclerosis. Sagittal FLAIR image magnetic resonance scan shows multiple lesions in corpus callosum (periventricular and perpendicular to corpus callosum, known as "Dawson's fingers") along with lesions in right frontal, occipital lobes. *(From Ferri FF: Ferri's Clinical Advisor 2012. Philadelphia, Mosby, 2012.)*

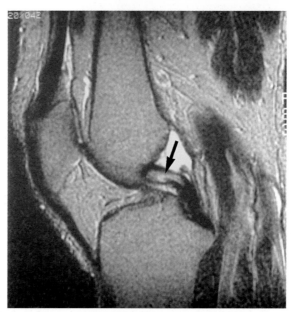

FIGURE 8-71 Posterior cruciate ligament tear. Sagittal T_2-weighted image shows abnormal bright signal *(arrow)* within normally dark posterior cruciate ligament. Fluid is also seen around proximal extent of partially torn posterior cruciate ligament. *(From Canale ST, Beaty JH: Campbell's Operative Orthopaedics, 11th ed. Philadelphia, Mosby, 2008.)*

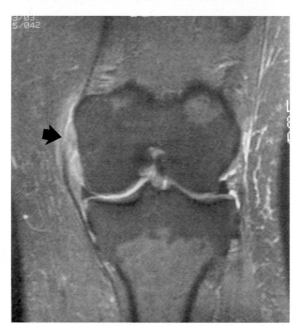

FIGURE 8-72 Medial collateral ligament tear. Complete disruption of proximal medial collateral ligament *(arrow)* is shown in coronal fat-suppressed, proton density–weighted image. *(From Canale ST, Beaty JH: Campbell's Operative Orthopaedics, 11th ed. Philadelphia, Mosby, 2008.)*

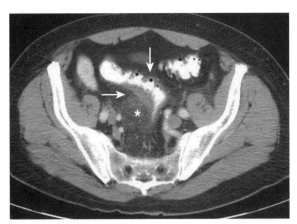

FIGURE 8-73 Diverticulitis. Computed tomography (CT) image demonstrates thickened wall of the sigmoid colon *(arrows)* with stranding in the adjacent fat *(*)*. *(From McNally PR: GI/Liver Secrets Plus, 4th ed., Philadelphia, Mosby, 2010.)*

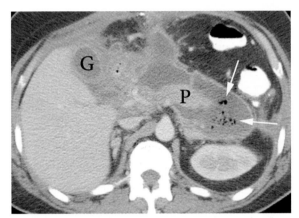

FIGURE 8-74 Acute necrotizing pancreatitis. Contrast-enhanced computed tomography (CT) scan that shows the pancreas (P) is surrounded by peripancreatic inflammation that contains bubbles of air *(arrows)* due to sterile necrosis. G, Gallbladder. *(From Feldman M, Friedman LS, Brandt LJ: Sleisenger and Fordtran's Gastrointestinal and Liver Disease, 8th ed. Philadelphia, Saunders, 2006.)*

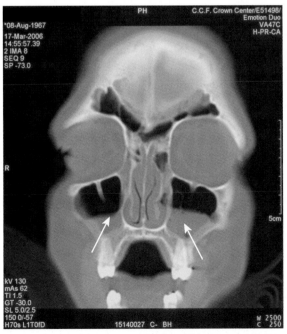

FIGURE 8-75 Computed tomography scan showing **acute sinusitis.** Note the fluid levels in the maxillary sinuses *(arrows)*. *(From Cleveland Clinic: Current Clinical Medicine, 2nd ed. Philadelphia, Saunders, 2010.)*

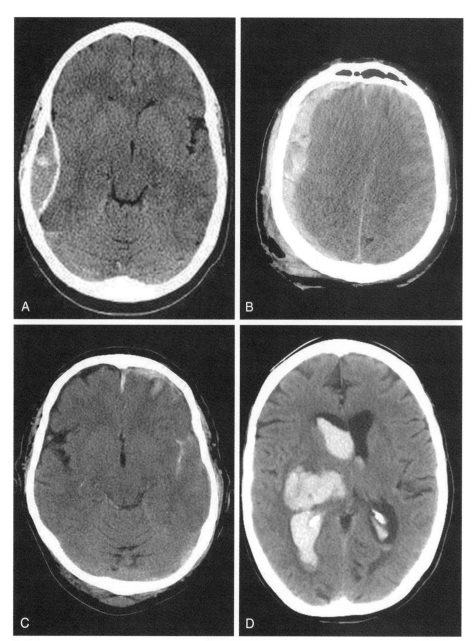

FIGURE 8-76 Computed tomographic scans of **intracranial hemorrhage. A**, Epidural hematoma; **B**, subdural hematoma; **C**, subarachnoid hematoma; **D**, intracerebral hematoma. *(From DeLee JC, Drez D, Miller MD: DeLee and Drez's Orthopaedic Sports Medicine, 3rd ed. Philadelphia, Saunders, 2009.)*

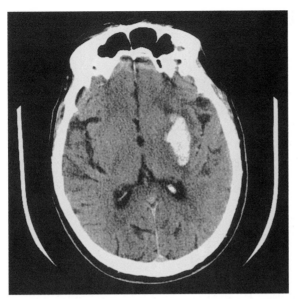

FIGURE 8-77 Computed tomography (CT) scan of the head showing **hemorrhage of the left basal ganglia.** *(From Layon J, Gabrielli A, Friedman W: Textbook of Neurointensive Care. Philadelphia, Saunders, 2004.)*

PATHOLOGY AND MICROSCOPY IMAGES

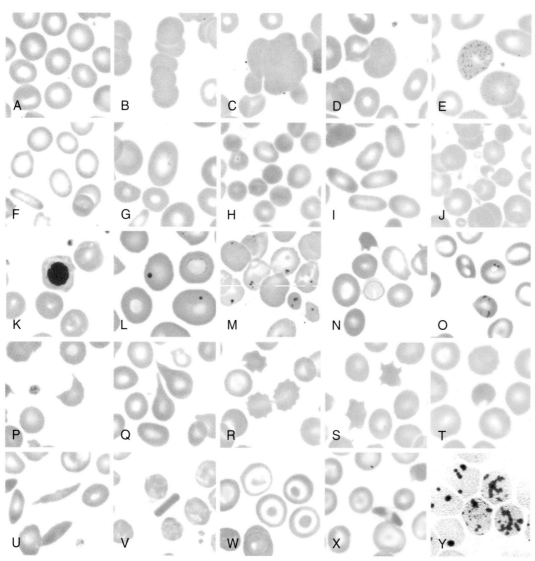

FIGURE 8-78 Classic red blood cell (RBC) morphology features and associated diseases. **A,** Normal RBCs. **B,** Rouleaux formation—multiple myeloma. **C,** Agglutination—cold agglutinin disease. **D,** Polychromasia—equivalent to a reticulocyte. **E,** Basophilic stippling—lead poisoning, thalassemia. **F,** Hypochromic microcytic cells—iron deficiency anemia. Note the widened central pallor and the "pencil" cell in lower left. **G,** Macrocytes—megaloblastic anemia (vitamin B_{12}, folate deficiency) or myelodysplastic syndrome. **H,** Spherocytes—hereditary spherocytosis. **I,** Elliptocytes—hereditary elliptocytosis. **J,** RBC fragments in a burn patient. **K,** Nucleated RBC marrow stress. **L,** Howell-Jolly bodies—splenic dysfunction or absence. **M,** Pappenheimer bodies—sideroblastic anemia. **N,** Cabot ring—megaloblastic anemia or MDS. **O,** Malarial parasites (*Plasmodium falciparum*). **P,** Schistocyte—TTP, DIC. **Q,** Tear drop cell—myelofibrosis. **R,** Echinocyte (burr cell)—uremia. **S,** Acanthocyte (spur cell)—abetalipoproteinemia, liver disease, artifact. **T,** "Bite" cell—G6PD deficiency. **U,** Sickle cell—sickle cell anemia. **V,** Hemoglobin C crystal. **W,** Target cells—liver disease, thalassemia, hemoglobin C disease. **X,** Hemoglobin SC. Note RBC in center has condensed hemoglobin at each pole. **Y,** Heinz body preparation (supravital stain) from a patient with G6PD deficiency. See Plate 30. *(From Hoffman R, Furie B, Benz EJ, et al: Hematology, 5th ed. Philadelphia, Churchill Livingstone, 2009.)*

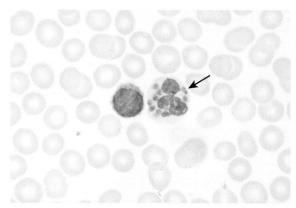

FIGURE 8-79 Neutrophil and lymphocyte from a patient with **Chédiak-Higashi syndrome.** Note the large dysmorphic cytoplasmic granules *(arrow)*. See Plate 31. *(From Mandell GL, Bennett JE, Dolin R: Mandell, Douglas, and Bennett's Principles and Practice of Infectious Diseases, 7th ed. Philadelphia, Churchill Livingstone, 2010.)*

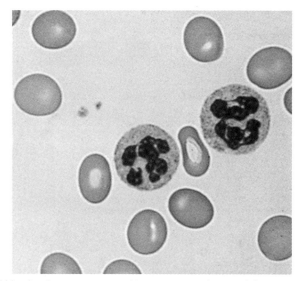

FIGURE 8-80 Peripheral blood with macrocytosis and hypersegmented neutrophils in **megaloblastic anemia.** See Plate 32. *(From Goldman L, Schafer AI: Goldman's Cecil Medicine, 24th ed. Philadelphia, Saunders, 2012.)*

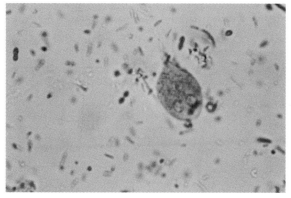

FIGURE 8-81 *Giardia lamblia* trophozoite seen by methylene blue wet mount staining under oil (×1000). The finding of cysts or trophozoites in a patient with diarrhea is sufficient to make a tentative diagnosis of giardiasis. See Plate 33. *(From Auerbach PS: Wilderness Medicine, 5th ed. Philadelphia, Mosby, 2007.)*

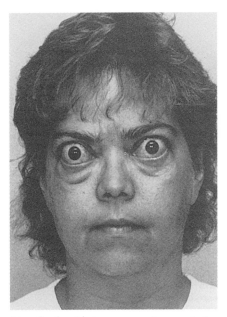

FIGURE 8-82 India ink preparations from cerebrospinal fluid of patient with **cryptococcal meningitis.** Note the encapsulated yeasts. See Plate 34. *(From Mandell GL, Bennett JE, Dolin R: Mandell, Douglas, and Bennett's Principles and Practice of Infectious Diseases, 7th ed. Philadelphia, Churchill Livingstone, 2010.)*

GROSS PHOTOGRAPHS AND OTHER IMAGES

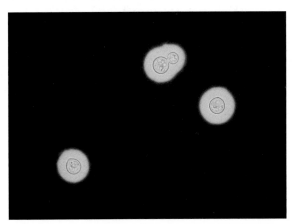

FIGURE 8-83 Graves disease: Note the thyroid stare, asymmetry, proptosis, and periorbital edema. *(From Ferri FF: Ferri's Clinical Advisor 2012. Philadelphia, Mosby, 2012.)*

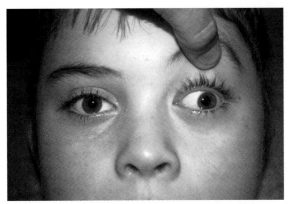

FIGURE 8-84 Third cranial nerve palsy of the left eye. See Plate 35. *(From Kliegman RM, Stanton BMD, St. Geme J, et al: Nelson Textbook of Pediatrics, 19th ed. Philadelphia, Saunders, 2011.)*

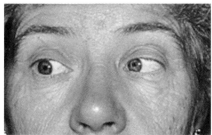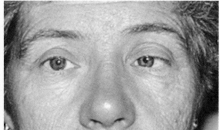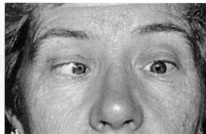

FIGURE 8-85 Left **sixth cranial nerve paresis.** Note the poor movement of the left eye in left gaze. See Plate 36. *(From Palay DA, Krachmer JH: Primary Care Ophthalmology, 2nd ed. Philadelphia, Mosby, 2005.)*

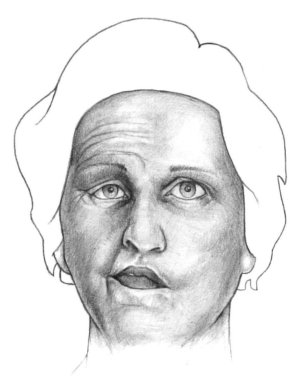

FIGURE 8-86 Bell's palsy (facial nerve palsy). Note unwrinkled forehead, widely opened eyes (with weakness of eyelid color), flattening of the nasolabial fold, and a droop of the corner of the mouth. *(From Remmel KS, Bunyan R, Brumback RA, et al: Handbook of symptom-oriented neurology, 3rd ed. St Louis, Mosby, 2002.)*

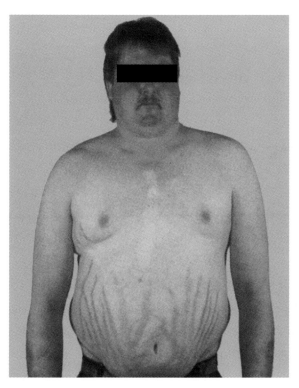

FIGURE 8-87 A patient with **Cushing syndrome** demonstrating central obesity, "moon facies," and abdominal striae. See Plate 37. *(Reproduced with permission from Lloyd RV, Douglas BR, Young WF, et al: Atlas of Nontumor Pathology: Endocrine Diseases. Washington, DC, American Registry of Pathology, 2002.)*

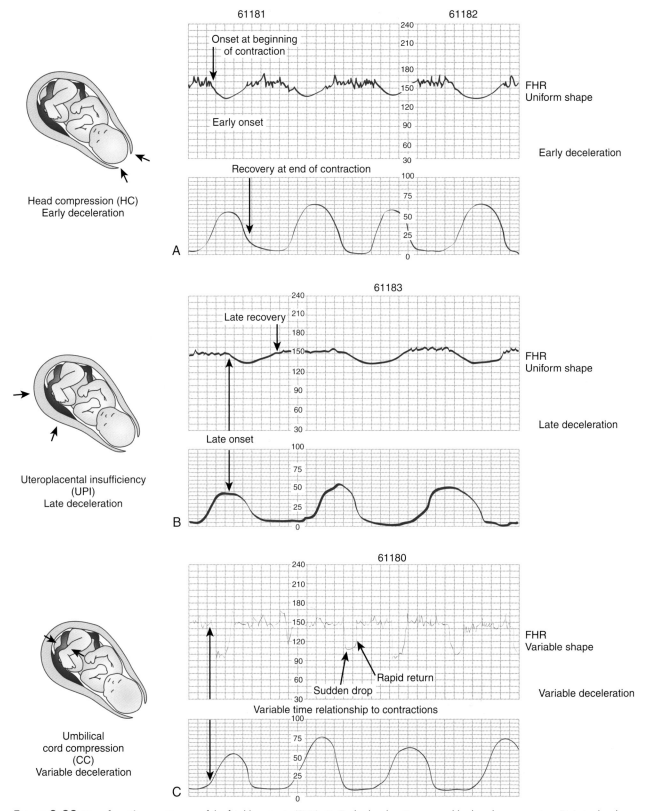

FIGURE 8-88 Deceleration patterns of the fetal heart rate (FHR). **A,** Early deceleration caused by head compression. **B,** Late deceleration caused by uteroplacental insufficiency. **C,** Variable deceleration caused by cord compression. *(From Marx J, Hockberger R, Walls R: Rosen's Emergency Medicine: Concepts and Clinical Practice, 7th ed. Philadelphia, Mosby, 2009.)*

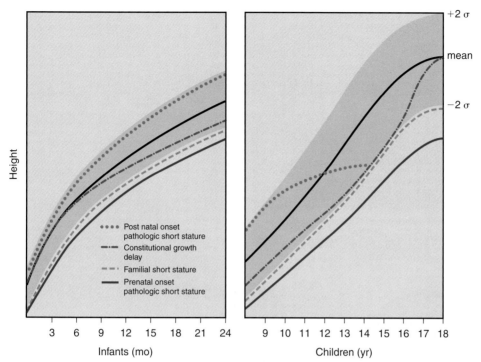

FIGURE 8-89 Height-for-age curves for the four general causes of proportional short stature: postnatal onset pathologic short stature, constitutional growth delay, familial short stature, and prenatal onset short stature. *(From Kliegman RM, Stanton BMD, St. Geme J, et al: Nelson Textbook of Pediatrics, 19th ed. Philadelphia, Saunders, 2011.)*

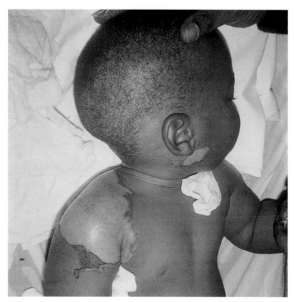

FIGURE 8-90 Burns in young children are often due to **child abuse,** especially if they are in atypical places. Although the body surface area of this burn is relatively small, the patient's age and the burn's location, coupled with the possibility of child abuse, require that this child be hospitalized. See Plate 38. *(From Roberts JR, Hedges JR: Clinical Procedures in Emergency Medicine, 5th ed. Philadelphia, Saunders, 2009.)*

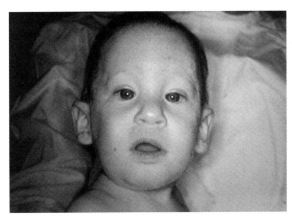

FIGURE 8-91 Infant with **fetal alcohol syndrome.** Note short palpebral fissures, mild ptosis, nostrils, smooth philtral area, and narrow vermilion of the upper lip. See Plate 39. *(From Gilbert-Barness E, Kapur RP, Oligny LL, Siebert JR: Potter's Pathology of the Fetus, Infant and Child, 2nd ed. Philadelphia, Mosby, 2007.)*

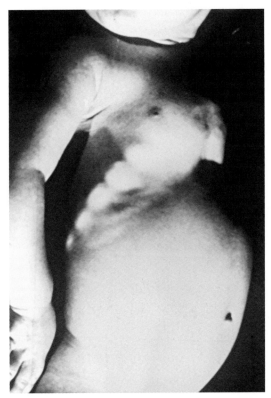

FIGURE 8-92 Rachitic rosary in a young infant with **rickets.** *(From Kliegman RM, Stanton BMD, St. Geme J, et al: Nelson Textbook of Pediatrics, 19th ed. Philadelphia, Saunders, 2011.)*

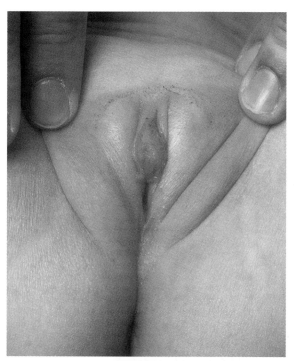

FIGURE 8-93 Ambiguous genitalia in a female infant. Virilization of the genitals, with an enlarged clitoris and fusion of the labia, can be seen. The underlying disorder was the 21-hydroxylase deficiency form of **congenital adrenal hyperplasia.** See Plate 40. *(From Wales JKH, Wit JM, Rogol AD: Pediatric Endocrinology and Growth, 2nd ed. Philadelphia, Saunders, 2003.)*

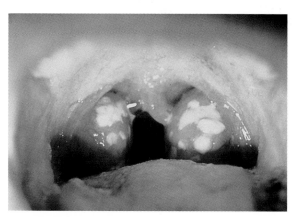

FIGURE 8-94 Acute streptococcal pharyngitis. Pus is present in the tonsillar crypts, and some palatal petechiae are evident. See Plate 41. *(From Forbes CD, Jackson WF: Color Atlas and Text of Clinical Medicine, 3rd ed. London, Mosby, 2003.)*

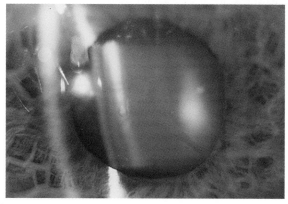

FIGURE 8-95 Age-related **cataract.** See Plate 42. *(From Yanoff M, Duker JS: Ophthalmology, 3rd ed. Philadelphia, Mosby, 2009.)*

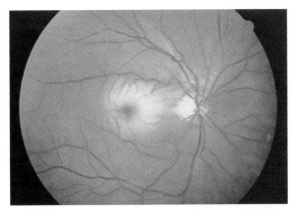

FIGURE 8-96 **Central retinal artery occlusion.** Note the cherry-red spot in the center of the macula, with surrounding whitening of the retina. See Plate 43. *(From Bradley WG, Daroff RB, Fenichel G, Jankovic J: Neurology in Clinical Practice, 5th ed. Philadelphia, Butterworth-Heinemann, 2008.)*

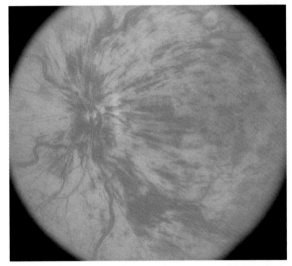

FIGURE 8-97 **Central retinal vein occlusion.** Note the dramatic retinal hemorrhages in all four quadrants. The veins are dilated and tortuous. The optic disc is blurred with blood from peripapillary hemorrhage. See Plate 44. *(From Palay DA, Krachmer JH: Primary Care Ophthalmology, 2nd ed. Philadelphia, Mosby, 2005.)*

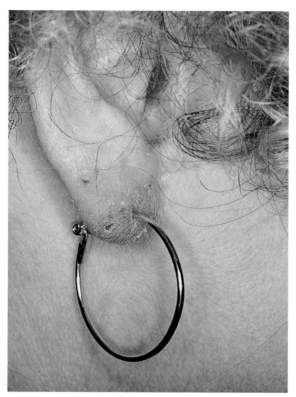

PLATE 1 Nickel dermatitis, the most common form of contact dermatitis in women, from nickel earrings. See Figure 8-1. *(From Habif TP: Clinical Dermatology, 5th ed. Philadelphia, Mosby, 2010.)*

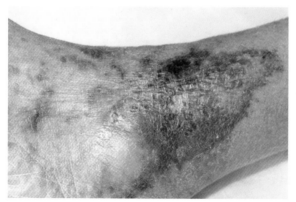

PLATE 2 Stasis dermatitis typically occurs on the lateral aspects of the shins. See Figure 8-2. *(From Cleveland Clinic: Current Clinical Medicine, 2nd ed. Philadelphia, Saunders, 2010.)*

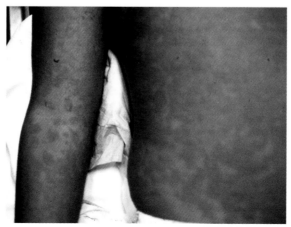

PLATE 3 Staphylococcal toxic shock syndrome showing diffuse erythrodermic rash. See Figure 8-3. *(From Baren JM, Rothrock SG, Brennan J, Brown L: Pediatric Emergency Medicine. Philadelphia, Saunders, 2008.)*

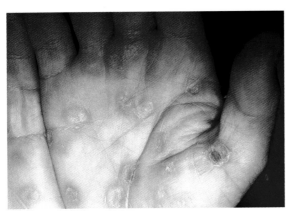

PLATE 4 Secondary syphilis: palmar lesions of secondary syphilis. See Figure 8-4. *(From Mandell GL, Bennett JE, Dolin R: Mandell, Douglas, and Bennett's Principles and Practice of Infectious Diseases, 7th ed. Philadelphia, Churchill Livingstone, 2010.)*

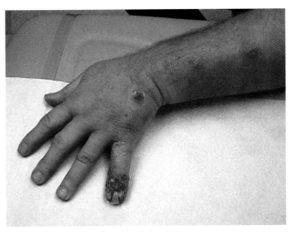

PLATE 5 Sporotrichosis of the fifth finger in a gardener. Three nodular lesions are visible on the hand and arm. See Figure 8-5. *(From Mandell GL, Bennett JE, Dolin R: Mandell, Douglas, and Bennett's Principles and Practice of Infectious Diseases, 7th ed. Philadelphia, Churchill Livingstone, 2010.)*

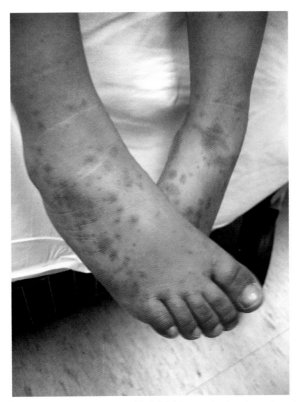

PLATE 6 Henoch-Schönlein purpura in a 7-year-old child. Note typical red-purple rash on the lower extremities. See Figure 8-6. *(From Marx J, Hockberger R, Walls R: Rosen's Emergency Medicine, 7th ed. Philadelphia, Mosby, 2010.)*

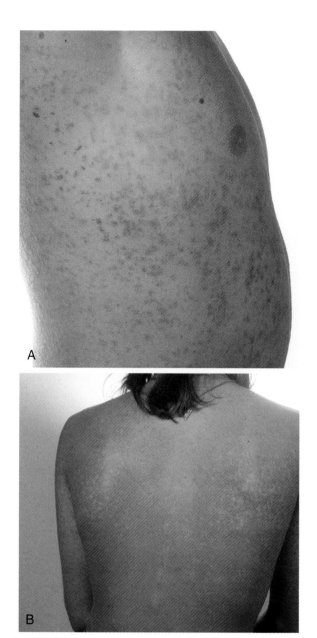

PLATE 7 Morbilliform drug rash secondary to amoxicillin. Adolescents (**A**, **B**) with Epstein-Barr virus mononucleosis who received amoxicillin and developed diffuse erythematous raised rashes. Note predominance on trunk and coalescence (**B**). See Figure 8-7. *(From Long SS, Pickering LK, Prober CG: Principles and Practice of Pediatric Infectious Diseases Revised Reprint, 3rd ed. Philadelphia, Saunders, 2009.)*

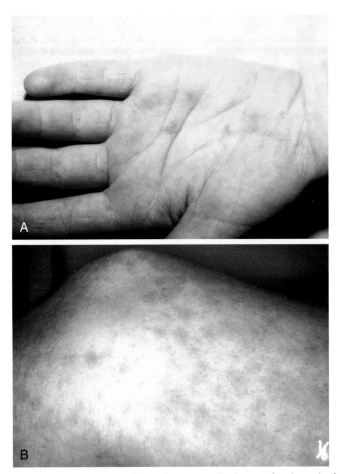

PLATE 8 Rocky Mountain spotted fever rash. A, The wrist and palm manifest the rash of Rocky Mountain spotted fever with central petechiae in some of the maculopapules. **B,** Early petechial rash on arm. See Figure 8-8. *(From Mandell GL, Bennett JE, Dolin R: Mandell, Douglas, and Bennett's Principles and Practice of Infectious Diseases, 7th ed. Philadelphia, Churchill Livingstone, 2010.)*

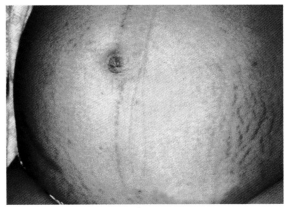

PLATE 9 Linea nigra. Hyperpigmentation of the linea alba and stretchmarks (striae gravidarum) on the lateral aspects of the abdomen. See Figure 8-9. *(From James DK, Steer PJ, Weiner CP, Gonik B: High Risk Pregnancy, 4th ed. Philadelphia, Saunders, 2011.)*

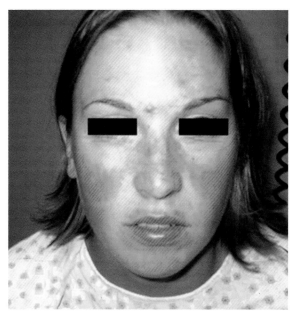

Plate 10 Melasma involving the cheeks, nose, upper lip, and forehead. See Figure 8-10. *(From Gabbe SG, Simpson JL, Niebyl JR, et al: Obstetrics: Normal and Problem Pregnancies, 5th ed. Philadelphia, Churchill Livingstone, 2007.)*

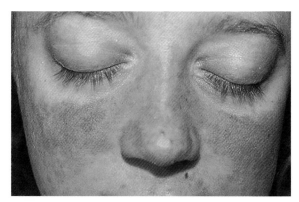

Plate 11 Malar rash of systemic lupus erythematous. See Figure 8-11. *(From Stern TA, Rosengaum AF, Fava M, et al: Massachusetts General Hospital Comprehensive Clinical Psychiatry. Philadelphia, Mosby, 2008.)*

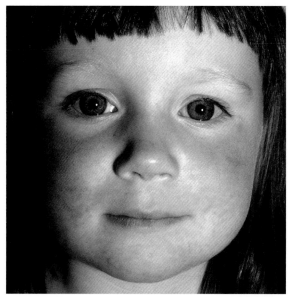

Plate 12 Erythema infectiosum. Facial erythema "slapped cheek." The red plaque covers the cheek and spares the nasolabial fold and the circumoral region. See Figure 8-12. *(From Habif TP: Clinical Dermatology, 5th ed. Philadelphia, Mosby, 2010.)*

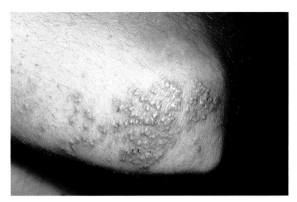

PLATE 13 **Cutaneous xanthomata** on the extensor surface of the elbow. Other classic and common locations include the knee and over the Achilles tendon. Most are located along tendons and extensor surfaces of joints. See Figure 8-13. *(From Kanski J: Clinical Diagnosis in Ophthalmology. Philadelphia, Mosby, 2006.)*

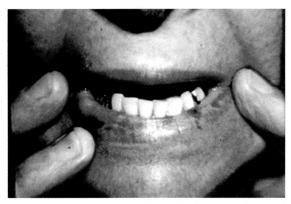

PLATE 14 Mucocutaneous pigmentation in a patient with **Peutz-Jeghers syndrome.** See Figure 8-14. *(From Feldman M, Friedman LS, Brandt LJ: Sleisenger and Fordtran's Gastrointestinal and Liver Disease, 9th ed. Philadelphia, Saunders, 2011.)*

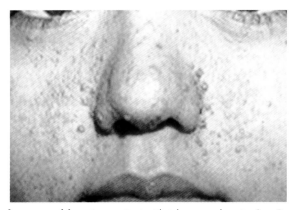

PLATE 15 **Adenoma sebaceum** of face in a patient with tuberous sclerosis. See Figure 8-15. *(From Yanoff M, Duker JS: Ophthalmology, 3rd ed. Philadelphia, Mosby, 2009.)*

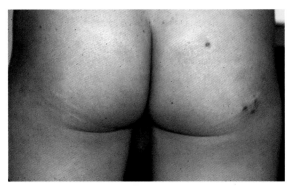

PLATE 16 Patches of **mycosis fungoides** often arise on double-clothed areas, and the lesions may recede with light exposure. See Figure 8-16. *(From Jaffe ES, Harris NL, Vardiman JW, et al: Hematopathology. Philadelphia, Saunders, 2011.)*

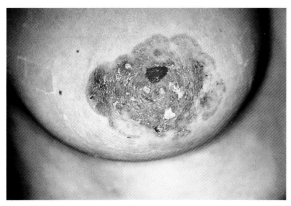

Plate 17 Paget's disease of the breast. Note the erythematous plaques around the nipple. See Figure 8-17. *(From Callen JP: Dermatologic signs of systemic disease. In Bolognia JL, Jorizzo JL, Rapini RP [eds]: Dermatology. Edinburgh, Mosby, 2003, p 714.)*

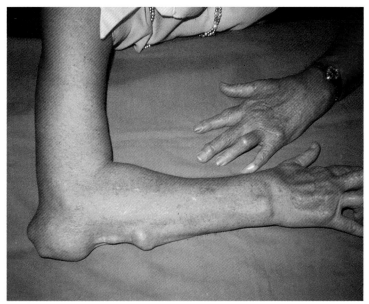

Plate 18 Rheumatoid nodules in the olecranon bursa and on subcutaneous surface of ulna. See Figure 8-18. *(From Canale ST, Beaty JH: Campbell's Operative Orthopaedics, 11th ed. Philadelphia, Mosby, 2008.)*

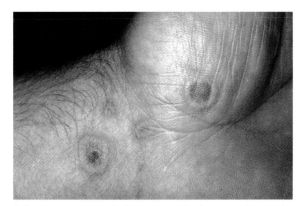

Plate 19 Erythema multiforme—target or "bull's-eye" annular lesions with central vesicles and bullae are characteristic. See Figure 8-19. *(From Goldman L, Schafer AI: Goldman's Cecil Medicine, 24th ed. Philadelphia, Saunders, 2012.)*

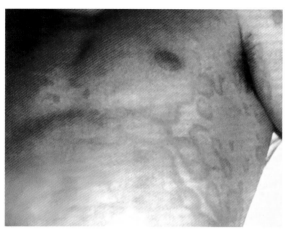

PLATE 20 Rash of **erythema marginatum** in an adolescent boy with acute rheumatic fever occurred with its characteristic serpiginous and erythematous margins are evident. See Figure 8-20. *(From Cassidy JT, Petty RE, Laxer R, Lindsley C: Textbook of Pediatric Rheumatology, 6th ed. Philadelphia, Saunders, 2011.)*

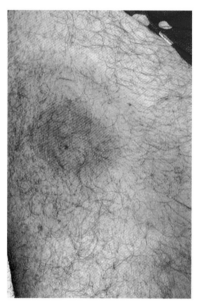

PLATE 21 The pathognomonic bull's eye rash of **erythema migrans**. This is the characteristic rash of Lyme disease. See Figure 8-21. *(From Cleveland Clinic: Current Clinical Medicine, 2nd ed. Philadelphia, Saunders, 2010.)*

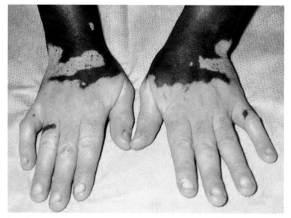

PLATE 22 Vitiligo on the hands. See Figure 8-22. *(From Cleveland Clinic: Current Clinical Medicine, 2nd ed. Philadelphia, Saunders, 2010.)*

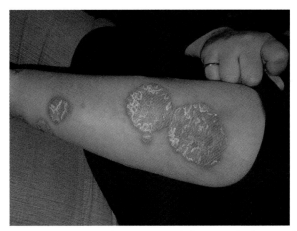

PLATE 23 Psoriasis demonstrating typical well-demarcated, red plaques with silvery scales. See Figure 8-23. *(From Rakel RE, Rakel D: Textbook of Family Medicine, 8th ed. Philadelphia, Saunders, 2011.)*

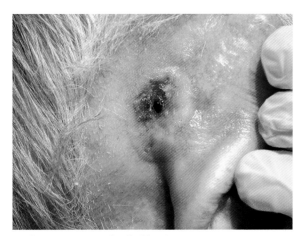

PLATE 24 Ulcerated **basal cell carcinoma** with rolled borders on posterior ear. See Figure 8-24. *(From Abeloff MD, Armitage JO, Niederhuber JE, et al: Abeloff's Clinical Oncology, 4th ed. Philadelphia, Churchill Livingstone, 2008.)*

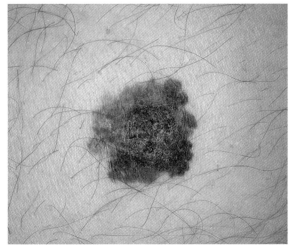

PLATE 25 Superficial spreading **melanoma.** This 2-cm diameter melanoma developed over a 2-year period. See Figure 8-25. *(From Townsend CM, Beauchamp D, Evers BM, Mattox KL: Sabiston Textbook of Surgery, 18th ed. Philadelphia, Saunders, 2008.)*

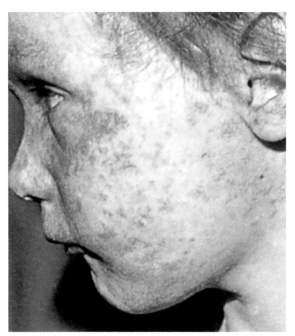

PLATE 26 Rash of **rubella** typically begins on the face and neck as small, irregular pink macules that coalesce, and it spreads centrifugally to involve the torso and extremities. See Figure 8-26. *(From Kliegman RM, Stanton BMD, St. Geme J, et al: Nelson Textbook of Pediatrics, 19th ed. Philadelphia, Saunders, 2011.)*

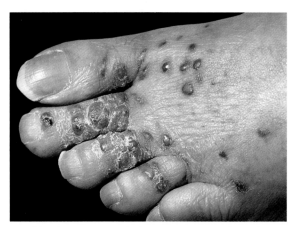

PLATE 27 Kaposi sarcoma. Most lesions are on the lower extremities. Shown here are plaques and tumors. See Figure 8-27. *(From Habif TP: Clinical Dermatology, 5th ed. Philadelphia, Mosby, 2010.)*

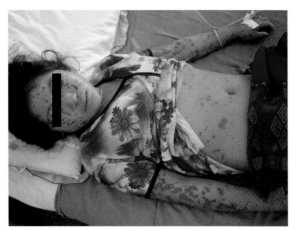

Plate 28 Classic rash of patient with **meningococcemia.** See Figure 8-28. *(From Cleveland Clinic: Current Clinical Medicine, 2nd ed. Philadelphia, Saunders, 2010.)*

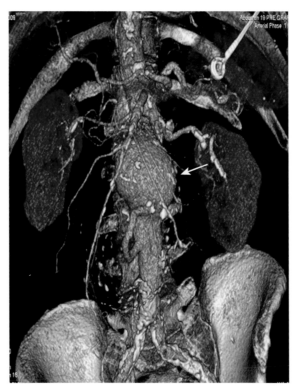

Plate 29 Three-dimensional reconstruction of a computed tomography (CT) scan in a patient with an infrarenal **abdominal aortic aneurysm** *(arrow)* See Figure 8-57. *(From Bonow RO, Mann DL, Zipes DP, Libby P: Braunwald's Heart Disease—A Textbook of Cardiovascular Medicine, 9th ed. Philadelphia, Saunders, 2012.)*

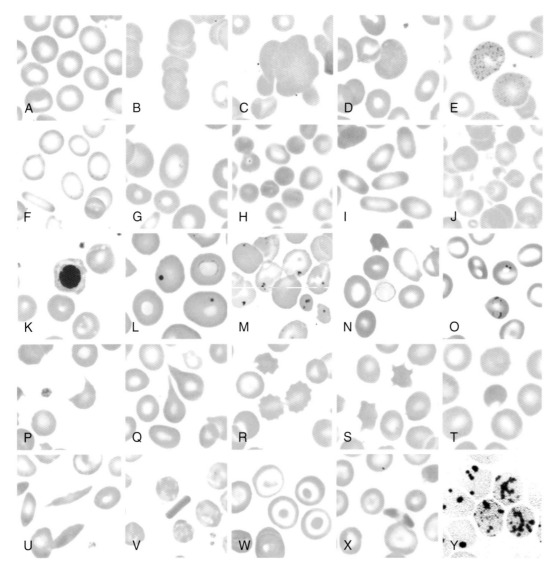

PLATE 30 Classic red blood cell (RBC) morphology features and associated diseases. **A,** Normal RBCs. **B,** Rouleaux formation—multiple myeloma. **C,** Agglutination—cold agglutinin disease. **D,** Polychromasia—equivalent to a reticulocyte. **E,** Basophilic stippling—lead poisoning, thalassemia. **F,** Hypochromic microcytic cells—iron deficiency anemia. Note the widened central pallor and the "pencil" cell in lower left. **G,** Macrocytes—megaloblastic anemia (vitamin B_{12}, folate deficiency) or myelodysplastic syndrome. **H,** Spherocytes—hereditary spherocytosis. **I,** Elliptocytes—hereditary elliptocytosis. **J,** RBC fragments in a burn patient. **K,** Nucleated RBC marrow stress. **L,** Howell-Jolly bodies—splenic dysfunction or absence. **M,** Pappenheimer bodies—sideroblastic anemia. **N,** Cabot ring—megaloblastic anemia or MDS. **O,** Malarial parasites (*Plasmodium falciparum*). **P,** Schistocyte—TTP, DIC. **Q,** Tear drop cell—myelofibrosis. **R,** Echinocyte (burr cell)—uremia. **S,** Acanthocyte (spur cell)—abetalipoproteinemia, liver disease, artifact. **T,** "Bite" cell—G6PD deficiency. **U,** Sickle cell—sickle cell anemia. **V,** Hemoglobin C crystal. **W,** Target cells—liver disease, thalassemia, hemoglobin C disease. **X,** Hemoglobin SC. Note RBC in center has condensed hemoglobin at each pole. **Y,** Heinz body preparation (supravital stain) from a patient with G6PD deficiency. See Figure 8-78. *(From Hoffman R, Furie B, Benz EJ, et al: Hematology, 5th ed. Philadelphia, Churchill Livingstone, 2009.)*

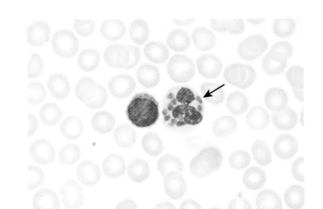

PLATE 31 Neutrophil and lymphocyte from a patient with **Chédiak-Higashi syndrome.** Note the large dysmorphic cytoplasmic granules *(arrow)*. See Figure 8-79. *(From Mandell GL, Bennett JE, Dolin R: Mandell, Douglas, and Bennett's Principles and Practice of Infectious Diseases, 7th ed. Philadelphia, Churchill Livingstone, 2010.)*

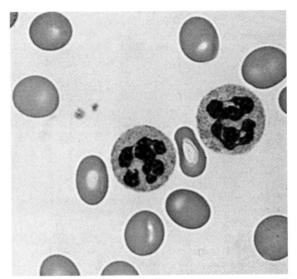

PLATE 32 Peripheral blood with macrocytosis and hypersegmented neutrophils in **megaloblastic anemia.** See Figure 8-80. *(From Goldman L, Schafer AI: Goldman's Cecil Medicine, 24th ed. Philadelphia, Saunders, 2012.)*

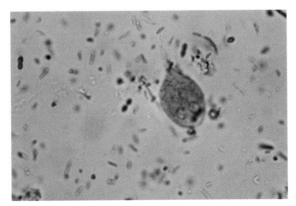

PLATE 33 *Giardia lamblia* trophozoite seen by methylene blue wet mount staining under oil (×1000). The finding of cysts or trophozoites in a patient with diarrhea is sufficient to make a tentative diagnosis of giardiasis. See Figure 8-81. *(From Auerbach PS: Wilderness Medicine, 5th ed. Philadelphia, Mosby, 2007.)*

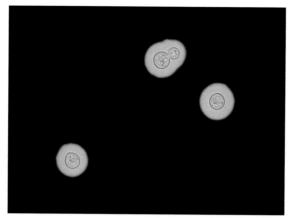

PLATE 34 India ink preparations from cerebrospinal fluid of patient with **cryptococcal meningitis.** Note the encapsulated yeasts. See Figure 8-82. *(From Mandell GL, Bennett JE, Dolin R: Mandell, Douglas, and Bennett's Principles and Practice of Infectious Diseases, 7th ed. Philadelphia, Churchill Livingstone, 2010.)*

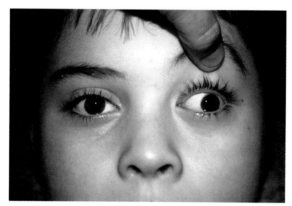

PLATE 35 Third cranial nerve palsy of the left eye. See Figure 8-84. *(From Kliegman RM, Stanton BMD, St. Geme J, et al: Nelson Textbook of Pediatrics, 19th ed. Philadelphia, Saunders, 2011.)*

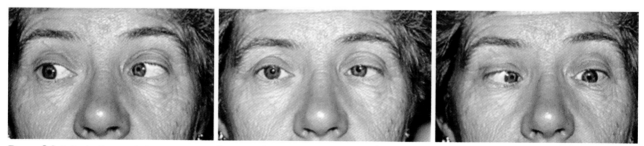

PLATE 36 Left **sixth cranial nerve paresis.** Note the poor movement of the left eye in left gaze. See Figure 8-85. *(From Palay DA, Krachmer JH: Primary Care Ophthalmology, 2nd ed. Philadelphia, Mosby, 2005.)*

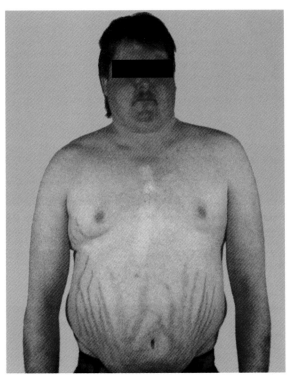

PLATE 37 A patient with **Cushing syndrome** demonstrating central obesity, "moon facies," and abdominal striae. See Figure 8-87. *(Reproduced with permission from Lloyd RV, Douglas BR, Young WF, et al: Atlas of Nontumor Pathology: Endocrine Diseases. Washington, DC, American Registry of Pathology, 2002.)*

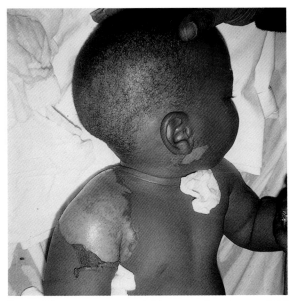

PLATE 38 Burns in young children are often due to **child abuse,** especially if they are in atypical places. Although the body surface area of this burn is relatively small, the patient's age and the burn's location, coupled with the possibility of child abuse, require that this child be hospitalized. See Figure 8-90. *(From Roberts JR, Hedges JR: Clinical Procedures in Emergency Medicine, 5th ed. Philadelphia, Saunders, 2009.)*

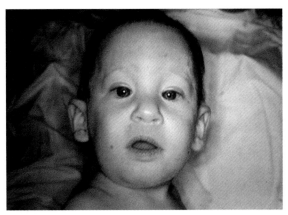

PLATE 39 Infant with **fetal alcohol syndrome.** Note short palpebral fissures, mild ptosis, nostrils, smooth philtral area, and narrow vermilion of the upper lip. See Figure 8-91. *(From Gilbert-Barness E, Kapur RP, Oligny LL, Siebert JR: Potter's Pathology of the Fetus, Infant and Child, 2nd ed. Philadelphia, Mosby, 2007.)*

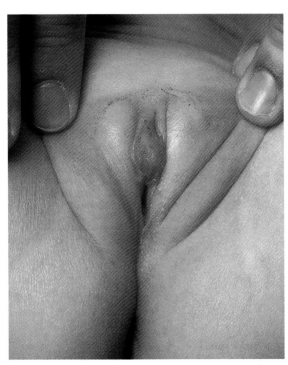

PLATE 40 Ambiguous genitalia in a female infant. Virilization of the genitals, with an enlarged clitoris and fusion of the labia, can be seen. The underlying disorder was the 21-hydroxylase deficiency form of **congenital adrenal hyperplasia.** See Figure 8-92. *(From Wales JKH, Wit JM, Rogol AD: Pediatric Endocrinology and Growth, 2nd ed. Philadelphia, Saunders, 2003.)*

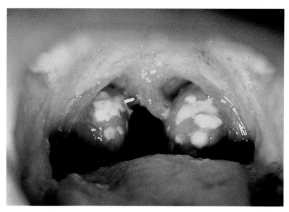

PLATE 41 Acute streptococcal pharyngitis. Pus is present in the tonsillar crypts, and some palatal petechiae are evident. See Figure 8-94. *(From Forbes CD, Jackson WF: Color Atlas and Text of Clinical Medicine, 3rd ed. London, Mosby, 2003.)*

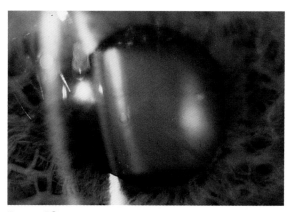

PLATE 42 Age-related **cataract.** See Figure 8-95. *(From Yanoff M, Duker JS: Ophthalmology, 3rd ed. Philadelphia, Mosby, 2009.)*

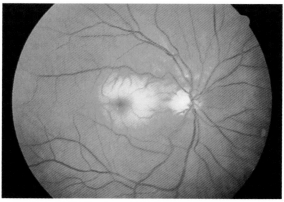

PLATE 43 Central retinal artery occlusion. Note the cherry-red spot in the center of the macula, with surrounding whitening of the retina. See Figure 8-96. *(From Bradley WG, Daroff RB, Fenichel G, Jankovic J: Neurology in Clinical Practice, 5th ed. Philadelphia, Butterworth-Heinemann, 2008.)*

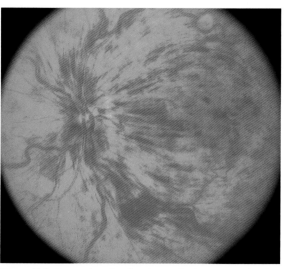

PLATE 44 Central retinal vein occlusion. Note the dramatic retinal hemorrhages in all four quadrants. The veins are dilated and tortuous. The optic disc is blurred with blood from peripapillary hemorrhage. See Figure 8-97. *(From Palay DA, Krachmer JH: Primary Care Ophthalmology, 2nd ed. Philadelphia, Mosby, 2005.)*

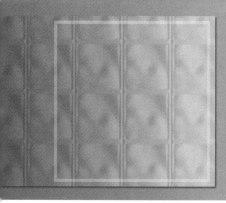

APPENDIX: ABBREVIATIONS

AAA	abdominal aortic aneurysm
Ab	antibody
ABC, ABCD, ABCDE	**a**irway, **b**reathing, **c**irculation, **d**isability, **e**xposure (trauma protocol)
ABG	arterial blood gas
ABO	blood types (A, B, AB, or O)
ACE	angiotensin-converting enzyme
ACL	anterior cruciate ligament
ACTH	adrenocorticotropic hormone
ACS	American Cancer Society
ADH	antidiuretic hormone
ADHD	attention-deficit hyperactivity disorder
AFP	alpha-fetoprotein
AIDS	acquired immunodeficiency syndrome
ALL	acute lymphoblastic leukemia
ALS	amyotrophic lateral sclerosis (aka Lou Gehrig disease)
ALT	alanine aminotransferase
AML	acute myeloid leukemia
ANA	antinuclear antibody
ANCA	antineutrophil cytoplasmic antibody
ANOVA	analysis of variance
ARDS	acute respiratory distress syndrome
ARF	acute renal failure
ASA	acetylsalicylic acid (aspirin)
ASD	atrial septal defect
AST	aspartate aminotransferase
ATG	antithymocyte globulin
AVM	arteriovenous malformation
AZT	azidothymidine (zidovudine)
B, β	beta
BP	blood pressure
BPH	benign prostatic hyperplasia/hypertrophy
BPP	biophysical profile
BT	bleeding time
BUN	blood urea nitrogen
C	centigrade (e.g., 37°C), complement (e.g., C1, C3, C4), or cervical (e.g., C5 vertebral body)
c-section	cesarean section
C of A	coarctation of the aorta
CA	cancer antigen (e.g., CA-125)
CAD	coronary artery disease
CBC	complete blood count
CD	cluster of differentiation (e.g., CD4$^+$, CD8$^+$)
CEA	carcinoembryonic antigen

CHD	coronary heart disease or congenital hip dysplasia
CHF	congestive heart failure
CK	creatine kinase
CLL	chronic lymphocytic leukemia
cm	centimeter
CML	chronic myelocytic (or myelogenous) leukemia
CMV	cytomegalovirus
CN	cranial nerve
CNS	central nervous system
CO	carbon monoxide or cardiac output
CO_2	carbon dioxide
COPD	chronic obstructive pulmonary disease
COX	cyclo oxygenase
CPD	cephalopelvic disproportion
Cr	creatinine
CRF	chronic renal failure
CSF	cerebrospinal fluid
CT	computed tomography scan
CVA	cerebrovascular accident (stroke)
CXR	chest x-ray
D&C	dilation and curettage
DDI	dideoxyinosine (HIV medication)
DES	diethylstilbestrol
DI	diabetes insipidus
DIC	disseminated intravascular coagulation
DIP	distal interphalangeal (joint)
DKA	diabetic ketoacidosis
dL	deciliter
DM	diabetes mellitus
DMSA	2,3-dimercaptosuccinic acid, succimer
DNA	deoxyribonucleic acid
DT	diphtheria and tetanus toxoids (age younger than 7)
DTaP	diphtheria, tetanus toxoids, and acellular pertussis vaccine
DTP	diphtheria, tetanus toxoids, and pertussis vaccine
DUB	dysfunctional uterine bleeding
DVT	deep venous thrombosis
EBV	Epstein-Barr virus
ECG	electrocardiogram
EDTA	edetate
EEG	electroencephalogram
ELISA	enzyme-linked immunosorbent assay
ELS	Eaton-Lambert syndrome
EMG	electromyography
ERCP	endoscopic retrograde cholangiopancreatography
ESR	erythrocyte sedimentation rate
F	fluoride or female
FAST	focused assessment with sonography for trauma
FDP	fibrin degradation products
Fe	iron
FEV	forced expiratory volume
FEV_1	forced expiratory volume in 1 second
FFP	fresh frozen plasma
FSH	follicle-stimulating hormone
FTA-ABS	fluorescent treponemal antibody-absorption test (for syphilis)
FVC	forced vital capacity
g, gm	gram

G6PD	glucose-6-phosphatase deficiency
GERD	gastroesophageal reflux disease
GGT	gamma-glutamyltranspeptidase
GI	gastrointestinal
GnRH	gonadotropin-releasing hormone
GU	genitourinary
GYN	gynecology or gynecologic
H$_2$	histamine type 2 receptor
H&P	history and physical examination
HAV	hepatitis A virus
HbA$_{1c}$	glycosylated hemoglobin
HBcAb/Ag	hepatitis B core antibody/antigen
HBeAb/Ag	hepatitis B "e" antibody/antigen
HBsAb/Ag	hepatitis B surface antibody/antigen
HBV	hepatitis B virus
HC	head circumference
HCG	human chorionic gonadotropin
HCV	hepatitis C virus
HDL	high-density lipoprotein
HELLP	**h**emolysis, **e**levated **l**iver enzymes, **l**ow **p**latelets (syndrome)
5-HIAA	5-hydroxyindoleacetic acid
HIV	human immunodeficiency virus
HLA	human leukocyte antigen
HPV	human papillomavirus
hr	hour/hours
HRT	hormone replacement therapy
HSP	Henoch-Schönlein purpura
HSV	herpes simplex virus
HTN	hypertension
HUS	hemolytic uremic syndrome
IBD	inflammatory bowel disease
IBS	irritable bowel syndrome
ICP	intracranial pressure
ICU	intensive care unit
Ig	immunoglobulin (e.g., IgA, IgM, IgG, IgE)
IIH	idiopathic intracranial hypertension
IL	interleukin (e.g., IL-2)
IM	intramuscular
IPV	inactivated poliovirus vaccine
IQ	intelligence quotient
IU	international units
IUD	intrauterine device
IUGR	intrauterine growth retardation
ITP	idiopathic thrombocytopenic purpura
IV	intravenous
IVC	inferior vena cava
IVF	intravenous fluid
IVP	intravenous pyelogram
K	potassium
kg	kilogram
KOH	potassium hydroxide
L	liter or lumbar (e.g., L5 nerve root)
LA	left atrium
LAE	left atrial enlargement
lb	pound
LCP	Legg-Calvé-Perthes disease

LDH	lactate dehydrogenase
LDL	low-density lipoprotein
LES	lower esophageal sphincter
LFT(s)	liver function test(s)
LGI	lower gastrointestinal (below the ligament of Treitz)
LH	luteinizing hormone
LLQ	left lower quadrant
LMN	lower motor neuron
LMP	last menstrual period
LR	lactated Ringer solution
L/S	lecithin-to-sphingomyelin ratio
LSD	lysergic acid diethylamide
LUQ	left upper quadrant
LV	left ventricle
LVH	left ventricular hypertrophy
M	male
MAI	*Mycobacterium avium-intracellulare* complex
MAOI	monoamine oxidase inhibitor
MCHC	mean corpuscular hemoglobin concentration
MCL	medial collateral ligament
MCP	metacarpophalangeal (hand joint)
MCV	mean corpuscular volume
MEN	multiple endocrine neoplasia
mg	milligram
MG	myasthenia gravis
MHA-TP	microhemagglutination assay for antibodies to *Treponema pallidum* (for syphilis)
MI	myocardial infarction
mL	milliliter
mm	millimeter
MMR	measles-mumps-rubella (vaccine)
mo	month/months
MRA	magnetic resonance angiography
MRI	magnetic resonance imaging
MRSA	methicillin-resistant *Staphylococcus aureus*
Na	sodium
NASH	nonalcoholic steatohepatitis
NPH	neutral protamine Hagedorn (isophane insulin suspension)
NPO	nothing by mouth
NPV	negative predictive value
NS	normal saline
NSAID	nonsteroidal antiinflammatory drug
O_2	oxygen
OA	osteoarthritis
OCP	oral contraceptive pill
OPV	oral poliovirus vaccine
P_1, P_2	heart sounds made by the pulmonary valve
PCN	penicillin
PCOS	polycystic ovary syndrome
PCP	*Pneumocystis (jirovecii, formerly carinii)* pneumonia
PCWP	pulmonary capillary wedge pressure
PDA	patent ductus arteriosus
PE	pulmonary embolism
PEEP	positive end-expiratory pressure
PG	prostaglandin (e.g., PGE_2, PGF) or phosphatidylglycerol
pH	hydrogen ion concentration scale (measures acidity)

PH	pulmonary hypertension
PID	pelvic inflammatory disease
PIP	proximal interphalangeal (joint)
PMN	polymorphonuclear leukocyte
PMS	premenstrual syndrome
PO$_4$	phosphate
PPD	purified protein derivative (tuberculosis skin test)
PPV	positive predictive value
prn	as needed
PROM	premature rupture of membranes
PSA	prostate-specific antigen
PT	prothrombin time
PTH	parathyroid hormone
PTT	partial thromboplastin time
PUD	peptic ulcer disease
PVC	premature ventricular contraction
PVD	peripheral vascular disease
RA	right atrium or rheumatoid arthritis
RAE	right atrial enlargement
RAI	radioactive iodine
RBC	red blood cells
RDW	red blood cell distribution width
REM	rapid eye movement (dream sleep)
RF	rheumatic fever
Rh	Rhesus blood group antigen
RI	reticulocyte index
RLQ	right lower quadrant
RNA	ribonucleic acid
RPR	rapid plasma reagin (test for syphilis)
RSV	respiratory syncytial virus
RUQ	right upper quadrant
RV	right ventricle
RVH	right ventricular hypertrophy
S	sacral (e.g., S1 nerve root)
S$_1$, S$_2$, S$_3$, S$_4$	heart sounds 1–4
SBO	small bowel obstruction
SCD	sickle cell disease
SCFE	slipped capital femoral epiphysis
SD	standard deviation
SIADH	syndrome of inappropriate antidiuretic hormone (secretion)
SIDS	sudden infant death syndrome
spp.	species
SSRI	selective serotonin reuptake inhibitors
STD	sexually transmitted disease
SVC	superior vena cava
SvO$_2$	systemic venous oxygen saturation
SVR	systemic vascular resistance
T$_3$	triiodothyronine
T$_4$	thyroxine
TB	tuberculosis
TCA	tricyclic antidepressant
Td	tetanus and diphtheria toxoids (age 7 and older)
Tdap	tetanus, diphtheria toxoids, and acellular pertussis vaccine
TE	tracheoesophageal
TIA	transient ischemic attack
TIBC	total iron-binding capacity

TIPS	transjugular intrahepatic portosystemic shunt
TMP-SMX	trimethoprim-sulfamethoxazole
ToF	tetralogy of Fallot
TORCH	**t**oxoplasma, **o**ther, **r**ubella, **c**ytomegalovirus, **h**erpes
tPA	tissue plasminogen activator
TRH	thyroid-releasing hormone
TSH	thyroid-stimulating hormone
TTP	thrombotic thrombocytopenic purpura
TURP	**t**rans**u**rethral **r**esection of the **p**rostate
UGI	upper gastrointestinal (proximal to the ligament of Treitz)
UMN	upper motor neuron
URI	upper respiratory infection
US	ultrasound
USPSTF	United States Preventive Services Task Force
UTI	urinary tract infection
VACTERL	**v**ertebral, **a**nal, **c**ardiac, **t**rach**e**oesophageal, **r**enal, **l**imb (malformations)
VDRL	Venereal Disease Research Laboratory (test for syphilis)
VFib or Vfib	ventricular fibrillation
VIPoma	pancreatic tumor that secretes vasoactive intestinal peptide
VMA	vanillylmandelic acid
V/Q	ventilation-perfusion (ratio)
VSD	ventricular septal defect
VTach or Vtach	ventricular tachycardia
vWF	von Willebrand factor
WBC	white blood cell
wk	week/weeks
WPW	Wolff-Parkinson-White syndrome
yr	year/years

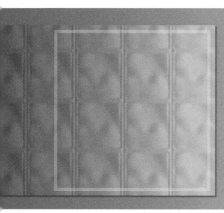

INDEX

Note: Pages numbers followed by *f* indicate figures; *t*, tables; *b*, boxes.

Backyard Bloodsuckers

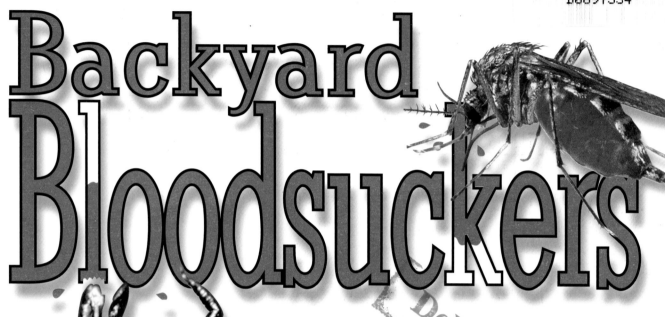

Questions,

Facts &

Tongue Twisters

About Creepy,

Crawly Creatures

Mike Artell

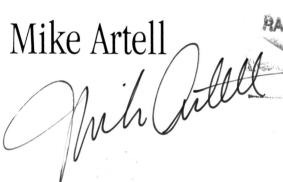

A GOOD YEAR BOOK™

Good Year Books
Tucson, Arizona

Photo credits:
Front cover: *t.* ©USDA/Science Source/Photo Researchers, Inc.; *m.* E.R. Degginger/Color-Pic, Inc.; *b.* James H. Robinson/Animals Animals. Back cover: Jack Clark/Animals Animals. Title page: *t.*©USDA/Science Source/Photo Researchers, Inc.; *m.* E.R. Degginger/Color-Pic, Inc. 3: ©Dr. Tony Brain/Science Photo Library/ Photo Researchers, Inc. 8: Jack Clark/Animals Animals. 9: Hans Pfletschinger/Peter Arnold, Inc. 10: C. James Webb/Phototake. 13: ©USDA/Science Source/Photo Researchers, Inc. 14: ©Dr. Tony Brain/ Science Photo Library/Photo Researchers, Inc. 18: *t.* David Scharf/Peter Arnold, Inc.; *b.* ©Syd Greenberg/ Photo Researchers, Inc. 21: Dwight R. Kuhn. 22: ©Stephen Dalton/Photo Researchers, Inc. 23: ©Gary Retherford/Photo Researchers, Inc. 26: James H. Robinson/Animals Animals. 27: Raymond C. Mendez/ Animals Animals. 28: E.R. Degginger/Color-Pic, Inc. 29: ©Noble Proctor/Photo Researchers, Inc. 31: Jane Burton/Bruce Coleman, Inc. 32: ©Ken Eward/Photo Researchers, Inc. 36: ©Oliver Meckes/Photo Researchers, Inc. 39: Tim Flach/Tony Stone Images. 41: David Scharf/Peter Arnold, Inc. 44: *t.*, *m.* Arthur M. Siegelman/Visuals Unlimited; *b.* Ken Lucas/Visuals Unlimited. 46: David Scharf/Peter Arnold, Inc. 47: Bill Beatty/Visuals Unlimited. 48: David Scharf/Peter Arnold, Inc. 53: S.J. Krasemann/Peter Arnold, Inc. 55: ©Martin Dohrn/Photo Researchers, Inc. 57: ©Meckes/Ottawa/Photo Researchers, Inc. 60: ©Gregory G. Dimijian/Photo Researchers, Inc. 62: Courtesy of The Pearson Museum, Southern Illinois University School of Medicine. 63: James H. Robinson/Animals Animals. 64: J. Paling/Animals Animals. 65: C. Milkins/Animals Animals. 67: ©Oliver Meckes/Photo Researchers, Inc. 71: Al Lamme/Phototake. 72: ©Rondi/Tani/Photo Researchers, Inc. 75: ©USDA/Science Source/Photo Researchers, Inc. 76: *t.*Dwight R. Kuhn; *b.*E.R. Degginger/Color-Pic, Inc. 77: David Scharf/Peter Arnold, Inc. 78: *t.* S.J. Krasemann/Peter Arnold, Inc.; *b.* James H. Robinson/Animals Animals.

Good Year Books

Our titles are available for most basic curriculum subjects plus many enrichment areas. For information on other Good Year Books and to place orders, contact your local bookseller or educational dealer, or visit our website at www.goodyearbooks.com. For a complete catalog, please contact:

Good Year Books
PO Box 91858
Tucson, AZ 85752-1858
www.goodyearbooks.com

Book Design: Sean O'Neill and Christine Ronan Design.
Drawings: Mike Artell

Copyright © 2000 Mike Artell.
Printed in the United States of America.
All Rights Reserved.

ISBN-10: 1-59647-271-5
ISBN-13: 978-1-59647-271-6
Previous ISBN: 0-673-59248-0

2 3 4 5 6 7 8 9   14 13 12 11 10 09 08

PREFACE

Most of the creatures described in this book are arthropods. Arthropods are creatures that have legs with joints and skeletons on the outside of their bodies. Some of the arthropods you'll meet in this book are mosquitoes, fleas, and ticks. You may think there are a lot of humans on Earth, but there are a lot more arthropods. In fact, approximately 80 percent of all the creatures in the animal kingdom are arthropods.

Other bloodsucking creatures in this book (such as leeches) are not arthropods. They're actually weird worms. The amazing thing about all of these creatures is that they feed on human and animal blood.

You're probably wondering why these backyard bloodsuckers want our blood. Why don't these creatures just eat other, smaller creatures, or plants? The reason is that bloodsucking creatures don't have all the chemicals in their bodies that they need to reproduce. They have to get those chemicals from human or animal blood. And since our blood is inside of us, bloodsuckers need to penetrate our skin to get to it. That means they have to bite us.

Human blood is made up of four basic ingredients: plasma, red blood cells, white blood cells, and platelets. Plasma is a light

yellow liquid. Plasma contains water, salt, and the proteins that bloodsucking animals need to reproduce.

Red blood cells are oxygen carriers. When you breathe, your lungs transfer the oxygen to the red blood cells, which deliver the oxygen to the rest of your body.

White blood cells are your body's "soldiers." They attack bacteria, viruses, and anything else that might be harmful to your body.

Platelets help you to stop bleeding if you get cut. They make your blood clot.

The blood cells in your body are very, very small. There are approximately 25 billion red blood cells, 35 million white blood cells, and 1.5 billion platelets in a single teaspoon of blood. You've probably seen a two-liter plastic soda bottle. If you drained the average human body of all of its blood, it would fill about two of those two-liter bottles. For more information about human blood, check out these Web sites:

http://www.bloodbook.com/facts.html
http://www.bloodcenters.org/aboutblood/bloodfacts.htm
http://www.pa.msu.edu/~sciencet/ask_st/061197.html

About the Author

Mike Artell has written and illustrated more than 30 books and has hosted his own television cartooning show. Mike likes to write and illustrate nonfiction books because he learns so much while doing the research for them. Mike also likes to write and illustrate joke books, riddle books, and tongue twister books because they make him laugh while he's writing them. Mike lives near New Orleans, Louisiana. He's married to Susan, a high school science teacher. They have two daughters (Stephanie and Joanna), a cat (Simba), a rabbit (Smokey), and two fish (Pisces and Aquarius).

TABLE of CONTENTS

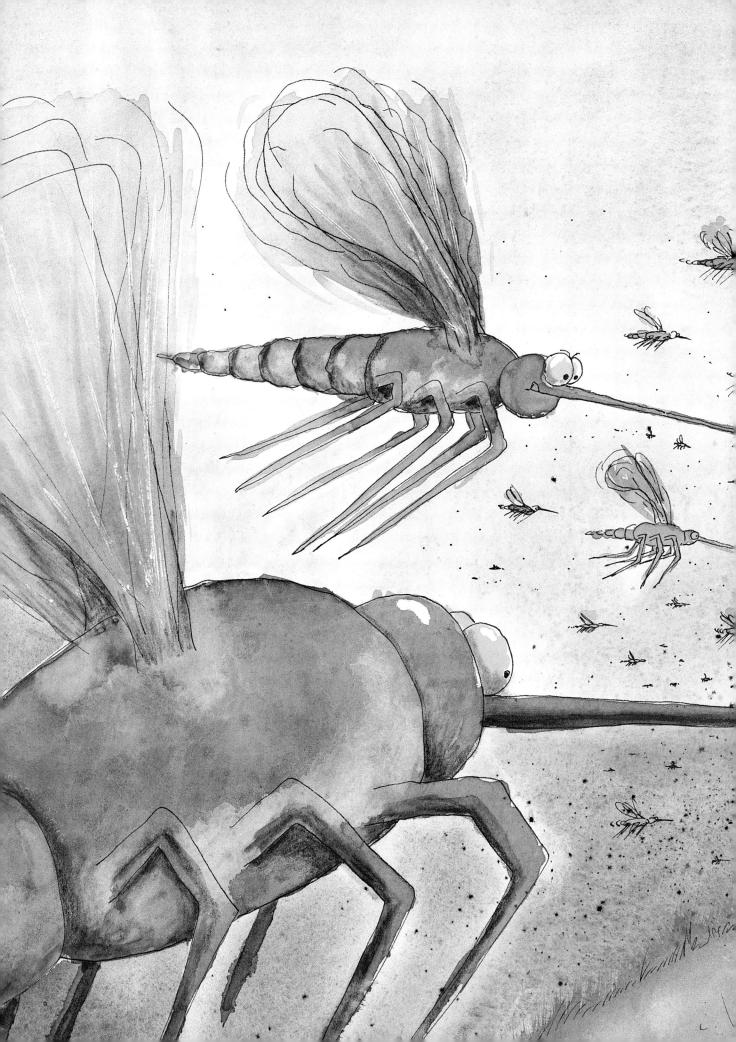

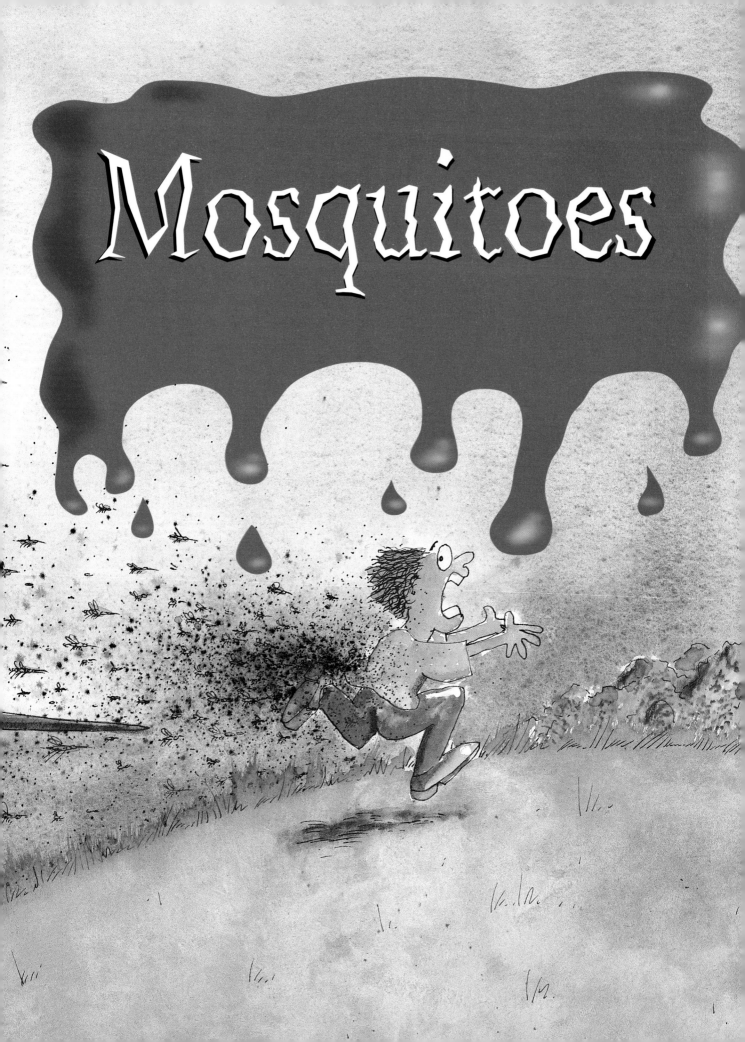

Mosquitoes

Bzzz. . . . Bzzz. . . .

Mosquitoes might be the most annoying insects on Earth. When they're not sticking you with their pointy little mouths and sucking your blood, they're buzzing around your ears while you're trying to sleep.

YO SOY... EL MUSKETA!

Backyard Bloodsuckers
Bulletin

The word *mosquitoes* comes from the Spanish word *musketas*, which means, "little flies." That's a very good name for them, because mosquitoes are actually a type of fly.

What Do They EAT?

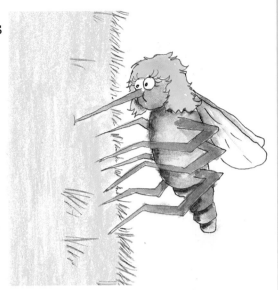

Is blood the only thing that mosquitoes drink? Nope. In fact, male mosquitoes never drink blood—they drink nectar from plants and flowers. Only female mosquitoes drink blood. Females usually drink nectar too, but when they are ready to reproduce, they need some of the chemicals that are contained in blood in order to produce eggs. So the next time you get a mosquito bite, you'll know that it was a girl mosquito that bit you.

Mosquitoes don't live very long. Some species live as long as 5 or 6 months, but most usually only live about 14 days. That doesn't count the ones that get eaten by animals or squished by people.

Why don't you see many mosquitoes during the winter? Do they hibernate? Mosquitoes don't go into a state of true hibernation, but their bodies do slow down a lot during the winter.

During their lifetimes, mosquitoes go through four separate stages. The first stage is the egg stage. Most mosquitoes lay their eggs on the surface of standing water, although some lay their eggs in damp soil and then wait for the soil to become flooded. The eggs are stuck together and form a little "raft," which floats on the surface of the water. In a day or so, the eggs hatch and mosquito larvae appears. This is the beginning of the second stage of the mosquito's life.

Mosquito LARVA

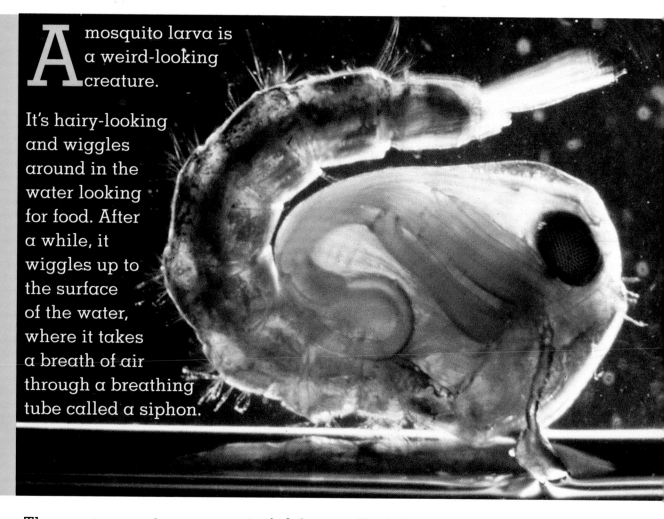

A mosquito larva is a weird-looking creature.

It's hairy-looking and wiggles around in the water looking for food. After a while, it wiggles up to the surface of the water, where it takes a breath of air through a breathing tube called a siphon.

The next stage in a mosquito's life is called the pupa stage. During this stage, mosquitoes begin to change. They stop eating and develop two breathing tubes called trumpets. They also change shape and develop a pupal case. It is in this case that they change into an adult mosquito.

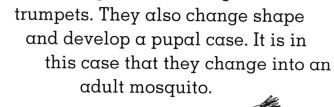

VERY COOL.

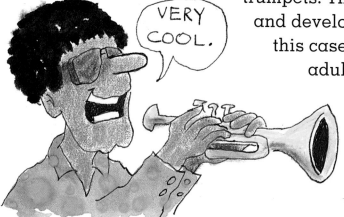

When the mosquito has changed into a fully formed adult, it splits out of the pupal case and stands on the surface of the water so its body can harden.

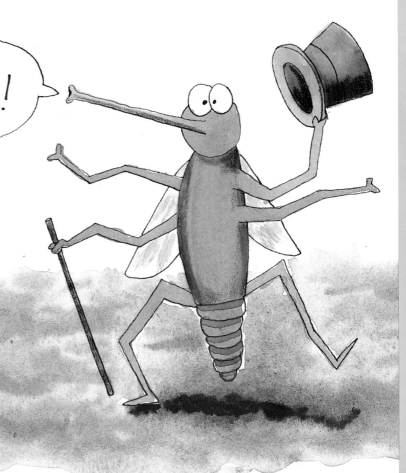

That's when the trouble starts.

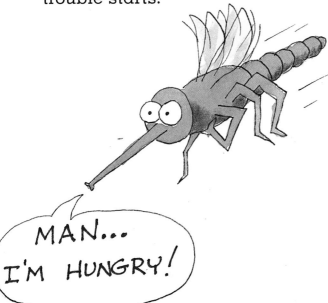

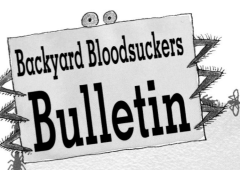

Backyard Bloodsuckers
Bulletin

If it's warm enough and conditions are right, it's possible for some species of mosquitoes to go from the egg stage to the adult stage in about 4 days.

How Do I Keep Them AWAY?

How can we control the mosquito population? The best way to control the number of mosquitoes in your area is to eliminate the mosquitoes' favorite breeding places. As you read earlier, mosquitoes' eggs, larvae, and pupae need water to grow. Almost any place outside that you find containers of water, you'll find mosquito eggs, larvae, and pupae. Here are some of the favorite places mosquitoes pick to lay their eggs:

- old tires
- birdbaths
- rain gutters
- wading pools
- barbeque grills
- water-filled tree holes
- pans under potted plants
- pet dishes

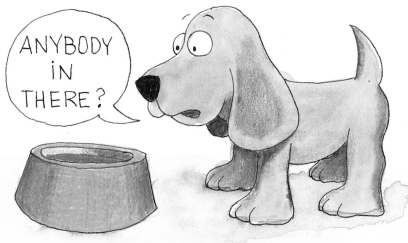

ANYBODY IN THERE?

It's important to clean up these mosquito breeding grounds if you want to cut down on the mosquito population.

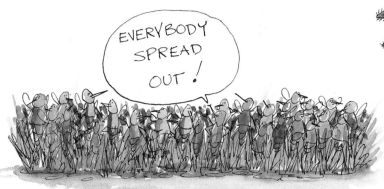

EVERYBODY SPREAD OUT!

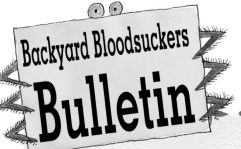

Backyard Bloodsuckers Bulletin

A wet, grassy area about the size of a page in this book can produce 1,000 mosquito larvae.

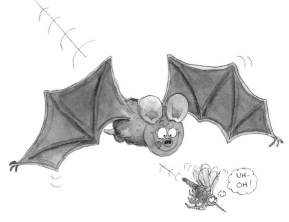

Another way to get rid of mosquitoes is to encourage mosquito predators, such as bats and dragonflies. Although you may think of bats as bloodsuckers too, not all bats drink blood. In fact, many species of bats are insect eaters. Did you know that one hungry bat can eat 600 mosquitoes in an hour?

You can also reduce the number of mosquitoes near you by adding turtles or mosquito-eating minnows to pools of water. Some minnows just love to eat mosquito eggs, larvae, and pupae.

Of course, another great way to get rid of mosquitoes is to wait until one lands on your skin, and then . . .

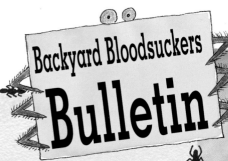

Backyard Bloodsuckers Bulletin

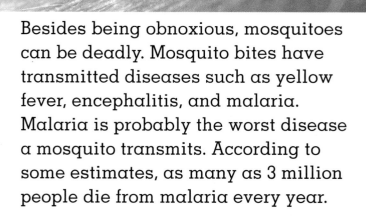

Most mosquitoes keep their bodies horizontal when they bite, but the Anopheles mosquito sticks its rear end up in the air when it bites.

Besides being obnoxious, mosquitoes can be deadly. Mosquito bites have transmitted diseases such as yellow fever, encephalitis, and malaria. Malaria is probably the worst disease a mosquito transmits. According to some estimates, as many as 3 million people die from malaria every year.

13

MORE on **Mosquitoes**

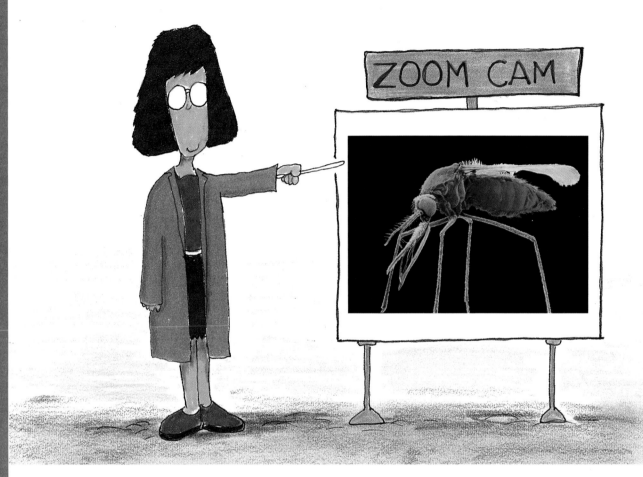

ZOOM CAM

- Most mosquitoes only live a couple of weeks.

- Only female mosquitoes bite.

- Mosquitoes go through four stages in their lives: egg, larva, pupa, and adult.

- Old tires and other containers are breeding grounds for mosquitoes.

- Mosquitoes can carry deadly diseases.

- A mosquito's wings flap 300 to 400 times each second.

- More than 2,700 species of mosquitoes have been identified.

Do You Want to Know MORE?

Log on to these Web sites to learn more about mosquitoes:

- http://www.mosquito.org/mosquito-information/faq.aspx
- http://www.ent.iastate.edu/imagegal/diptera/culicidae/
- http://www-rci.rutgers.edu/~insects/njmos.htm
- http://www.gurnee.il.us/public_works/mosquitoes.html
- http://ohioline.osu.edu/hyg-fact/2000/2148.html
- http://www.control-mosquitoes.com/
- http://www.ivyhall.district96.k12.il.us/4TH/KKHP/1INSECTS/mosquito.html
- http://www.mosquito.org/mosquito-information/index.aspx
- http://www.tinymosquito.com/mosquitofacts.html
- http://www.shastamosquito.org/Mosquito_Facts/mosquito_facts.htm
- http://mosquitotraps.net/mosquito-facts.htm

Also, look in your local phone book to see if your state or county has a "mosquito abatement" organization. Often, these people visit schools and talk about the ways you can reduce the number of mosquitoes where you live.

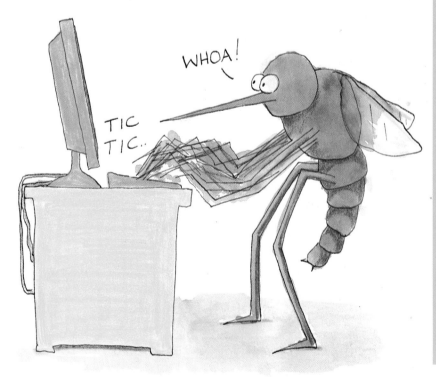

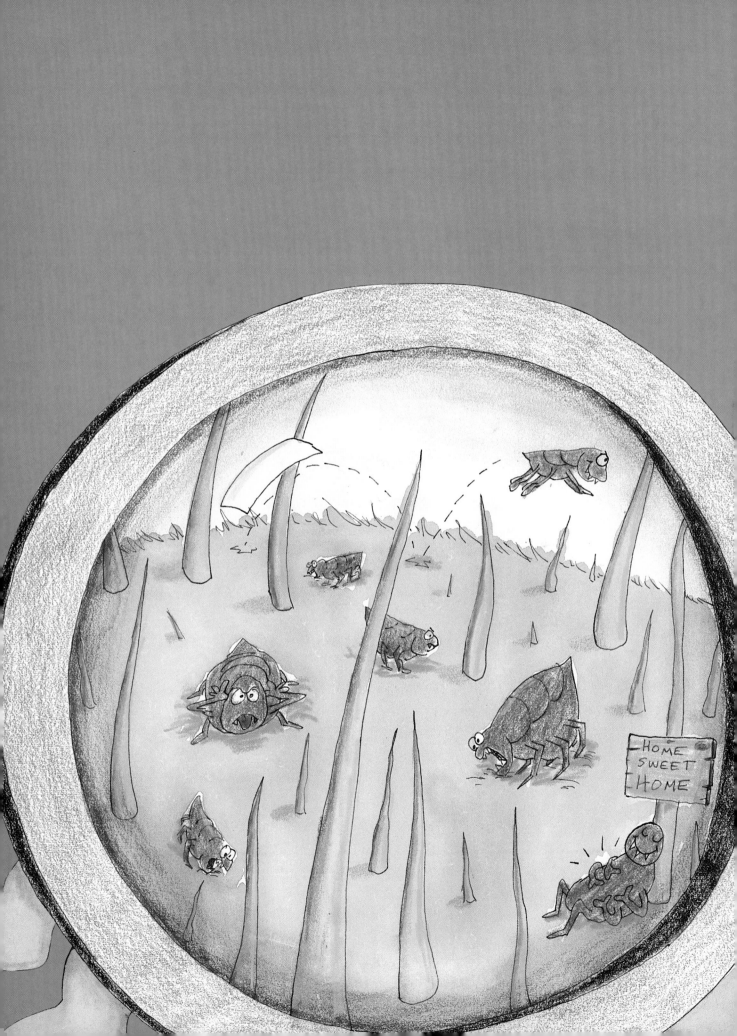

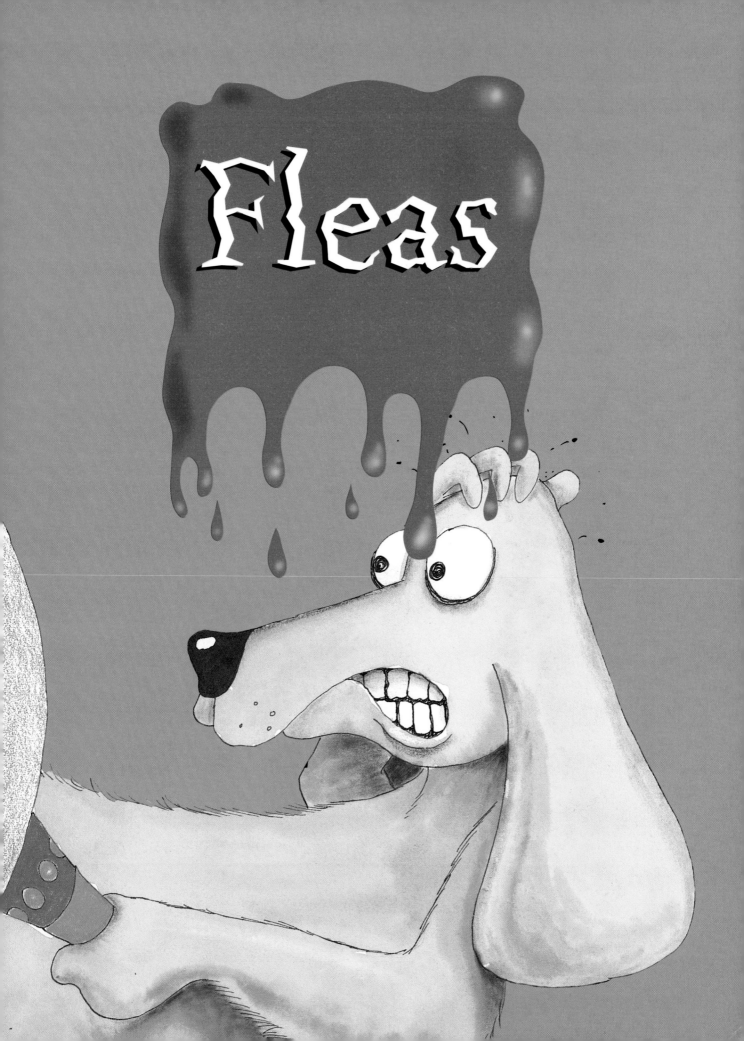

YUK!

Can you imagine a nastier creature than a flea? There are lots of different kinds of fleas. There are dog fleas and cat fleas and rabbit fleas and rat fleas, but all of them are a bother to humans and their pets. Like mosquitoes, fleas go through four life-cycle stages: egg, larva, pupa, and adult. Flea eggs are smooth and white. Eggs may take anywhere from two days to two weeks to hatch into larvae.

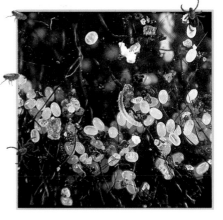

The larvae look like little hairy worms. They're about 1/4 inch long and have brown heads and yellowish bodies. Although the larvae are blind, they prefer dark places where they can hide.

Backyard Bloodsuckers Bulletin

One way to tell if your house has fleas is to place a plate with a little water and some dishwashing detergent on the floor. If you place a lamp with a long neck over the plate,

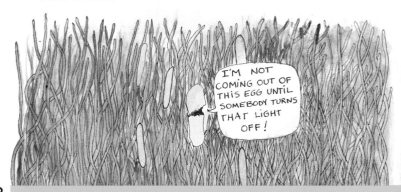

I'M NOT COMING OUT OF THIS EGG UNTIL SOMEBODY TURNS THAT LIGHT OFF!

What Do They EAT?

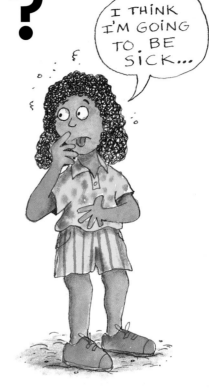

I THINK I'M GOING TO BE SICK...

The larvae have a most disgusting diet. They do not suck blood, but instead eat dead skin, hair, digested blood from the adult fleas' feces, and other nauseating stuff.

After a while, each larva spins a little silken cocoon around itself and becomes a pupa. Most of the time, the pupa remains in its cocoon for a week or two. But if there is no food source around (such as an animal or human being), the pupa may stay in its cocoon for months.

the adult fleas will be attracted to the light from the lamp. When they jump toward the light, some of them will fall back into the plate. The dishwashing detergent makes it hard for the fleas to stay on the surface of the water and they drown. If you find dead fleas in the plate, your house has fleas.

When the pupa detects movement or carbon dioxide from a living creature's breath, it will emerge from the cocoon as an adult flea. And after all that time in its cocoon, it is very hungry! Once the young adult fleas emerge from their cocoons, they need to drink some blood within a few days or they'll die.

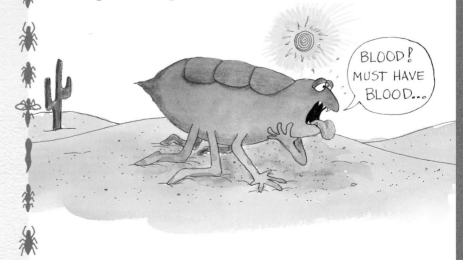

BLOOD! MUST HAVE BLOOD...

How Do I Keep Them AWAY?

If there are fleas in your house, chances are only about 5 percent of them are biting adults. Usually, about half of the population are eggs, 30 percent are larvae and about 15 percent are pupae.

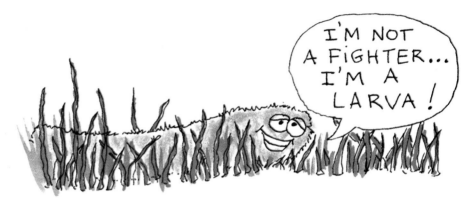

I'M NOT A FIGHTER... I'M A LARVA!

THAT TICKLES!

Do you know why it's hard to squish a flea? Fleas are small and have hard bodies. Human fingers are soft on the ends. Fleas are just too hard and your fingers are too soft. What makes squishing a flea even harder is the shape of the flea's body. It's flattened vertically, sort of like a fish. Fleas are shaped this way so they can move through animal and human hair easily. When you squeeze it, the flea's body just gets a little skinnier.

Tongue Twister

Try saying this tongue twister three times fast: **Freddie found fifty filthy fleas in Fido's fur.**

The best way to control fleas is to make sure your pets are free of them. Check pet areas regularly and vacuum around the places where they sleep and lie.

How Do They MOVE?

When it comes to jumping, fleas are hard to beat. A typical flea can jump as high as 7 inches and as far as 13 inches.

If that doesn't seem like a lot to you, think about this: if you could jump as high and as far as a flea, you could jump 250 feet in the air and 450 feet down the street.

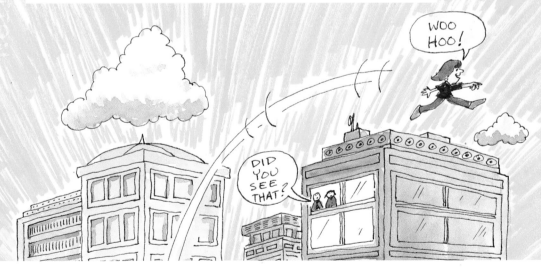

Fleas have made a lot of people and animals sick. Because fleas jump around a lot, they often bite one animal or person, then jump to another animal or person and bite them. In doing this, they can spread lots of diseases. In the fourteenth century, fleas spread a disease in Europe called "the plague" or "Black Death," and millions of people died. Fleas are also known to spread typhus and tapeworms in animals.

WHEN Will I See Them?

Fleas like warm weather. That's why you see them most often in the summer. They like temperatures between 70 and 85 degrees Fahrenheit. They also like humid weather. When the humidity is around 70 percent, fleas are the happiest.

Sometimes people talk about "sand fleas," but there's really no such thing. Sand and gravel are excellent breeding places for fleas, so they like to live there. A sand flea is just a regular flea that lives in sand.

Some people believe that feeding their pets garlic will keep fleas away. Since garlic has such a strong smell, they think that the fleas will try to get away from the odor. It would be great if it worked, but there's no scientific proof that it does work. If it did, all we would have to do is feed Fido some garlic bread with his pesto, and presto! No more fleas!

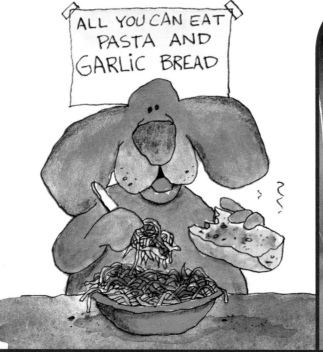

ALL YOU CAN EAT PASTA AND GARLIC BREAD

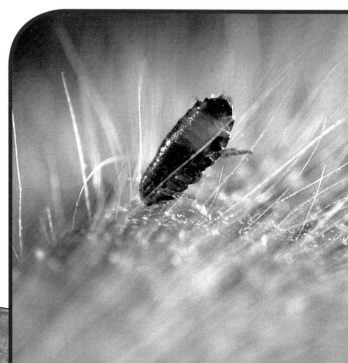

FLEA Facts

- A flea that lives 6 to 8 weeks can lay 2,000 eggs in her life span.

- Americans spend more than $1 billion each year fighting fleas.

- Vibrations can make a flea hatch.

- A flea's life cycle can stretch from 2 weeks to 2 years.

- Most fleas attack mammals, such as humans, dogs, and cats. Some attack birds.

- In 30 days, 10 female fleas can multiply to more than 250,000 fleas in various stages.

- There are more than 250 species of fleas in North America.

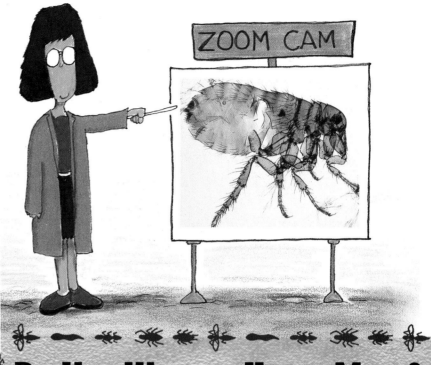

ZOOM CAM

Do You Want to Know More?

Log on to these Web sites to learn more about fleas:

- http://www.greensmiths.com/fleas.htm
- http://ohioline.osu.edu/hyg-fact/2000/2081.html
- http://www.ext.colostate.edu/Pubs/insect/05600.html
- http://www.orkin.com/fleas/fleas.html
- http://www.ianr.unl.edu/ianr/lanco/enviro/ pest/factsheets/fleas.html
- http://www.stopthefleas.com/flea-facts-flea-information.html
- http://www.ca.uky.edu/entomology/entfacts/ef602.asp
- http://www.hartz.com/cats/ArticlePreview.asp?Animal=2&Article=83
- http://vetmedicine.about.com/od/parasites/a/fleaticktips04.htm
- http://www.fleafree.co.uk/flea_facts/en/bites.shtml

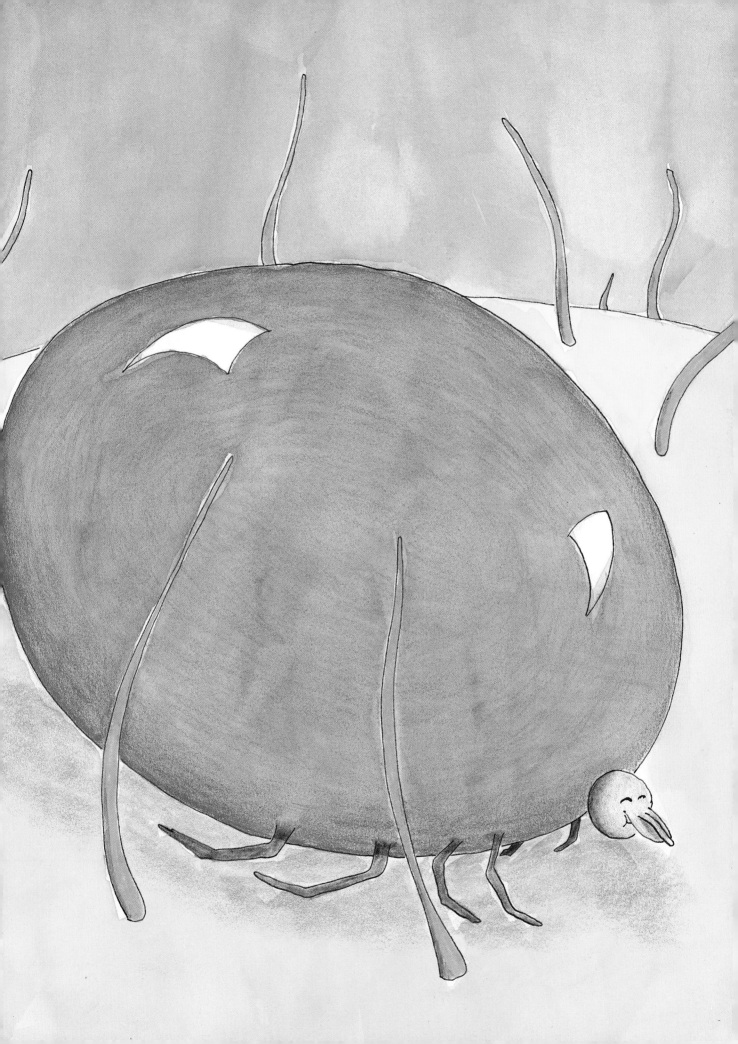

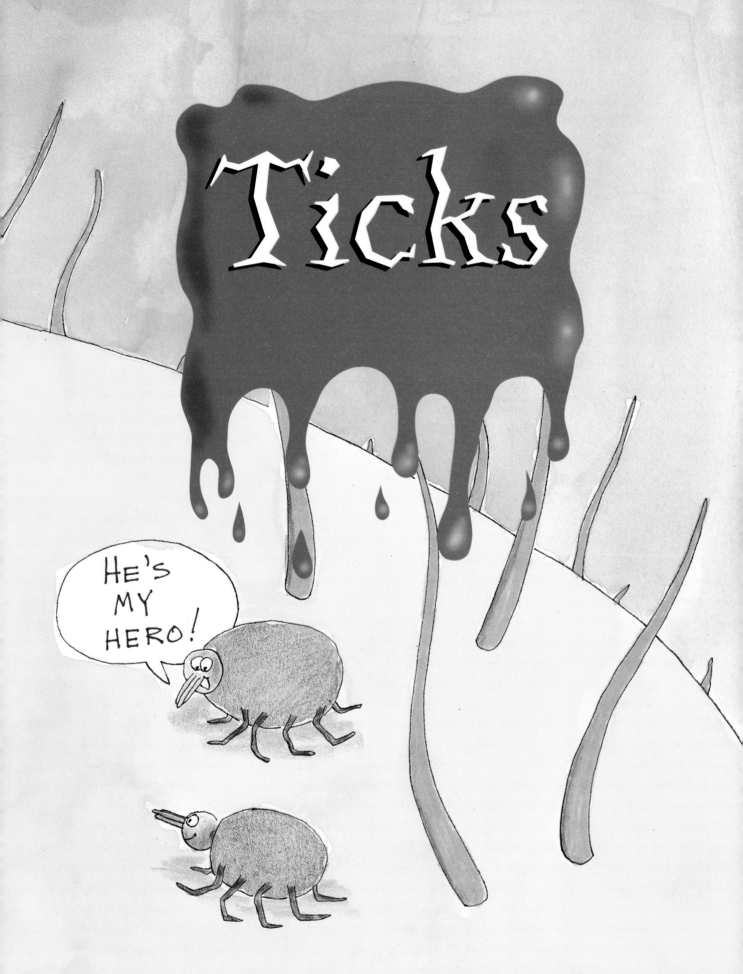

Types of TICKS

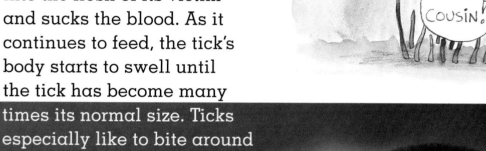

T here are more than 800 species of ticks, and they are divided into two basic families: hard ticks and soft ticks. Unlike mosquitoes and fleas, ticks are not insects. They are more closely related to spiders. A tick digs its mouth parts into the flesh of its victim and sucks the blood. As it continues to feed, the tick's body starts to swell until the tick has become many times its normal size. Ticks especially like to bite around the victim's head, neck, and ears.

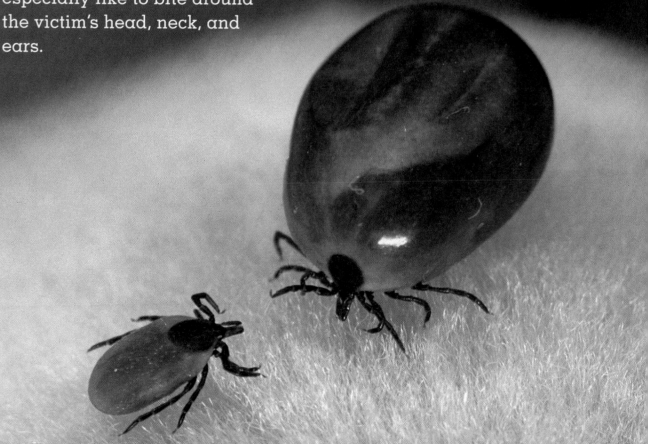

DISEASE

icks are the champs when it comes to carrying diseases. You might say:

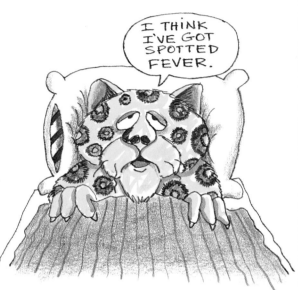

"When it comes to making people sick, Nothing's better than a tick."

Ticks transmit lots of different bacteria and viruses. You may have heard of Lyme disease and Rocky Mountain Spotted Fever. Ticks spread both of those diseases.

Ticks undergo a number of changes during their lifetimes. Like the other creatures we've seen, ticks start out as eggs. One of the amazing things about female ticks is the number of eggs they lay. Usually it's thousands at a time!

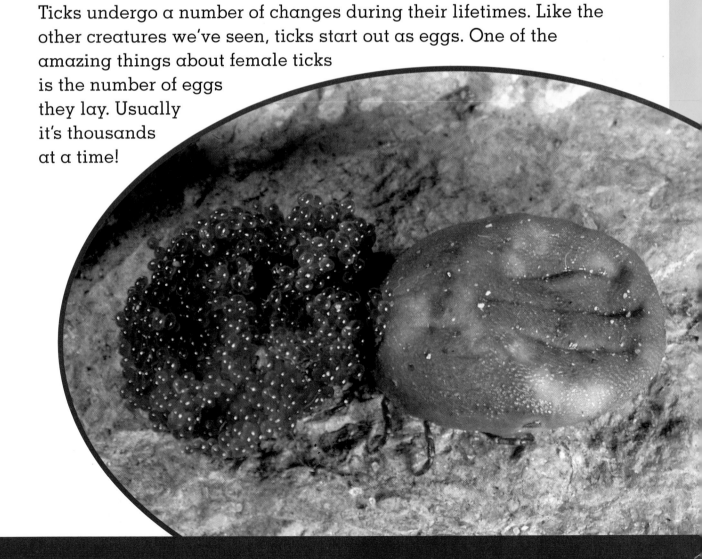

Life Stages of a TICK

When the tick emerges from its egg, it begins its life as a larva. Unlike some of the other bloodsucking creatures we've seen, tick larvae are not wormlike. Instead, they have six legs. This is really weird, because in all future stages of a tick's life, the tick has eight legs, like a spider! After a brief stage as a nymph, the tick becomes a full-grown adult.

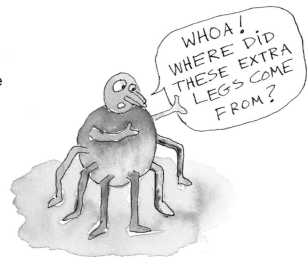

WHOA! WHERE DID THESE EXTRA LEGS COME FROM?

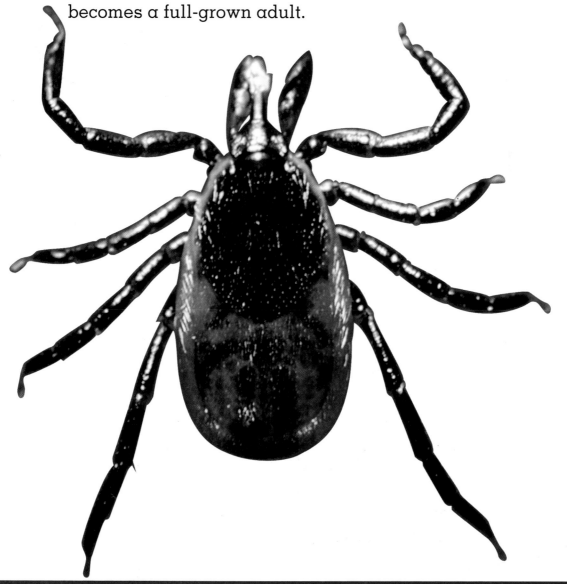

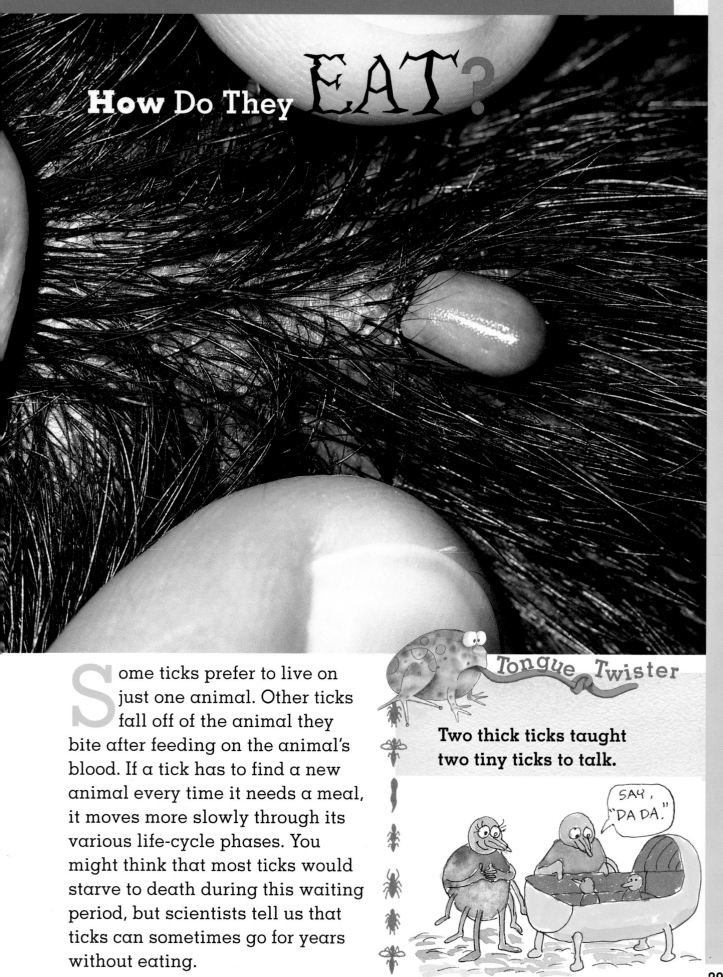

How Do They EAT?

Some ticks prefer to live on just one animal. Other ticks fall off of the animal they bite after feeding on the animal's blood. If a tick has to find a new animal every time it needs a meal, it moves more slowly through its various life-cycle phases. You might think that most ticks would starve to death during this waiting period, but scientists tell us that ticks can sometimes go for years without eating.

Tongue Twister

Two thick ticks taught two tiny ticks to talk.

SAY, "DA DA."

How Do They Find FOOD?

If you breathe, a tick can find you. How? Mammals such as humans, dogs, and rabbits all breathe air into their lungs and breathe out carbon dioxide. Ticks can sense carbon dioxide in the air. And when they get a whiff of carbon dioxide, they know that "dinner" is nearby.

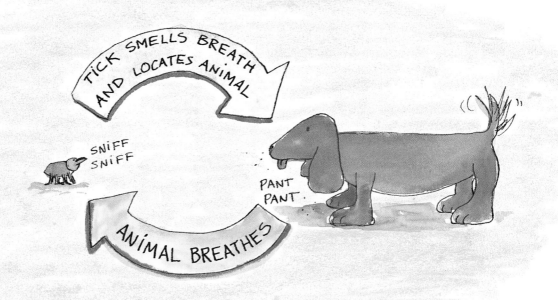

Ticks are often found in places where the grass is tall and there's lots of shade. People and animals that walk through tall grass or brush often pick up tick "hitchhikers" that attach themselves to clothing, skin, and fur.

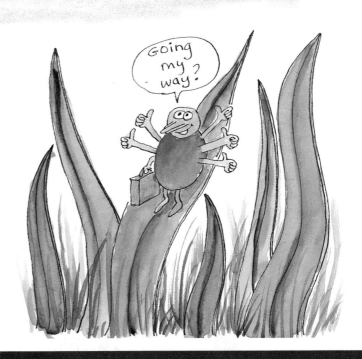

Removing a TICK Can Be a Trick

The trick to removing a tick is to go slowly. You'll probably want some adult help if you need to remove a tick. First, take a pair of small tweezers and dip the end of them in alcohol. The head of the tick will be under the skin, so you'll have to grasp just the body of the tick with the tweezers. Try to grasp the tick's body as close as possible to the place where it meets the victim's skin. Pull the tick gently until the skin starts to pucker a little. Be careful not to squish the tick. All this pulling on its body makes the tick very uncomfortable, so in a minute or so, the tick will probably pull out of the victim's skin. If it doesn't, drip one or two drops of alcohol on the tick's body. Make every effort to remove the tick in one piece. If the head breaks off under the skin, it can cause an infection.

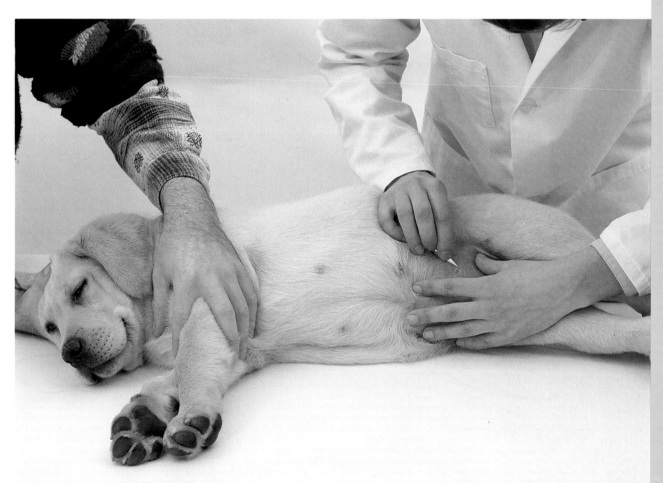

TICK Tidbits

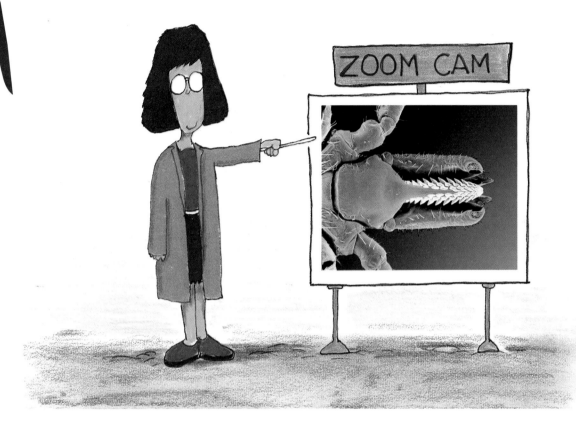

- Ticks are not insects. Adult insects have six legs, and adult ticks have eight legs.

- Female ticks lay thousands of eggs at a time.

- Ticks can detect victims by the carbon dioxide in the victim's breath.

- Ticks do not reproduce well indoors. They prefer outdoors.

- A tick should be removed carefully or its head can break off and remain under the skin, causing infection.

- Ticks inject a chemical that keeps the victim's blood from clotting. That way, the tick can keep sucking blood until it is full.

- It's easier to find ticks on you if you wear light-colored clothing.

Do You Want to Know MORE?

Log on to these Web sites to learn more about ticks:

- http://www.hartz.com/dogs/ArticlePreview.asp?Animal=1&Article=125

- http://www.lyme.org/ticks/facts.html

- http://www.petco.com/Content/Article.aspx?id=2552&Nav=153

- http://animals.nationalgeographic.com/animals/bugs/deer-tick.html

- http://www.fleatickfacts.com/ticktrouble.asp

- http://www.sickofticks.com/facts.html

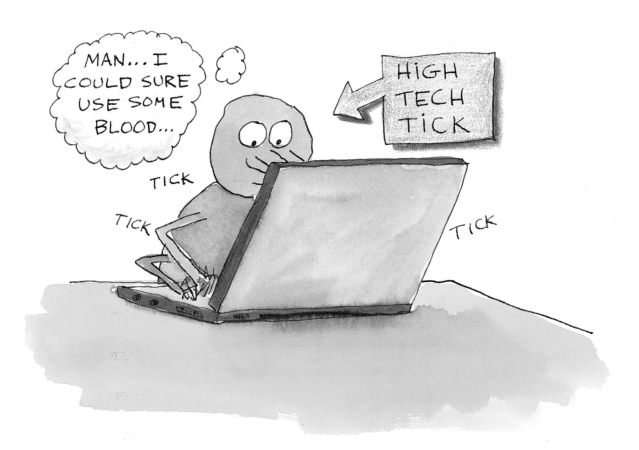

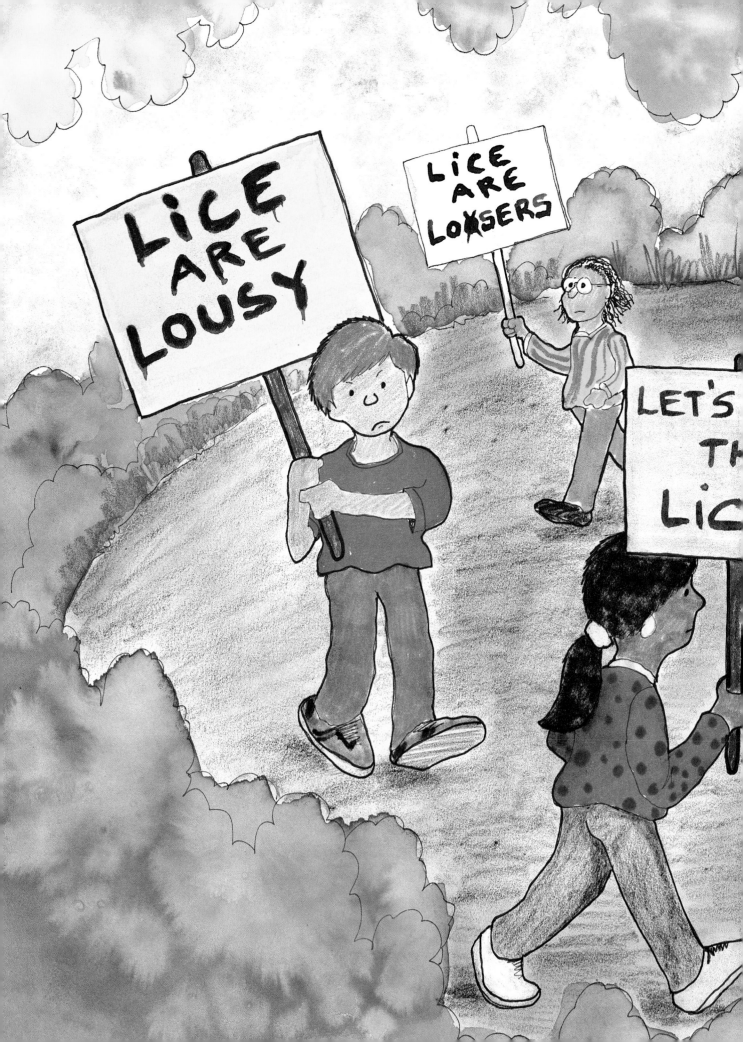

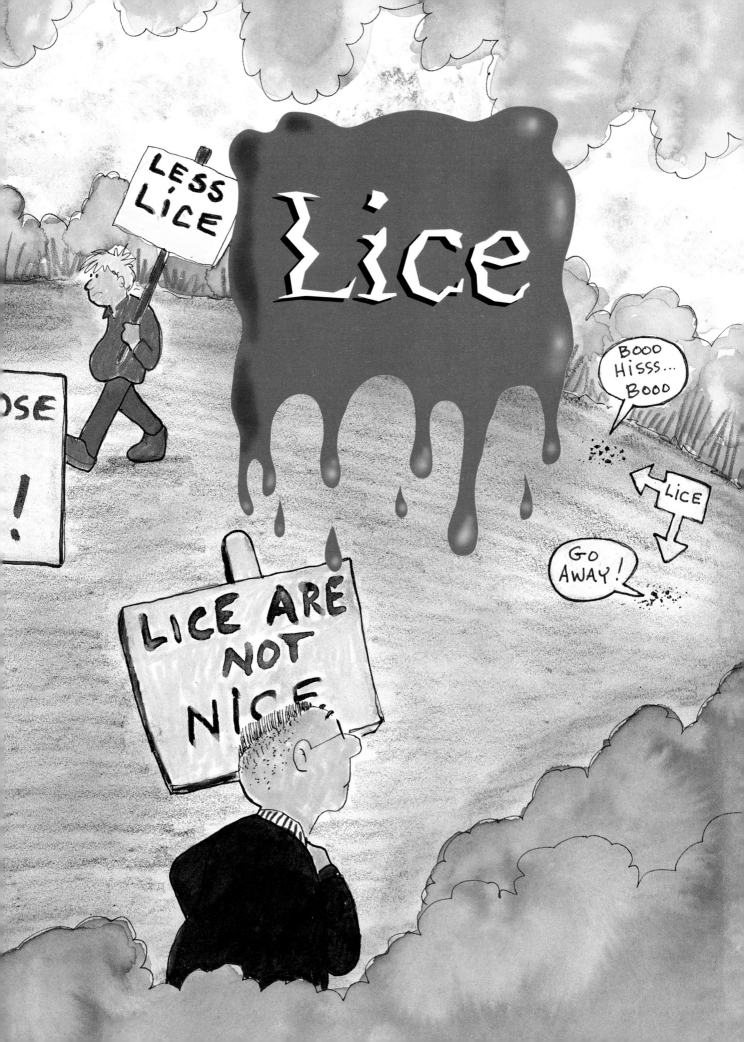

Lots of LICE

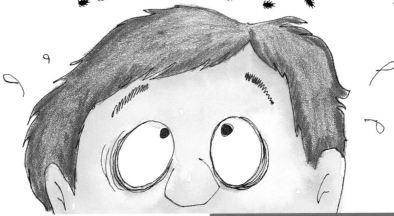

There are about 200 species of sucking lice, but only 3 species attack humans. The species that people know best is called "head lice." Head lice live in your hair and suck your blood. Then they attach their eggs to your hair and let the heat from your body keep the eggs nice and warm until they're ready to hatch. Pretty soon, the whole lice family is having a party on your head!

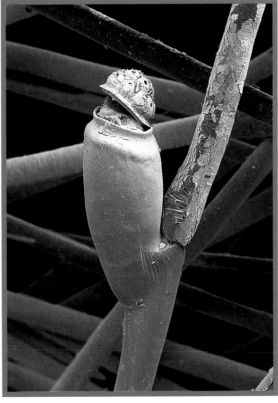

Backyard Bloodsuckers Bulletin

Head lice can crawl fast, but they can't jump or hop. They can't fly either. They don't have wings.

An itchy scalp might be a sign that lice have made a home on your head. As the louse digs into a human scalp, chemicals in its saliva (spit) irritate the skin and cause itching. It can sometimes even cause a rash.

How Do They SPREAD?

Just because someone has head lice doesn't mean that person is dirty. In fact, anybody can get head lice. Lice get passed from person to person by direct contact. That means if you share a comb, a brush, or even a hat, the lice could move from another person's head to yours, even if your head is perfectly clean.

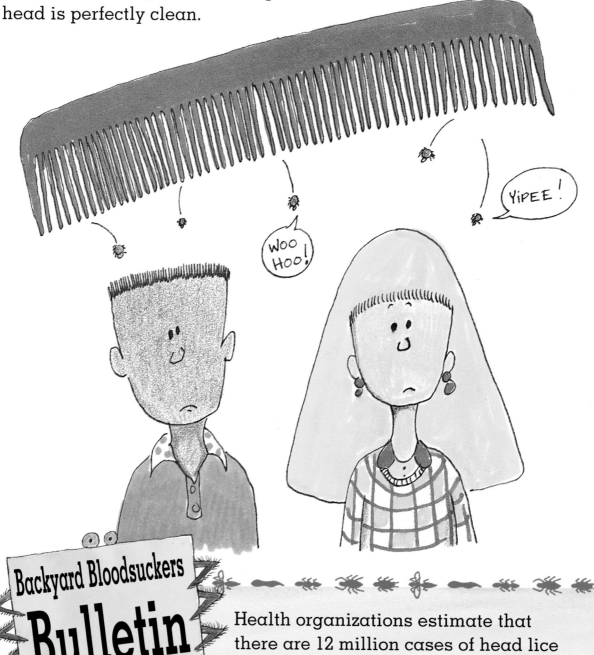

WOO HOO!

YIPEE!

Backyard Bloodsuckers Bulletin

Health organizations estimate that there are 12 million cases of head lice each year.

How Do I REMOVE Them?

One of the best ways to remove the nits (eggs) is to comb the hair with a fine-toothed comb. As the comb is pulled through the hair, the teeth of the comb will break the glue that sticks the nit to the hair shaft.

Some people use strong chemicals to kill nits, but others think this is a bad idea since the chemicals have to be placed on the heads of children.

The normal life span of a louse is about 30 days. The female louse lays about 150 eggs in a month. It's easy to mistake other things in the hair for nits. Sometimes dandruff and dead skin can look a lot like nits. But if a person shampoos his or her hair and there's still some little whitish-tan specks sticking to the hair shaft, it's a good bet that that person has head lice.

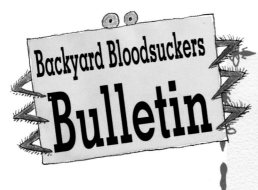

Backyard Bloodsuckers Bulletin

In World War I, the soldiers nicknamed head lice "galloping dandruff."

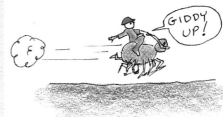

GIDDY UP!

Life Stages of a LOUSE

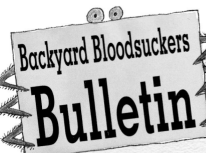

It takes about 10 days for the nits to hatch. When they do, a nymph emerges. Nymphs are hungry little critters. As soon as they emerge from the egg, they're ready to eat. They generally need to feed on some blood about every 3 to 6 hours. Over the next 2 weeks, the nymph goes through three stages before it becomes an adult and is ready to reproduce.

Most of the time, lice are found where humans have hair. Body lice, however, actually live in the seams of clothing and bedding. They come out to eat, then go back into the clothing. If your clothes are washed regularly, you probably don't have to worry too much about body lice.

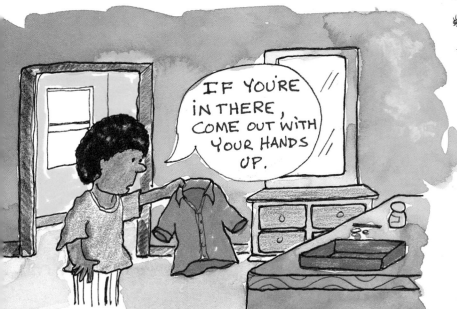

IF YOU'RE IN THERE, COME OUT WITH YOUR HANDS UP.

Backyard Bloodsuckers
Bulletin

Lice have strong claws that they use to hold onto hair shafts and clothing fabric.

Other Kinds of LICE

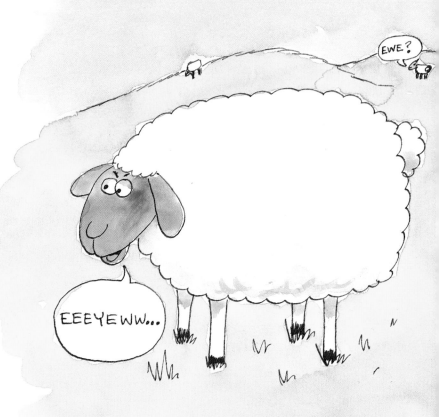

Some lice live only on animals. For instance, the sheep louse lives only on (you guessed it!) sheep. The sheep louse is very small and lays only 3 eggs every 5 days. The sheep body louse is different from the kind of louse that sucks human blood. In fact, sheep body lice don't suck blood at all. They just live on the small stuff they can scrounge off the skin of the sheep.

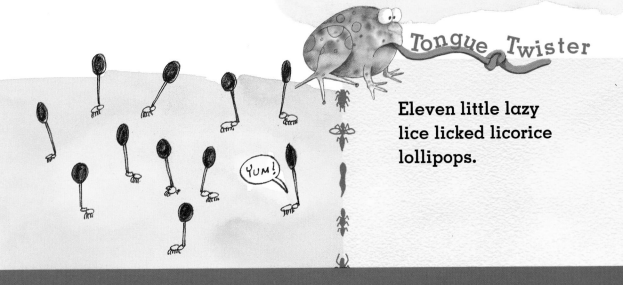

Tongue Twister

Eleven little lazy lice licked licorice lollipops.

Leads on LICE

- Head lice live in your hair.

- The eggs of head lice are called nits.

- Anyone can get head lice.

- Once lice hatch, they need to feed on blood about every 3 to 6 hours.

- Lice use their strong claws to hold onto hair shafts.

- Some lice live on humans; some live on animals.

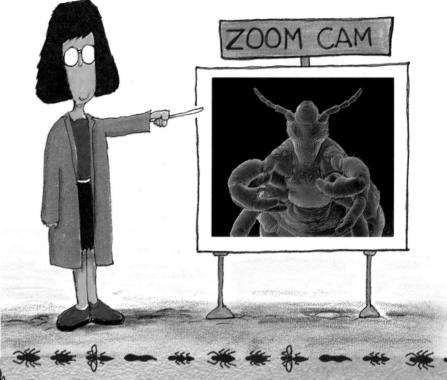

Do You Want to Know More?

Log on to these Web sites to learn more about lice:

- http://www.newton.dep.anl.gov/natbltn/200-299/nb292.htm

- http://www.headlice.org/

- http://www.mdchoice.com/pt/ptinfo/pedi.asp

- http://www.drgreene.com/21_640.html

- http://www.dhpe.org/infect/lice.html

- http://www.headliceinfo.com/20facts.htm

- http://www.in.gov/isdh/healthinfo/HeadLice.htm

- http://www.wordconstructions.com/articles/health/licefact.html

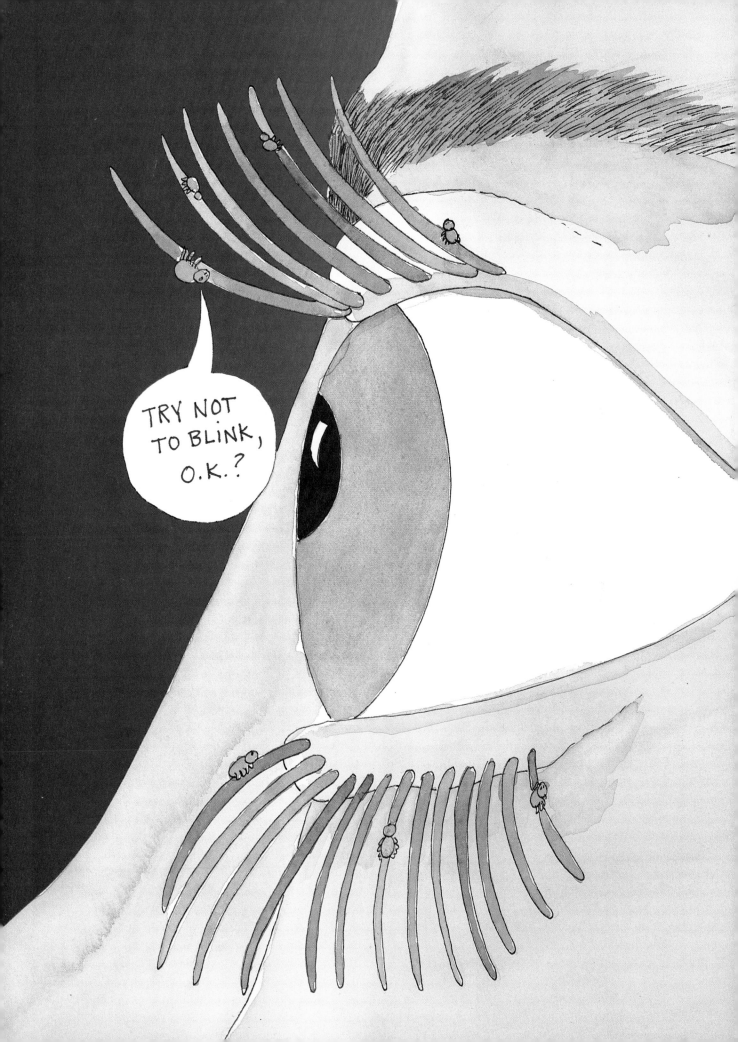

Mites and Chiggers

MITES

Technically, mites aren't bloodsuckers. They're more like "dissolved-tissue suckers." Why? Because as they dig into human or animal skin, they inject saliva (spit), which contains chemicals that dissolve the tissues of the victim. Then they suck up the juicy dissolved tissue for a tasty meal.

Like many other parasites in this book, mites go through four stages of life: egg, larva, nymph, and adult.

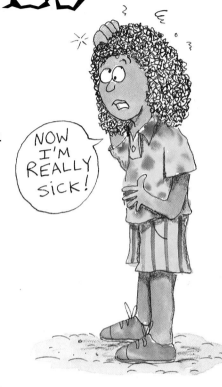

Although most mites are found on the surface of the skin, some live inside the bodies of animals.

Mites are not insects. They're more like ticks and spiders. In fact, when mites hatch from their eggs, they have six legs, just like tick larvae. Later, they develop two more legs, for a total of eight.

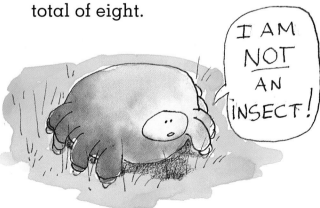

SCABIES Mites

One particularly irritating mite is the scabies mite. The female scabies mite chews into the skin of its host and feeds on the body fluids. After she feeds, she lays about 3 eggs in the little tunnel she dug. In 3 or 4 days the larvae emerge from the eggs. Soon the larvae molt and become nymphs.

When the nymphs start burrowing into the skin and feeding, they can cause an itchy rash. That's generally the first sign that scabies mites have found a home on somebody's body. After the nymphs have been feeding a while, they molt again and become adults. The entire life cycle of the mite normally takes about 2 weeks.

A scabies mite is "host-specific." That means that it doesn't move from one kind of creature to another during its life cycle. It may "hitch a ride" for a while and cause some itching, but it won't raise its family there.

Like many other backyard bloodsuckers, scabies mites need to eat every few hours. In fact, a scabies mite will die if it is separated from its food source for more than 24 hours.

Backyard Bloodsuckers Bulletin

When a creature molts, it sheds its outer layer of skin or shell so it can grow. Lots of creatures molt, even snakes and crabs!

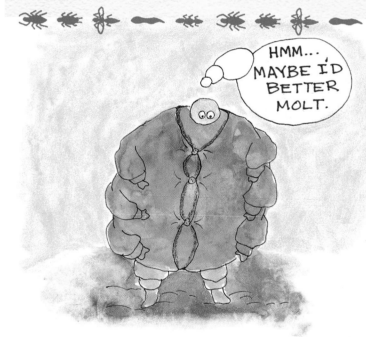

HMM... MAYBE I'D BETTER MOLT.

Microscopic MITES

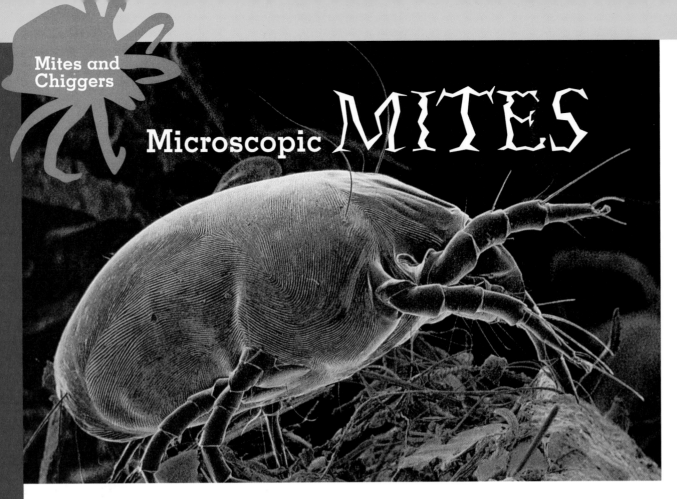

Although many mites can be seen easily, some are so tiny you need a microscope to see them. Here are two examples:

House Dust Mites

These little guys live in your carpet and mattresses at home and can cause you some big problems if you have allergies. About half of the homes in the United States are infested with dust mites. In the average mattress, there could be 1 million to 2 million dust mites. They're very tiny critters that live off of dead skin cells and other yummy stuff. Unfortunately, their feces can cause asthma and allergic reactions in many people. Steam-cleaning carpets can help keep their numbers down.

Follicle Mites

You're not going to like this next sentence. At this very moment, there is an excellent chance that you have follicle mites crawling all over your eyelashes. That's right. Most people have follicle mites living on the hairs of their eyelids or on the glands near the surface. Even though you can't see them, they're there. But don't worry. They don't bite and they won't bother you.

CHIGGERS

Chiggers are a type of very small, reddish mites. They're only about 1/150 of an inch long. That's about this big: ⟶

Chiggers are a little lazy. Rather than dig a hole into the skin to get food, they often feed at the base of a hair shaft or in a pore in the skin. Most often, chiggers can be found where clothing fits tightly. Typical chigger sites would include the skin near the tops of socks and skin around a person's waist.

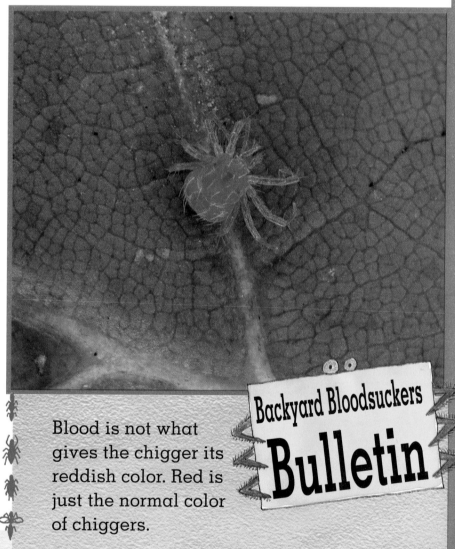

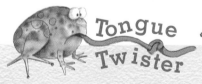

Tongue Twister

The chigger-checkers checked the trail-trekkers for chiggers chewing on their chins.

Blood is not what gives the chigger its reddish color. Red is just the normal color of chiggers.

After a chigger begins to feed off of its victim, the skin around the feeding area becomes hard. Then it becomes irritated and itchy. Chiggers are pests, but fortunately, they do not transmit any diseases to humans.

Backyard Bloodsuckers Bulletin

MORE on **Mites** and **Chiggers**

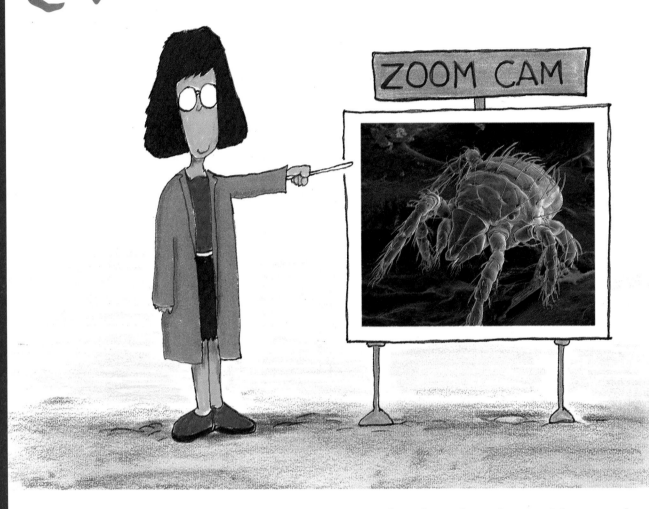

- Mites are not insects. They're more closely related to spiders and ticks.

- Mites are small. Some cannot be seen without a magnifying glass or microscope.

- Mite larvae shed their skin as they grow. This is called molting.

- Dust mites live in carpeting and can cause allergies.

- Follicle mites live on and around human eyelashes.

- Chiggers are small red mites. They do not transmit diseases to humans.

Do You Want to Know MORE?

Log on to these Web sites to learn more about mites and chiggers:

- http://www.uky.edu/Agriculture/Entomology/entfacts/struct/ef630.htm

- http://www.skinsite.com/info_chiggers.htm

- http://mdc.mo.gov/nathis/arthopo/chiggers/

- http://www.entomon.net/mites-scabies-chiggersfacts.htm

- http://www.deh.enr.state.nc.us/phpm/CHIGGERS.PDF

- http://en.wikipedia.org/?title=Chigger

- http://www.dupagehealth.org/misc/itchmitefactsheet.pdf

- http://cybersleuth-kids.com/sleuth/Science/Animals/Arachnids/Ticks_and_Mites/index.htm

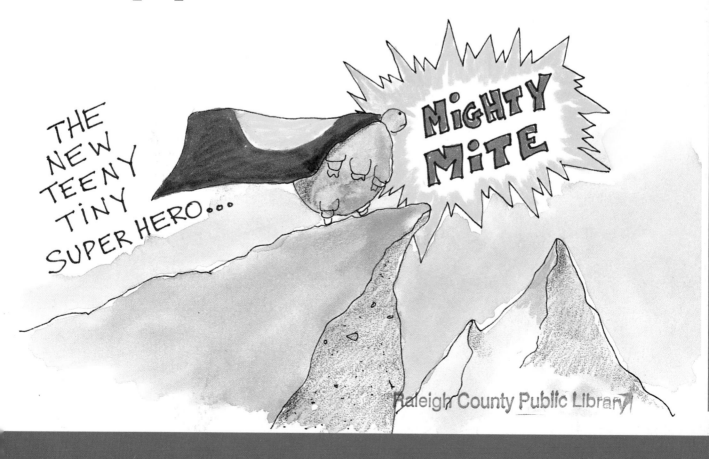

THE NEW TEENY TINY SUPER HERO...

MiGHTY MiTE

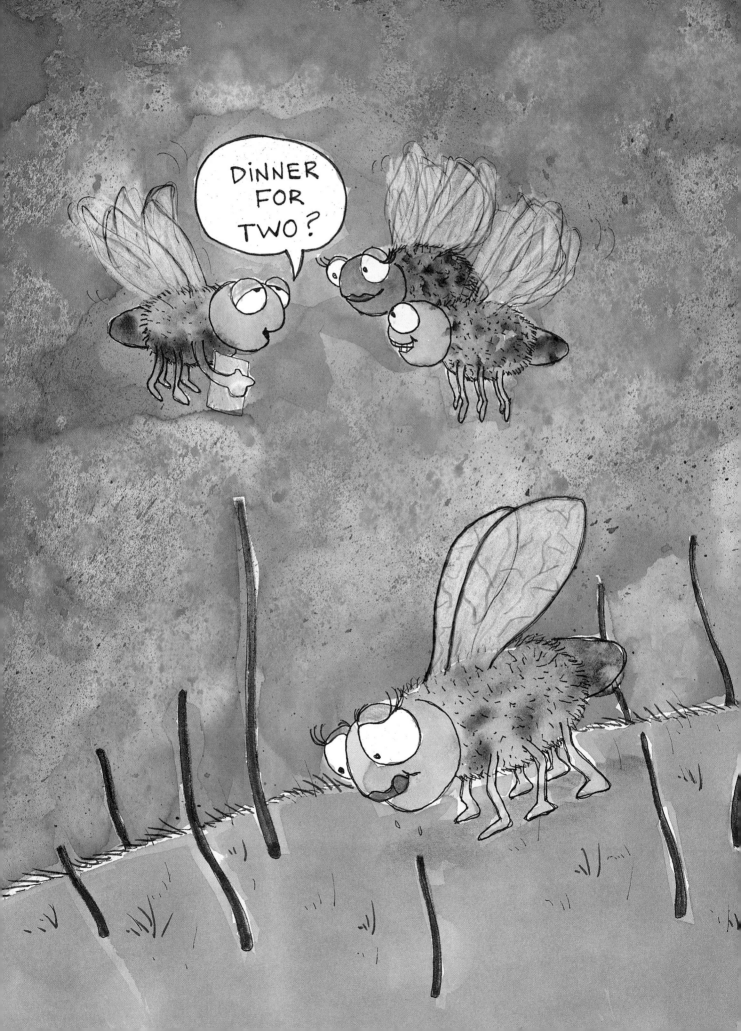

Bloodsucking Flies

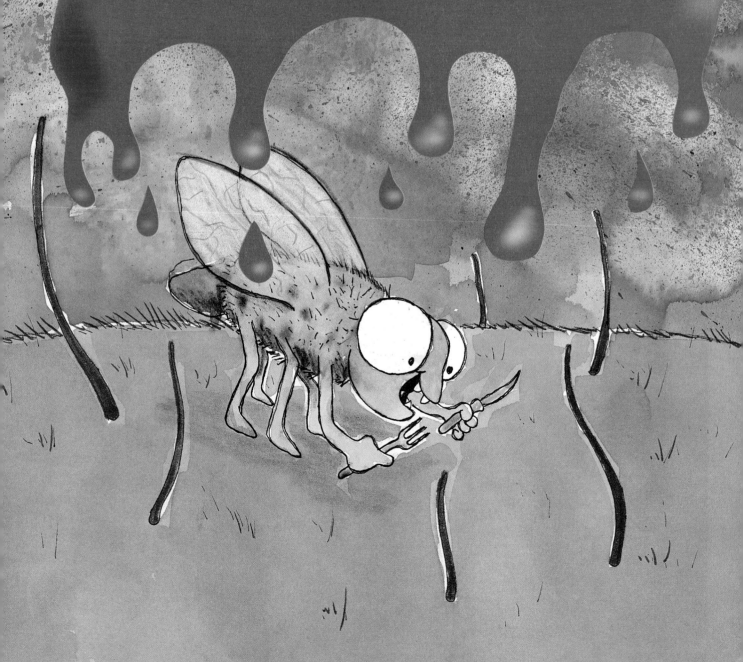

Types of Bloodsucking FLIES

There are lots of bloodsucking flies that are real pests to humans and animals. Here are just a few:

Stable Flies

As you can guess by its name, the stable fly can be found in stables, barns, and other places where animals are sheltered. But they can also be found in open areas such

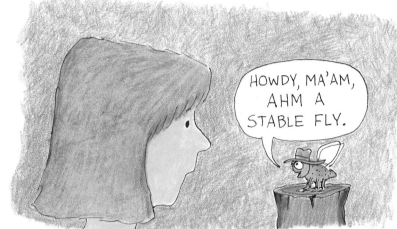

HOWDY, MA'AM, AHM A STABLE FLY.

as pastures. Unlike some of the other bloodsuckers we've seen, it's not only the female stable fly that sucks blood. The males do too. Their bites can be very painful.

Females must have a blood meal before they can produce eggs. They like to lay their eggs in some rotting vegetation mixed with manure. Within a few days, the eggs hatch into larvae. The larvae grow through several larval stages until they become pupae. In a week or two, they become adults. The entire life cycle takes about 2 to 5 weeks.

Stable flies don't actually live on animals and people. They just visit them when they get hungry. Stable flies are a real bother to cattle. Dairy farmers and ranchers work hard to keep the stables and barns clean so stable flies don't have places to breed.

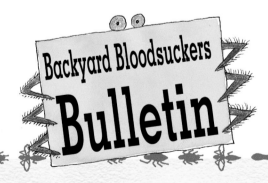

Backyard Bloodsuckers
Bulletin

A female stable fly may lay as many as 400 eggs during her short lifetime.

Horn Flies

Unlike stable flies, horn flies do not bite people, but they love to bite horses and cows! You can tell how irritating these little pests are by their scientific name: *Haematobia irritans*.

When it's hot outside, you can sometimes see horn flies on the backs, shoulders, and undersides of cattle. That's where they live . . . in the hair of the animal. The really bad news is that both male and female horn flies bite and they can feed as many as 40 times each day. Ouch!

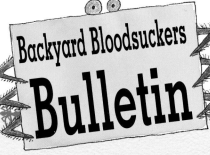

It's not unusual to see 500 or more horn flies on a single cow or horse infested with horn flies.

After the females feed, they leave the animal and lay their eggs in fresh manure. The eggs hatch into larvae that grow into pupae in 1 or 2 weeks. The pupae take another week or two to grow into adults and the cycle begins again.

Face Flies

Can you imagine your face covered with biting flies? Blaaah! Disgusting! In the southern United States there's a fly called the face fly that likes to feed on blood and other fluids around the eyes and noses of cattle.

You can imagine how irritating this is to cattle. Often, when there are lots of face flies around, cattle will crowd together to try to protect themselves.

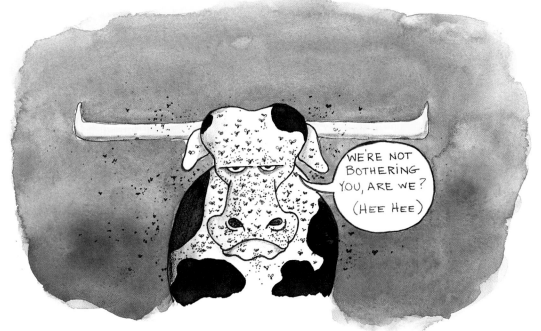

Like the horn fly, the face fly prefers to stay outside, although it will seek shelter indoors during winter months. Also like the horn fly, the face fly goes through four stages: egg, larva, pupa, and adult. The entire life cycle of the face fly takes only about 3 weeks to complete.

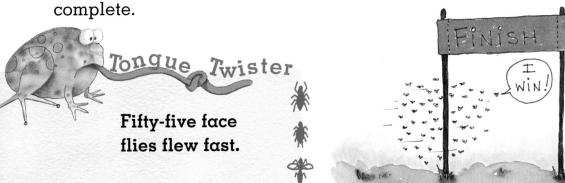

Tongue Twister

**Fifty-five face
flies flew fast.**

Tsetse (pronounced "SEAT see") Flies

In some parts of the world, tsetse flies kill tens of thousands of people each year. The good news is you're not likely to see any tsetse flies unless you visit the tropical regions of Africa.

Tsetse flies live only on blood and can transmit a disease called "sleeping sickness." It's a very serious disease, but it can be treated if the person who is bitten can get to a doctor quickly.

Female tsetse flies do not lay eggs, but instead give birth to a single full-grown larva. The larva immediately turns into a pupa. A short time later, it becomes a full-grown adult.

One of the ways scientists are controlling the population of tsetse flies is by exposing male tsetse flies to radiation. This makes the males unable to reproduce. Since tsetse flies usually only mate once before they die, many female tsetse flies mate with these males and then die without producing any offspring. Scientists have also used traps to catch tsetse flies, but these haven't been as effective. In addition to making humans sick, tsetse flies also transmit diseases to cattle.

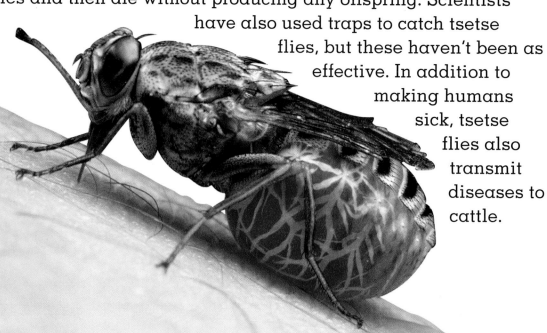

Insect MUSEUMS

Are you interested in seeing some critters up close? If so, you might try to visit some of these insect museums:

If you're in the Philadelphia area, you may want to visit the Philadelphia Insectarium. It has a cockroach kitchen, a live termite tunnel, and other cool exhibits. Call (215) 335-9500 for more information.

The Bohart Museum of Entomology is located on the campus of the University of California in Davis, CA. The museum has an arthropod petting zoo as well as their "Oh My!" collection. Call (530) 752-0493 for more information.

The Museum of Biological Diversity on the campus of The Ohio State University has more than 3.5 million specimens. They do allow visitors, but it's best to call before you visit. Phone: (614) 292-7773.

The University of Wyoming in Laramie, WY, has an Insect Museum that houses the world's largest collection (60,000 specimens) of a specific parasitic wasp that lives in Costa Rica. They also have a live insect zoo, insect hand stamps, insect models, and lots more. Call the University of Wyoming for more information. Phone: (307) 766-1121.

If you live in the central United States, you might want to visit the Enns Entomology Museum on the campus of the University of Missouri in Columbia, MO. This museum has been around for more than 100 years and currently holds almost 6 million specimens of insects, arachnids, and fossils. The collection can be seen, but be sure you call first. Sometimes the scientists are outside tracking down new bugs for their collection. Phone: (573) 882-2410.

If you're in Canada, the Newfoundland Insectarium is a great place to see insects and arachnids up close. This place has lots of giant things—giant water bugs, giant beetles, and giant scorpions. Great fun! Phone: (709) 635-4545.

Buckets of Info on Bloodsucking Flies

- Both male and female stable flies suck blood.

- Horn flies can feed as many as 40 times each day.

- Face flies feed on the fluids around the faces of cattle.

- Tsetse flies are found in Africa.

- Tsetse flies do not lay eggs.

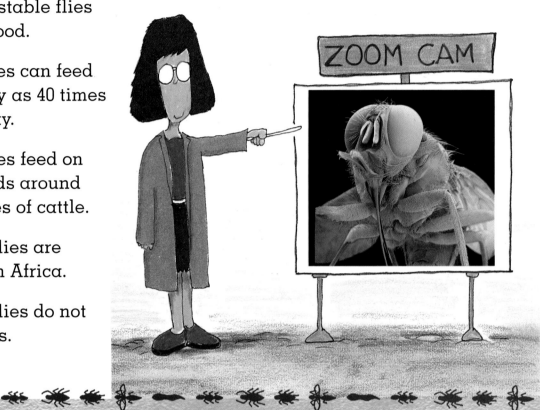

Do You Want to Know More?

Log on to these Web sites to learn more about biting flies:

- http://www.fao.org/NEWS/1998/980505-e.htm

- http://wihort.uwex.edu/gardenfacts/XHT1049.pdf

- http://kids.yahoo.com/animals/insects/3653--Black+Horse+Fly

- http://www.mass.gov/agr/pesticides/pestfacts/bitingflies.htm

- http://www.ext.colostate.edu/PUBS/INSECT/05582.html

- http://www.urbanshield.co.uk/html/flies.html

- http://www.ridmax.com/flies.htm

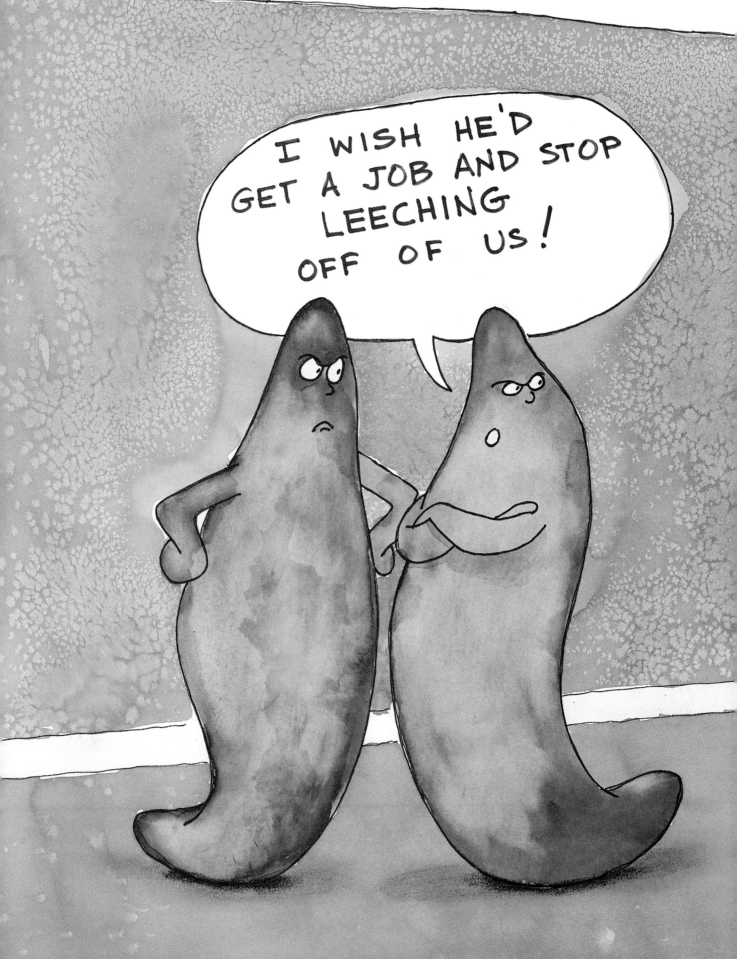

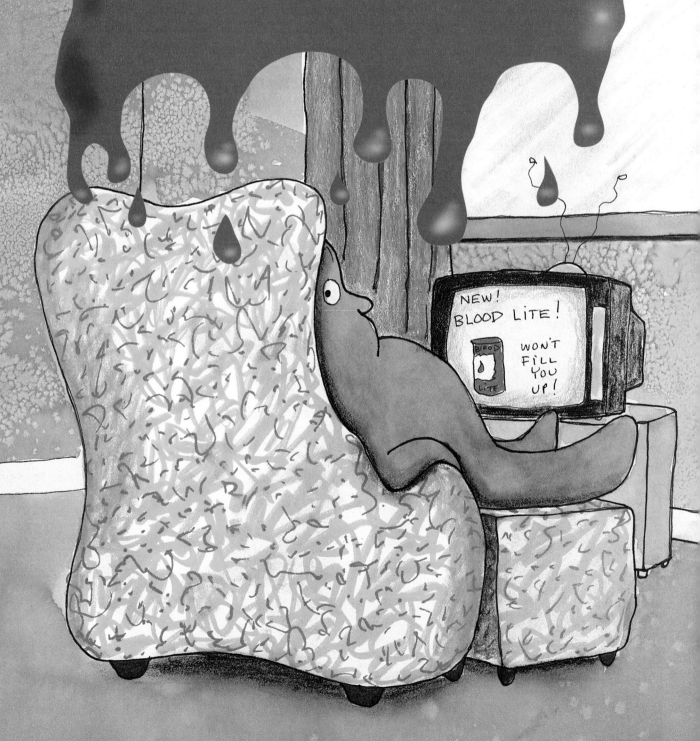

Loads of LEECHES

Unlike some of the other bloodsuckers we've seen, leeches are not insects. And they're not related to ticks and spiders. Leeches are actually worms. And even though leeches are hungry bloodsuckers, they can be very helpful to humans. Here's how: When a leech bites a person, it injects fluids that open the person's blood vessels and keep the blood flowing. This makes the job of sucking blood easier for the leech. These fluids are so effective that blood from a leech bite will continue to flow as long as 2 days after the leech has bitten the person (although 6 hours is the average). Knowing this, doctors have used leeches to help people whose ear, finger, or other body part has been cut off and reattached. Doctors attach leeches to the injured area and let the leeches feed. As they feed, the leeches keep the blood flowing to the area. This makes it possible for the body part to heal and become healthy again.

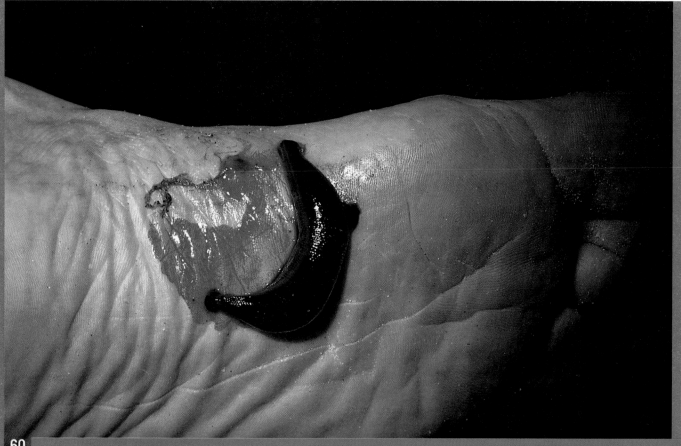

Medical Uses of LEECHES

Doctors also use leeches to remove "pools" of blood that are not flowing well under the skin of humans. Leeches have become so popular for medical uses that one company in England ships more than 20,000 leeches a year to doctors and hospitals.

Long ago, doctors believed that people could be cured of many different illnesses if some of their blood was removed. It sounds crazy to us today, but they didn't know all we know about how the human body works. When it came time to remove the blood, doctors would sometimes make a cut in the person's arm and let the blood drain. Other times, the doctor would stick hungry leeches on the person's arm and let the leeches feed until the leeches were nice and fat.

Backyard Bloodsuckers Bulletin

Some scientists in Europe discovered that leeches were attracted by garlic. Unfortunately (for the leeches), the garlic killed the leeches after a couple of hours.

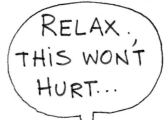

RELAX, THIS WON'T HURT...

MUCH.

Leech MUSEUM

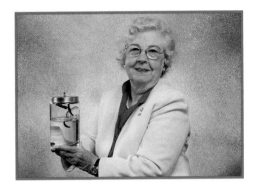

Would you like to spend a little "quality time" with some real live leeches? In Illinois, there's a lady who spends time with live leeches every day. Her name is Barbara Mason, and she is the curator of the Pearson Museum.

The Pearson Museum is part of the Southern Illinois School of Medicine in Springfield, Illinois, and it contains some pretty strange stuff. In the "Bloodsuckers" department, there are plenty of leeches, and Ms. Mason will be happy to show you her live specimens. There are also other medical exhibits that deal with blood-letting. Blood-letting was the practice of draining the blood from people who were ill or bothered by physical ailments. People used to believe that if they drained blood from sick people, they could make the sick people feel better. Pretty weird, huh?

While you're at the museum, don't forget to ask Ms. Mason to show you the mummified human hand too!

You can contact Ms. Mason at the Pearson Museum by phoning (217) 785-2128. The museum is located at 801 North Rutlidge Street in Springfield, Illinois.

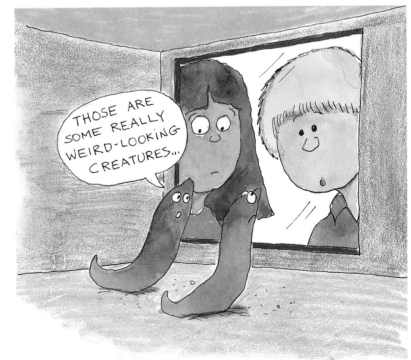

What Do They EAT?

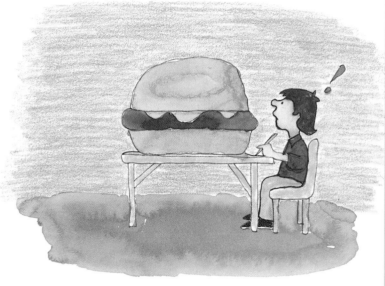

How much do you weigh? Imagine eating five times your weight in food at one meal! That's what leeches do. It's true! A typical leech can eat five times its body weight in blood at one "meal." When leeches are in the water, their bodies ripple up and down like a wave. When they are out of the water, they use their suckers (one on each end of their bodies) to grab hold and pull themselves forward.

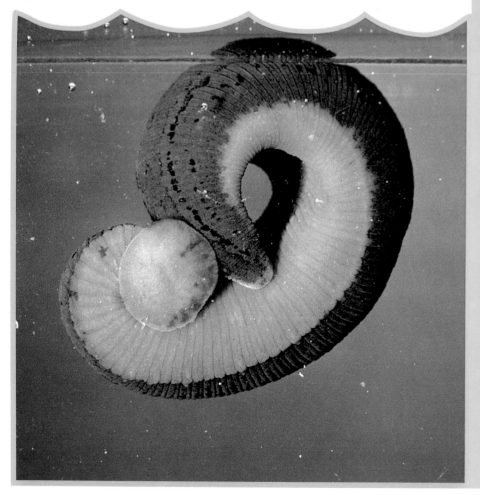

One of the reasons why people generally don't feel a leech bite them is because the leech's saliva (spit) contains a chemical that deadens the skin where it's biting. Generally, it's only after the leech has been feeding a while that the victim realizes that he or she has become the leech's dinner.

How Do I REMOVE It?

As repulsive as a leech is, it's probably not a good idea to tear it off of your skin if you find one on you. That's because the leech has strong "grabbers" in its mouth, and you might leave the "grabbers" in your skin if you rip the leech off too hard. The mouth parts could then become infected. It's better to put some salt or something hot (but not too hot) on the leech to make it let go.

And be prepared for some bleeding if you remove a leech. Remember, one of the things it does best is keep the blood flowing. If you remove a leech, your blood will probably flow for a short while.

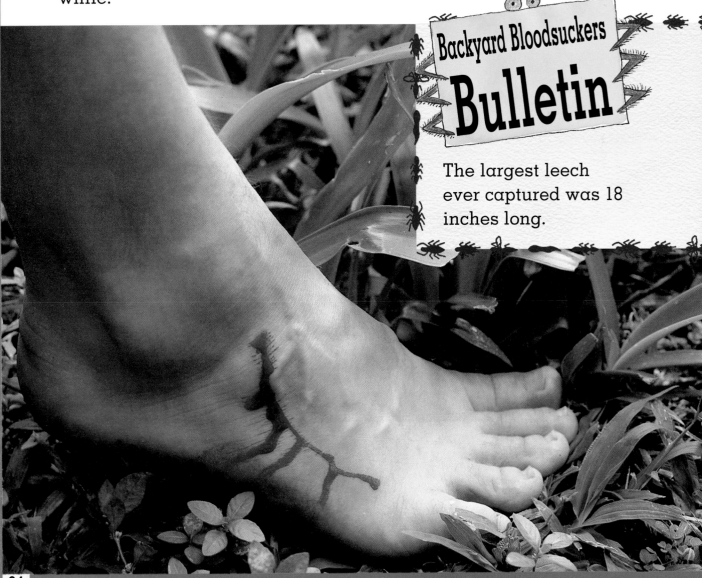

Backyard Bloodsuckers Bulletin

The largest leech ever captured was 18 inches long.

Where Do They **LIVE?**

Leeches are most often found in ponds, lakes, and rivers, but about 20 percent of the leech species live in the sea, where they attach themselves to fish and feed off of the fish's blood.

Even though we think of leeches as bloodsucking creatures, not all leeches suck blood. Many leeches are predators and live by eating earthworms and other small creatures.

In some parts of the United States, people who like to fish buy leeches as bait.

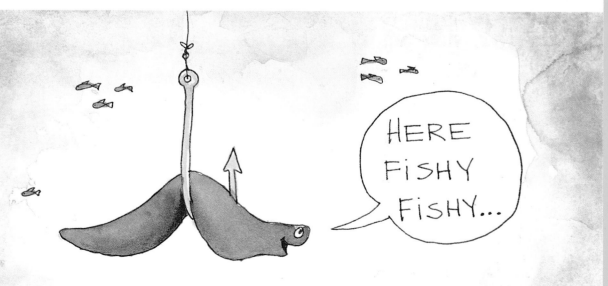

What Kind of ANIMAL Is a Leech?

Do you know what some leeches and frogs have in common? They're amphibious! That means they can live on land or on water. Even though some leeches are amphibious, that doesn't mean they're amphibians. Amphibians are animals, such as frogs, salamanders, and newts. Amphibians have backbones. Leeches are a kind of weird worm called annelids . . . they don't have backbones.

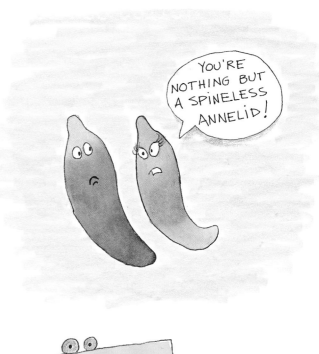

YOU'RE NOTHING BUT A SPINELESS ANNELID!

Backyard Bloodsuckers
Bulletin

Leeches aren't just warm-weather creatures. Some leeches have been found in waters near the Antarctic!

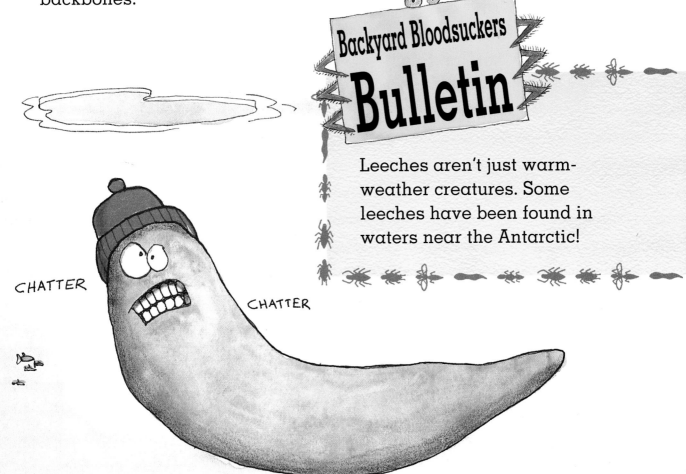

CHATTER

CHATTER

Lots of Info on LEECHES

- Leeches are worms.

- Leeches can be helpful to humans.

- A leech can eat five times its weight in blood.

- A chemical in a leech's saliva deadens human skin.

- After a leech is removed, blood will continue to flow for a while.

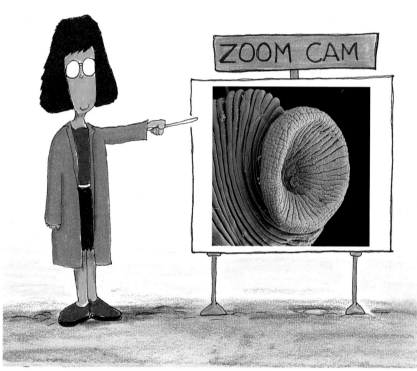

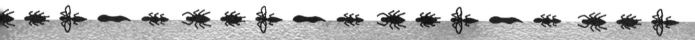

Do You Want to Know More?

Log on to these Web sites to learn more about leeches:

- http://www.accessexcellence.org/LC/SS/leechlove.html

- http://www.uib.no/isf/surprise.htm

- http://www.leechesusa.com

- http://www.leeches.biz/about-leeches.htm

- http://www.bugsurvey.nsw.gov.au/html/popups/bpedia_29_vtol_le.html

- http://www.austmus.gov.au/factSheets/leeches.htm

- http://www.biopharm-leeches.com/leech_facts.htm

- http://www.bristolzoo.org.uk/learning/animals/invertebrates/leech

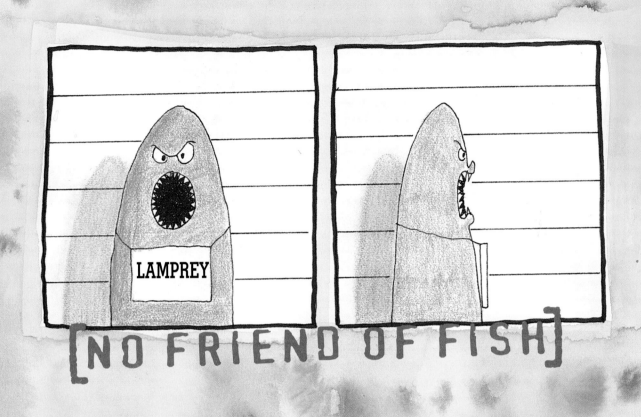

[NO FRIEND OF FISH]

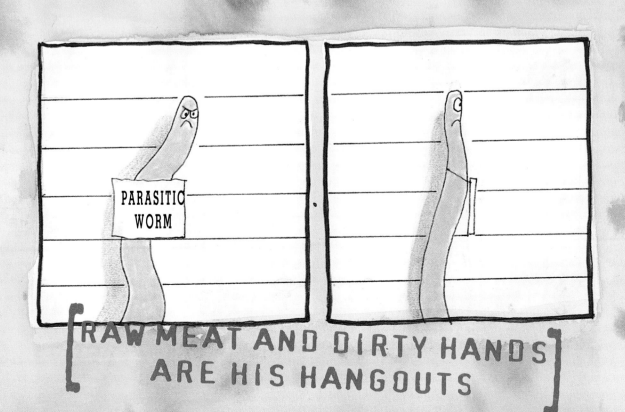

[RAW MEAT AND DIRTY HANDS
ARE HIS HANGOUTS]

Other Bloodsuckers

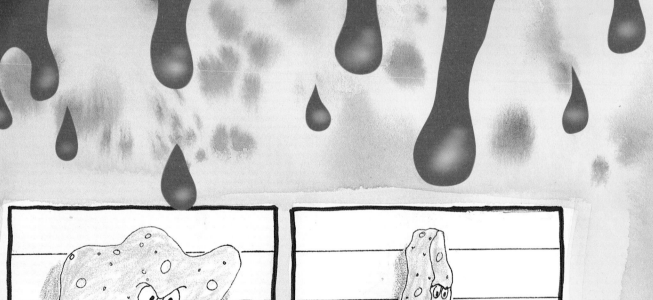

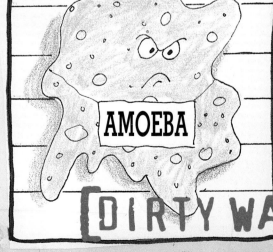

AMOEBA

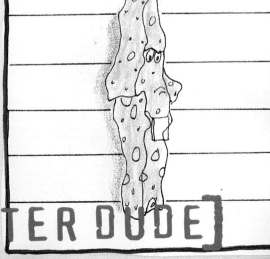

[DIRTY WATER DUDE]

Parasitic WORMS

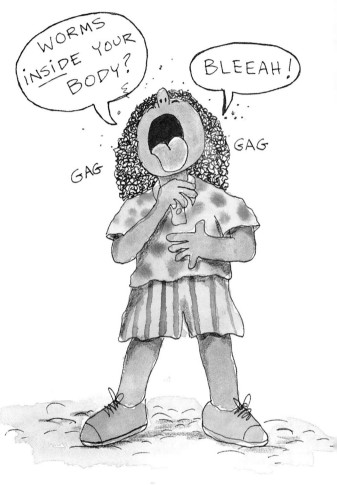

Parasites are creatures that live off of the bodies of other creatures. So far, the creatures we've seen all live on the outside of humans and animals. They only bite and dig into our skin when they want to eat. But some creatures actually live inside of humans and animals. As you might imagine, these animals are very small. They include tapeworms and pinworms. These little pests can really upset your stomach, and millions of people around the world get sick every year because of them. The best way to avoid these critters is to wash your hands regularly and make sure your food is cooked well.

Log on to these Web sites to learn more about these creatures:

- http://www.cdc.gov/ncidod/dpd/aboutparasites.htm
- http://www.nhc.ed.ac.uk/index.php?page=24.25.333
- http://www.chem.gla.ac.uk/staff/alanc/research/worms.htm
- http://www.micrographia.com/specbiol/helmint/nematod/nema0100.htm
- http://www.kidshealth.org/parent/infections/parasitic/pinworm.html

The TINIEST Bloodsuckers

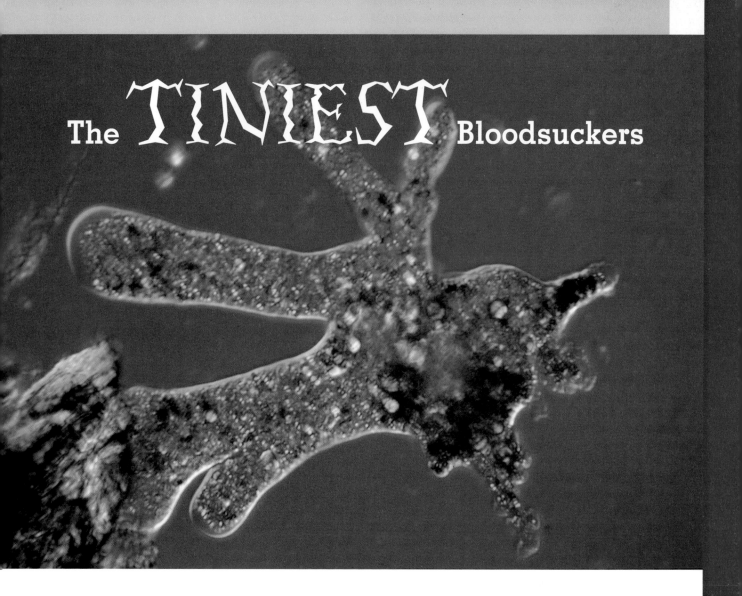

Amoebas and protozoans are very tiny, microscopic creatures that can cause a lot of trouble. They can give people dysentery and other nasty diseases. In poorer countries where the people don't have clean drinking water, they may drink water that has these parasites in it. This can make the people very sick. Sometimes, even in the United States, after a flood or a hurricane, there's not enough clean drinking water in certain places. When this happens, people can avoid amoebas and protozoans by drinking bottled water. Since our bodies are mostly water, it's important that the water we drink is clean and healthy.

LAMPREYS

If you were a fish, you would not like to see a lamprey headed your way. Lampreys have a large mouth that's like a vacuum cleaner. When a fish swims by, the lamprey attaches itself to the fish with its big vacuum-cleaner mouth.

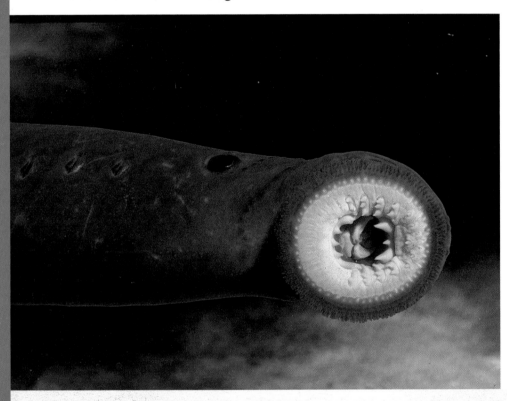

Then, the lamprey uses its rough, sharp tongue to cut a hole in the side of the fish (ouch!) and begins sucking out the fish's fluids. Yuck! A single lamprey can kill many fish this way.

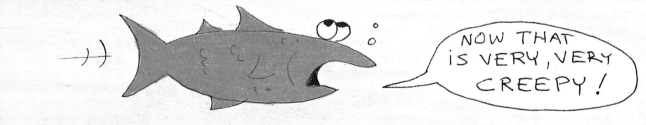

NOW THAT IS VERY, VERY CREEPY!

Log on to these Web sites to learn more about lampreys:

- http://www.adfg.state.ak.us/pubs/notebook/fish/lampreys.php
- http://etc.usf.edu/clipart/galleries/Animals/lampreys.htm
- http://en.wikipedia.org/wiki/Lamprey
- http://www.fisheries.vims.edu/lamprey.htm

Studying INSECTS

Many insects eat smaller insects. Those insects in turn are eaten by birds, fish, and other creatures. Then larger animals eat the birds and fish. This cycle of larger creatures eating smaller creatures is called "the food chain." Even though most of the creatures in this book are pesky to humans, they are very important in the food chain.

If there are too many pests in an area, humans and their pets can become sick. If there are not enough pests for other animals to eat, those animals might starve. Scientists are working hard to help nature maintain its "pest" balance. If you're interested in this kind of work, you may think about becoming an entomologist. An entomologist studies insects. Some entomologists are interested in finding safe ways to reduce the number of insects. Others study the ways insects reproduce and spread disease. To learn more, ask the media specialist at your library for information about the work that entomologists do.

Your school library or public library has some other great books about insects, arachnids, and other parasites. If you'd like to visit some interesting Web sites, try these:

- http://www.pestweb.com
This site has information about insects and other creatures. It's a good place to start.

- http://www.ent.iastate.edu/list/158/vid/5
This site has great info and ways to contact insect experts.

- http://www.eatbug.com/
Hungry? There are more than 1,400 insects that you can eat!

- http://www.ento.vt.edu/~sharov/3d/virtual.html
3D insects! Very cool.

- http://www.insects.org
Good general insect site.

- http://www.enchantedlearning.com/subjects/insects/printouts.shtml
Printouts of insects.

- http://www.earthlife.net/insects/six.html
Cool insect facts.

- http://www.astrographics.com/cgi-bin/search/search.pl
Incredible insect images.

GLOSSARY
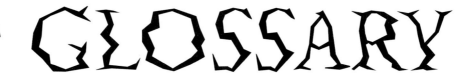

Amoebas Microscopic creatures that live inside animals and may cause disease.

Arachnids Creatures, such as ticks and spiders, who have eight legs.

Arthropods Creatures whose skeletons are on the outside of their bodies and who have legs with joints.

Carbon Dioxide The gas that humans and animals breathe out of their lungs.

Cocoon A tube or container spun by a pupa; used as protection for continued growth.

Dysentery A disease caused by amoebas.

Entomologist A scientist that studies insects.

Feces Animal waste; also known as manure or droppings.

Follicle A shaft of hair.

Insects Creatures, such as mosquitoes, flies, and fleas, who have six legs.

Larva The stage of development that follows the egg stage.

Lyme disease A disease spread by ticks, characterized by fever, joint pain, and red, circular spots on the skin.

Malaria One of the diseases transmitted by mosquitoes.

Molt Process during which an animal sheds its outer layer of skin or skeleton so it can grow.

Nits Another word for lice eggs.

Nymph A young insect or other small creature that has not fully developed into an adult but looks very much like the adult in shape.

Parasite A creature that lives off of another creature.

Pesticides Chemicals designed to kill pests.

Plague A disease spread by fleas in the fourteenth century; also called the "Black Death."

Plasma A substance in human blood that contains the proteins some bloodsuckers need to reproduce.

Platelets The substance in blood that stops bleeding and helps blood clot.

Predator An animal that eats other animals.

Pupa The stage of development that follows the larva stage.

Red blood cells Blood cells that carry oxygen to the rest of the body.

Saliva Another word for "spit."

Trumpets Breathing tubes used by mosquito pupae.

White blood cells Blood cells that fight infection.

Yellow fever A disease transmitted by mosquitoes.

Photocopy these "backyard bloodsucker" silhouettes, cut out each one, and project the image on the overhead projector in your classroom as you discuss each creature.

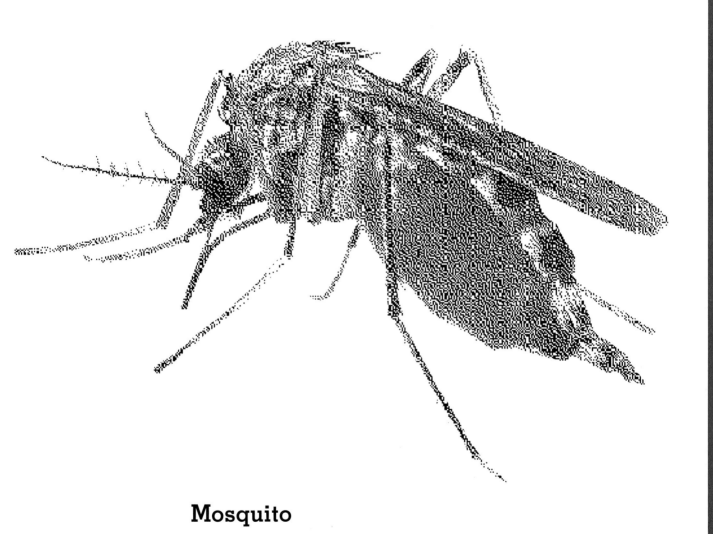

Mosquito

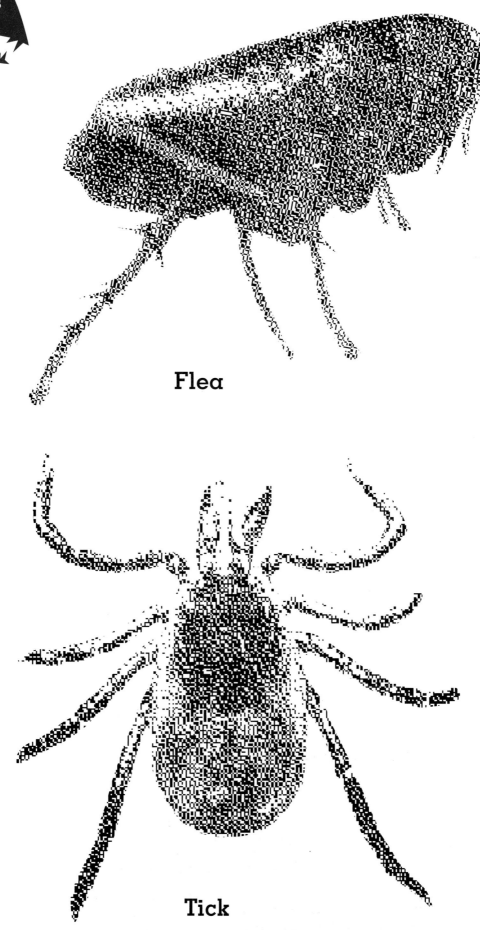

Flea

Tick

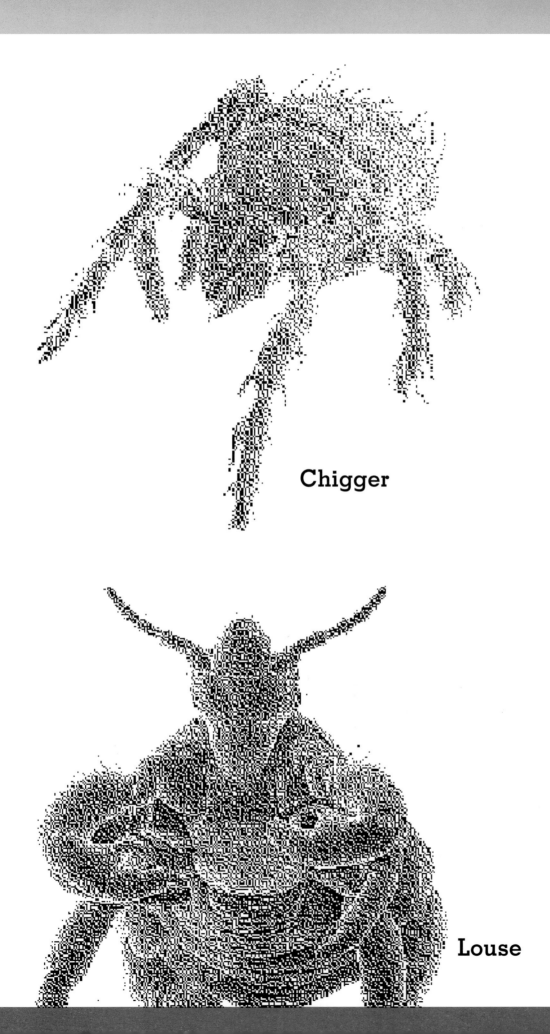

Chigger

Louse

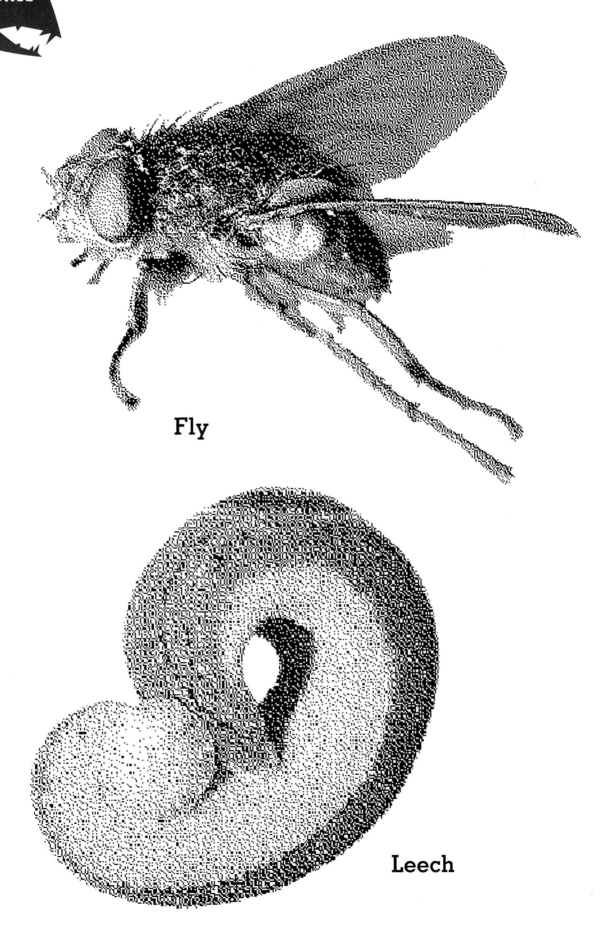

Fly

Leech

FINAL NOTE

You don't have to go on a long field trip to see interesting sights. You can find lots of interesting creatures in your own backyard or in a nearby park. The next time you're outside, sit on the ground, move the grass around a little, and see if you can find any little critters moving around. Check near the bottoms of nearby trees for other creatures too. Then look on the underside of leaves and flowers. Roll a rock over and look underneath. You'll be amazed by all the life you'll find.

Don't just watch the world on television. Get out and explore! If you're lucky, you may find some backyard bloodsuckers. Good luck!

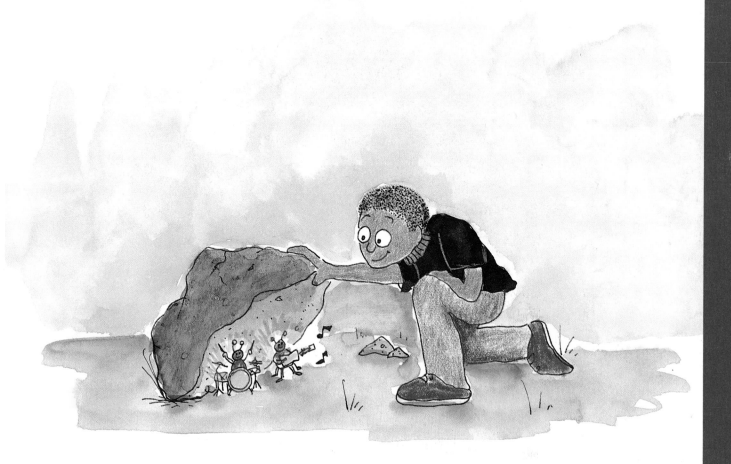

Other Science Books by Mike Artell
The Earth & Me (with Pam Schiller)
Starry Skies
Weather Whys
Pee-Yew!

Some Nonscience Books by Mike Artell
Awesome Alphabets
Classroom Cartooning

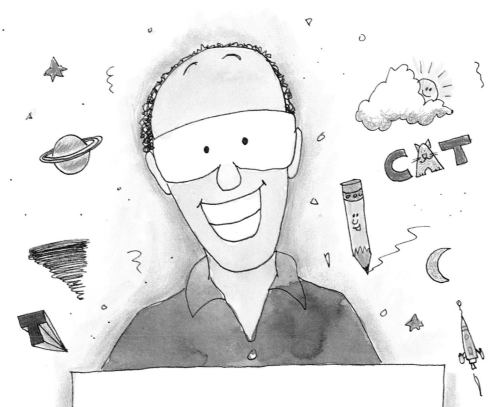

Would you like to contact Mike? Send him an e-mail:

mike@mikeartell.com